Biosensors - Current and Novel Strategies for Biosensing

Edited by Luis Jesús Villarreal-Gómez and Ana Leticia Iglesias

Published in London, United Kingdom

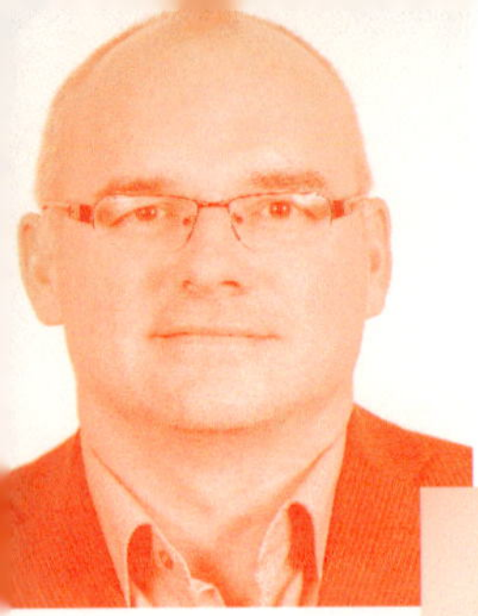
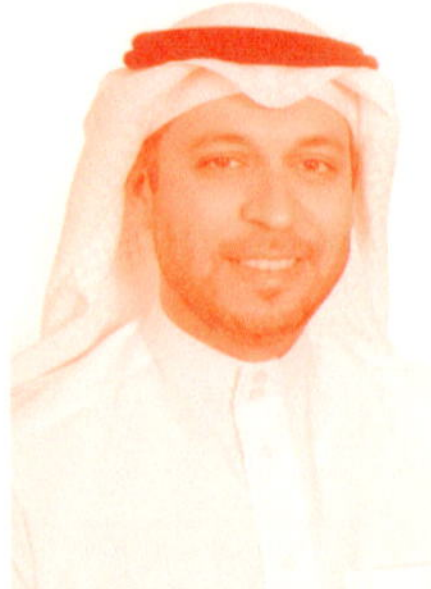
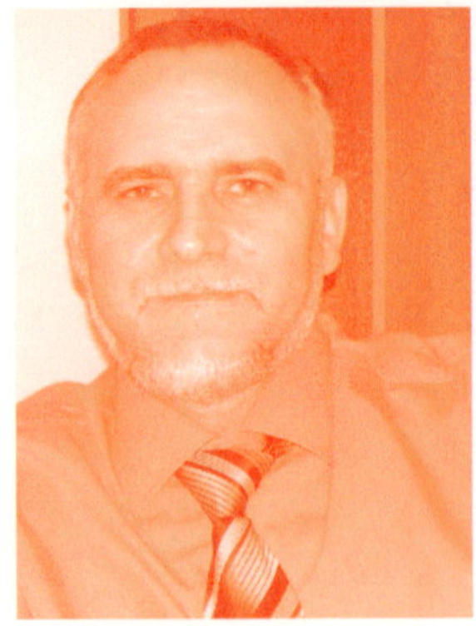
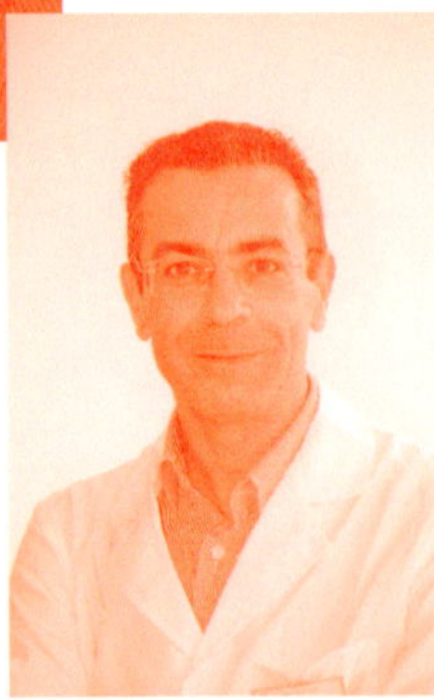
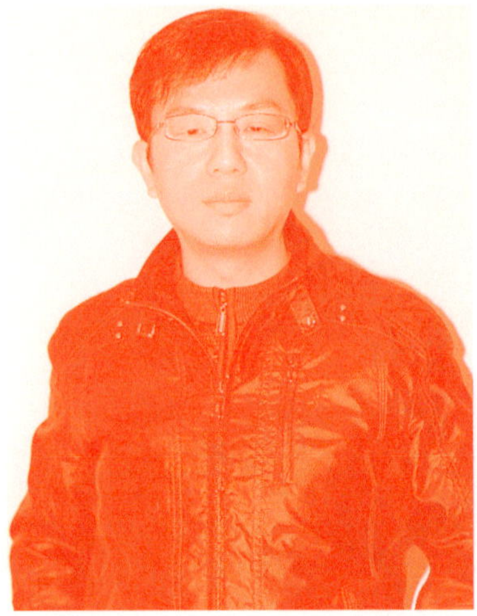
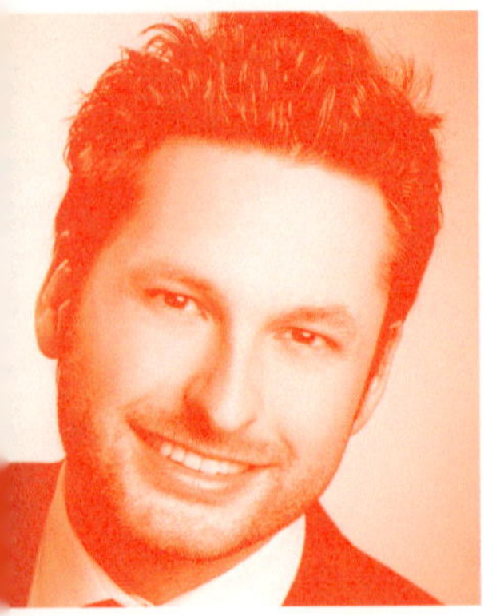
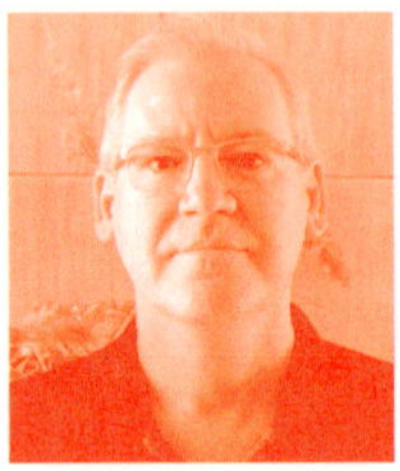

IntechOpen

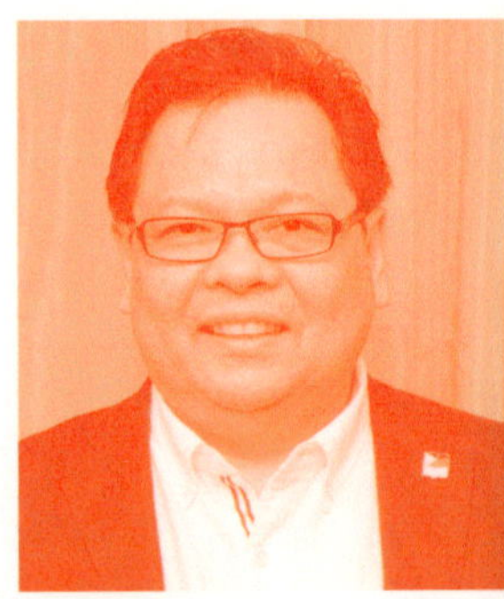
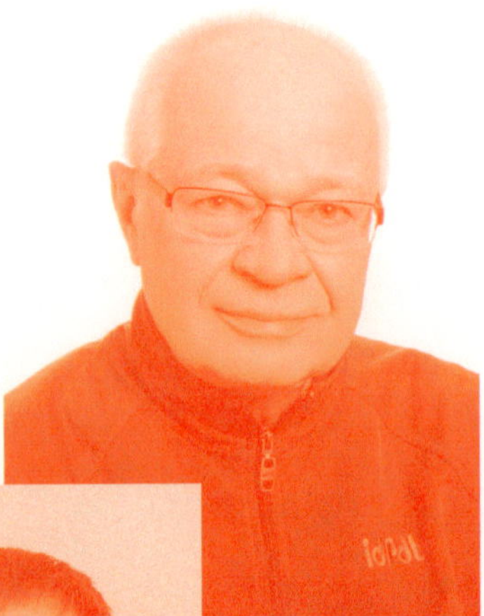
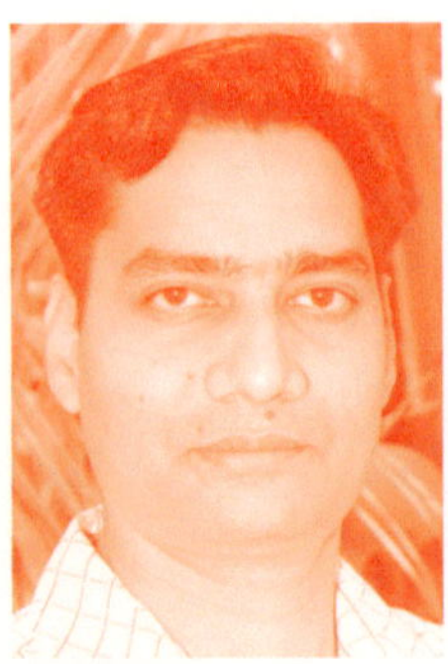
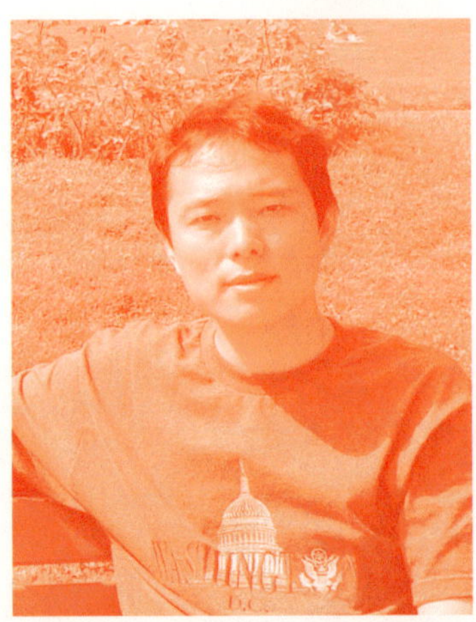
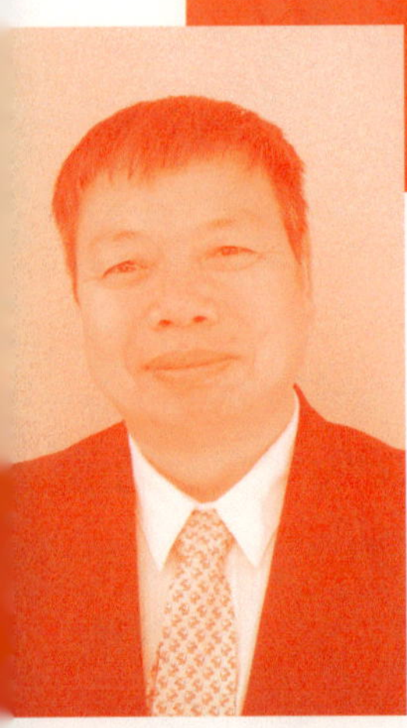
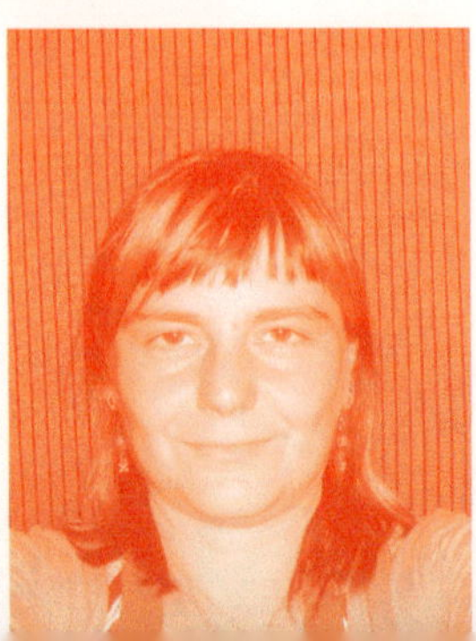

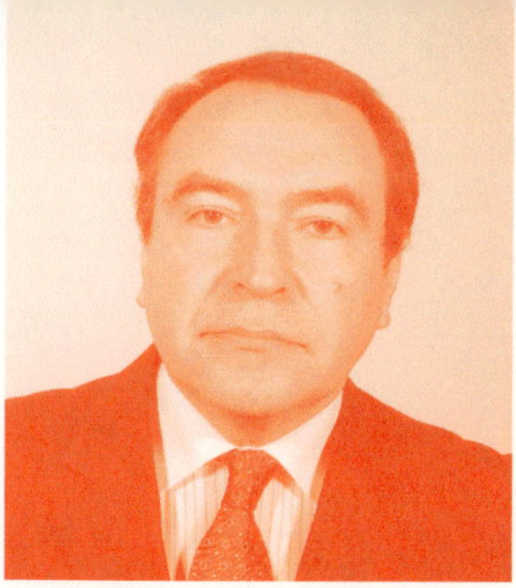

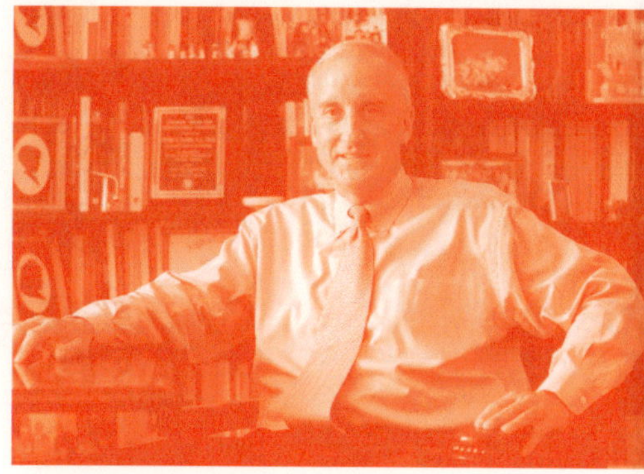

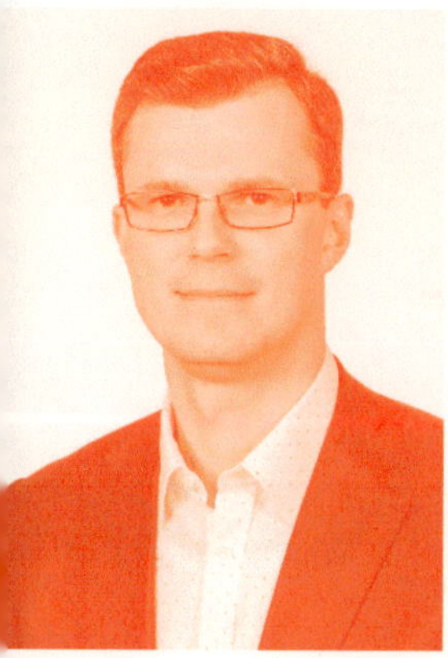

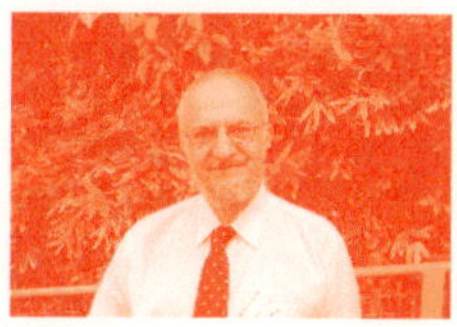

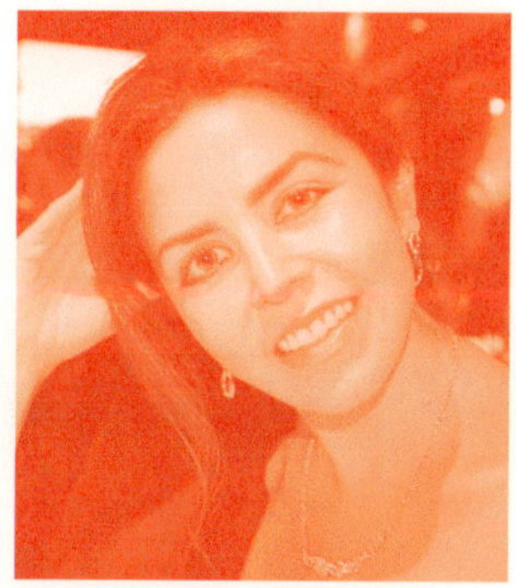

Supporting open minds since 2005

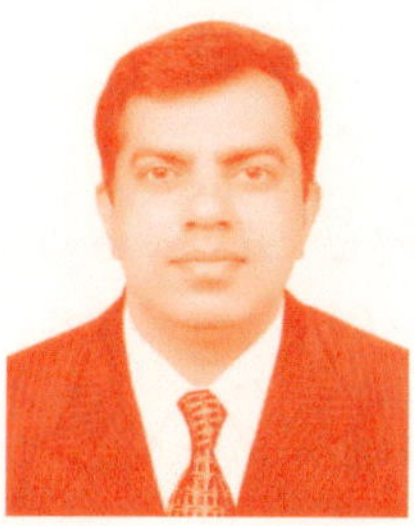

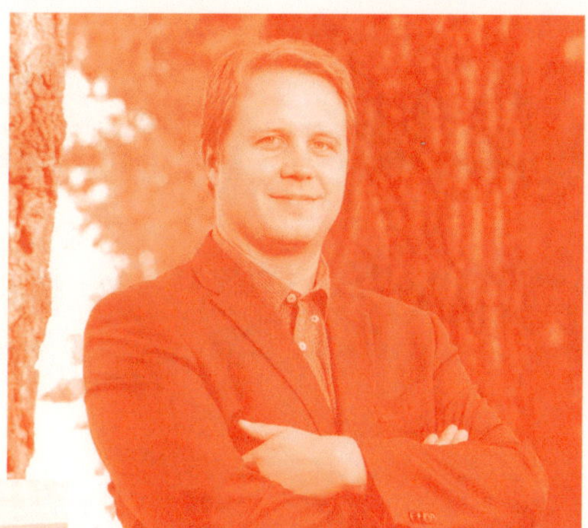

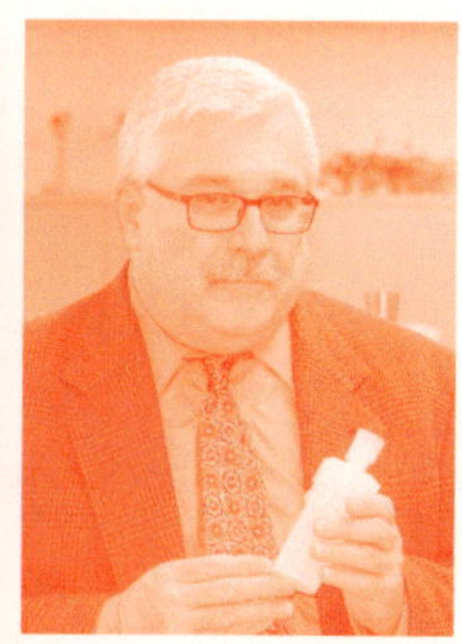

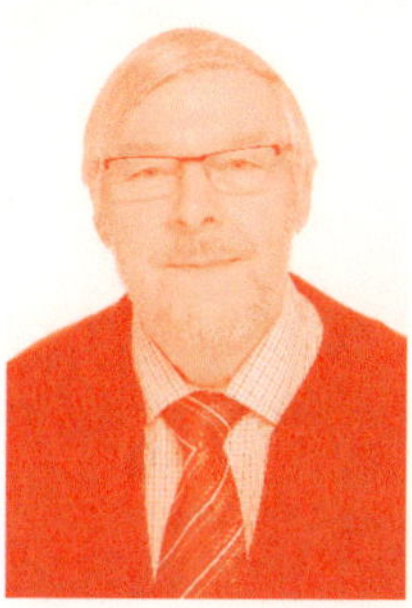

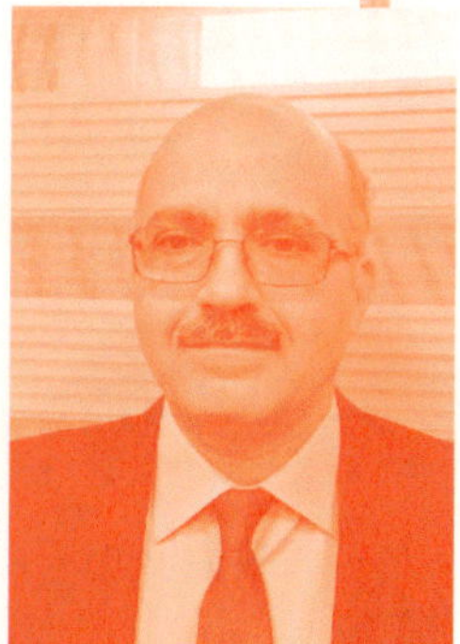

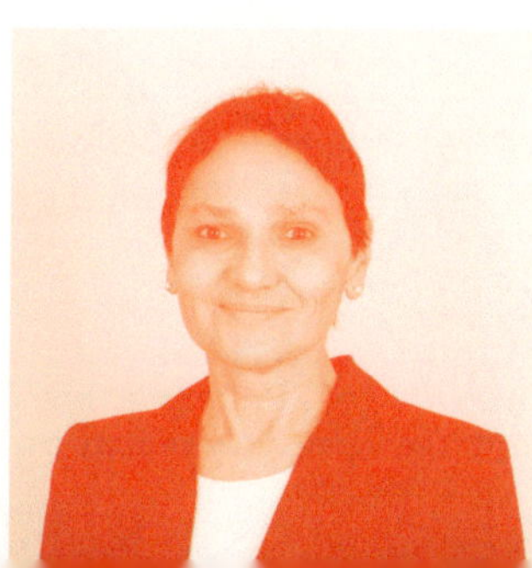

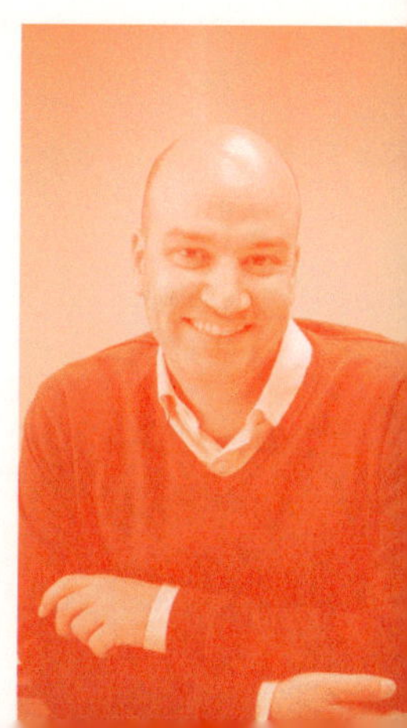

Biosensors - Current and Novel Strategies for Biosensing
http://dx.doi.org/10.5772/intechopen.87692
Edited by Luis Jesús Villarreal-Gómez and Ana Leticia Iglesias

Part of IntechOpen Book Series: Biomedical Engineering, Volume 11
Book Series Editor: Robert Koprowski

Contributors
Alex Simonian, Lang Zhou, Pengyu Chen, Ruthber Rodriguez, Roberto Sagaro Zamora, Enrique Marañón, Zihni Onur Onur Uygun, Hilmiye Deniz Ertuğrul Uygun, Ferhan Girgin Sağın, Chi Hwan Lee, Eun Kwang Lee, Hocheon Yoo, Ivana Jokić, Jikui Wu, Principia Dardano, Luca De Stefano, Ilaria Rea, Mario Battisti, Selene De Martino, Luigi Nicolais, Bruno Miranda, Timothy Anton Okhai, Azeez Idris, Usisipho Feleni, Lukas Willem Snyman, Vinayak Pachkawade, Md. Shamim Anower, Md. Mahabubur Rahman, M. Saifur Rahman, Elvis Kwason Tiburu, Bernard O. Asimeng, Richard Asiamah, Samuel Kojo Kwofie, Emmanuel Nyankson, William N. Gblerkpor

First published in London, United Kingdom, 2021 by IntechOpen
IntechOpen is the global imprint of INTECHOPEN LIMITED, registered in England and Wales, registration number: 11086078, 5 Princes Gate Court, London, SW7 2QJ, United Kingdom
Printed in Croatia

British Library Cataloguing-in-Publication Data
A catalogue record for this book is available from the British Library

Additional hard and PDF copies can be obtained from orders@intechopen.com

Biosensors - Current and Novel Strategies for Biosensing
Edited by Luis Jesús Villarreal-Gómez and Ana Leticia Iglesias
p. cm.
Print ISBN 978-1-83962-431-5
Online ISBN 978-1-83962-438-4
eBook (PDF) ISBN 978-1-83962-439-1
ISSN 2631-5343

For EU product safety concerns:
IN TECH d.o.o., Prolaz Marije Krucifikse Kozulić 3, 51000 Rijeka, Croatia,
info@intechopen.com or visit our website at intechopen.com.

IntechOpen Book Series

Biomedical Engineering

Volume 11

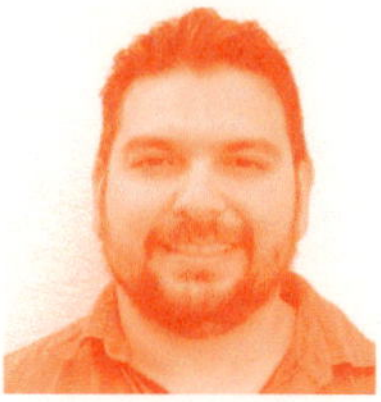

Dr. Luis Villarreal is a research professor from the Facultad de Ciencias de la Ingeniería y Tecnología, Universidad Autónoma de Baja California, Tijuana, Baja California, México. Dr. Villarreal is the editor in chief and founder of the *Revista de Ciencias Tecnológicas* (RECIT) (https://recit.uabc.mx/) and is a member of several editorial and reviewer boards for numerous international journals. He has published more than thirty international papers and reviewed more than eight-five manuscripts. His research interests include biomaterials, nanomaterials, bioengineering, biosensors, drug delivery systems, and tissue engineering.

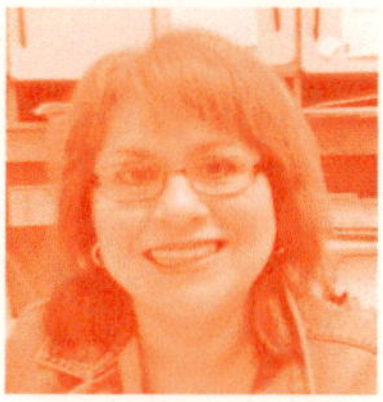

Dr. Iglesias is a research professor at Facultad de Ciencias de la Ingeniería y Tecnología, Universidad Autónoma de Baja California, Tijuana, Baja California, where she has been teaching for the past twelve years undergraduate courses in the Bioengineering program. Her research interests include organometallic and coordination compounds, the biological activity of metallodrugs, catalysis, biomaterials, and biosensors.

Editors of Volume 11:
Luis Jesús Villarreal Gómez and Ana Leticia Iglesias
Facultad de Ciencias de la Ingeniería y Tecnología
Universidad Autónoma de Baja California
Tijuana, Baja California, México

Book Series Editor:
Robert Koprowski
University of Silesia, Poland

Scope of the Series

Biomedical engineering is one of the fastest-growing interdisciplinary branches of science and industry. The combination of electronics and computer science with biology and medicine has resulted in improved patient diagnosis, reduced rehabilitation time, and better quality of life. Nowadays, all medical imaging devices, medical instruments, or new laboratory techniques are the result of the cooperation of specialists in various fields. The series of biomedical engineering books covers such areas of knowledge as chemistry, physics, electronics, medicine and biology. This series is intended for doctors, engineers and scientists involved in biomedical engineering or those wanting to start working in this field.

Contents

Preface XI

Section 1
Nanomaterials in Biosensing 1

Chapter 1 3
Nanomaterial-Enhanced Receptor Technology for Silicon On-Chip Biosensing Application
by Timothy Anton Okhai, Azeez O. Idris, Usisipho Feleni and Lukas W. Snyman

Chapter 2 21
Nucleic Acids for Electrochemical Biosensor Technology
by Zihni Onur Uygun, Hilmiye Deniz Ertuğrul Uygun and Ferhan Girgin Sağin

Section 2
Wearable Biosensors 37

Chapter 3 39
Theranostic Microneedle Devices: Innovative Biosensing and Transdermal Drugs Administration
by Principia Dardano, Mario Battisti, Selene De Martino, Ilaria Rea, Bruno Miranda, Luigi Nicolais and Luca De Stefano

Chapter 4 59
Control Strategy for Underactuated Multi-Fingered Robot Hand Movement Using Electromyography Signal with Wearable Myo Armband
by Ruthber Rodríguez Serrezuela, Roberto Sagaro Zamora and Enrique Marañón Reyes

Chapter 5 83
Advanced Materials and Assembly Strategies for Wearable Biosensors: A Review
by Eun Kwang Lee, Hocheon Yoo and Chi Hwan Lee

Section 3
Mathematical Assessment on Biosensors **111**

Chapter 6 **113**
Ultra-Precise MEMS Based Bio-Sensors
by Vinayak Pachkawade

Chapter 7 **131**
Microfluidic Adsorption-Based Biosensors: Mathematical Models of Time Response and Noise, Considering Mass Transfer and Surface Heterogeneity
by Ivana Jokić

Chapter 8 **157**
Hybrid Heterostructures for SPR Biosensor
by Md. Shamim Anower, Md. Mahabubur Rahman and M. Saifur Rahman

Section 4
Biological Monitoring with Biosensors **173**

Chapter 9 **175**
Advanced Biosensing towards Real-Time Imaging of Protein Secretion from Single Cells
by Lang Zhou, Pengyu Chen and Aleksandr Simonian

Chapter 10 **203**
Novel Biosensing Strategies for the *in Vivo* Detection of microRNA
by Junling Zhang, Shanshan Zhao and Jikui Wu

Chapter 11 **221**
Electrochemical Response of Cells Using Bioactive Plant Isolates
by Elvis K. Tiburu, Richard Asiamah, Bernard O. Asimeng, Samuel Kojo Kwofie, Emmanuel Nyankson and William N. Gblerkpor

Preface

Biosensors are analytical devices that convert a biological stimulus into an electrical signal [1]. Biosensors have been utilized in a wide range of applications across various fields, such as in biomedicine (drug discovery, diagnosis, etc.), food safety, processing, environmental monitoring, defense, security, and the marine sector, among others. Biosensors provide better stability and sensitivity compared with conventional methods [2].

This book includes eleven chapters organized into four sections. Together they present the state of the art in current and novel strategies for biosensing.

Section 1 "Nanomaterials in Biosensing"

Section 2 "Wearable Biosensors"

Section 3 "Mathematical Assessment on Biosensors"

Section 4 "Biological Monitoring with Biosensors"

Section 1 includes two chapters. Chapter 1, "Nanomaterial-Enhanced Receptor Technology for Silicon On-Chip Biosensing Application", explains how integrating nanomaterials into biosensor design enhances sensing capabilities due to the large surface area and intrinsic reactivity of nanomaterials owing to their distinctive optical, chemical, electrical, and catalytic properties. The chapter examines the incorporation of silver nanoparticles (AgNPs) into a silicon-on-a-chip biosensor platform to detect cancer biomarkers such as prostate-specific antigen (PSA). Chapter 2, "Nucleic Acids for Electrochemical Biosensor Technology", explains how nucleic acids are used as both recognition agents and target molecules, the way they are used in biosensor technology, and their electrical properties.

Nanomaterials are relevant in several areas. In the case of biosensors, they increase sensitivities and low detection limits, allowing the detection of even individual molecules. Also, nanomaterials can immobilize a greater quantity of bioreceptor units at reduced volumes and act as transduction elements [3].

Section 2 includes three chapters that address wearable biosensors, which are devices that provide continuous, real-time physiological information via dynamic, noninvasive measurements of biochemical markers in body fluids, such as blood, sweat, tears, saliva, and interstitial fluid. Recent developments have focused on electrochemical and optical biosensors, together with advances in the noninvasive monitoring of biomarkers including metabolites, bacteria, and hormones [4].

Chapter 3, "Theranostic Microneedle Devices: Innovative Biosensing and Transdermal Drugs Administration", explains the use of microneedles, how can they be used as biosensors, and their usefulness in drug release. Moreover, the chapter authors claim that microneedle devices allow the continuous monitoring of physiological parameters with very low invasiveness, together with sustained administration of local drugs for long surgical procedures.

Chapter 4, "Control Strategy for Underactuated Multi-Fingered Robot Hand Movement Using Electromyography Signal with Wearable Myo Armband", develops a control strategy for an underactuated robotic hand, based on surface electromyography (sEMG) signal obtained from a wireless Myo gesture armband to distinguish six several hand movements.

Chapter 5, "Advanced Materials and Assembly Strategies for Wearable Biosensors: A Review", discusses various types of wearable biosensors within the context of human health monitoring with a focus on their constituent materials, mechanics designs, and large-scale assembly strategies. The chapter also addresses current challenges and potential future research directions.

Section 3 includes three chapters that examine processes that occur in sensors' layers and at their interface. Chapters also provide analytical and numerical methods to solve equations of conjugated enzymatic (chemical) and diffusion processes. Thus, digital modeling is important for both proximal analytical solutions and experimental data [5].

Chapter 6, "Ultra-Precise MEMS Based Bio-Sensors", discusses state-of-the-art micro-electro-mechanical system (MEMS) sensors used for biosensing applications. It studies a new class of resonant microsensors and presents the device architecture/s based on an array of weakly coupled resonators.

Chapter 7, "Microfluidic Adsorption-Based Biosensors: Mathematical Models of Time Response and Noise, Considering Mass Transfer and Surface Heterogeneity", gives advanced mathematical models of time response and noise of such devices, which are needed to improve the interpretation of empirical measurement results, to achieve the optimal sensor performance. It presents the mathematical models and considers the coupling of processes that generate the sensor signal: adsorption-desorption (AD) of the target analyte particles on the heterogeneous sensing surface, and mass transfer (MT) in a microfluidic chamber.

Chapter 8, "Hybrid Heterostructures for SPR Biosensor", demonstrates the details of surface plasmon resonance (SPR) technology with two recently studied prism-based hybrid heterostructures. These heterostructures are made up of conventional SPR biosensors with two additional layers of recently invented transition metal dichalcogenides, platinum di-selenide (PtSe2), and highly sensitive 2D material, tungsten di-sulfide (WS2).

Section 4 includes three chapters that provide a comprehensive glimpse of different biosensors and their characteristics, operating principles, and designs, based on transduction types and biological components [6].

Chapter 9, "Advanced Biosensing towards Real-Time Imaging of Protein Secretion from Single Cells", summarizes recent advances in real-time imaging of single cellular protein secretion, including label-free and labeling techniques, to unravel the direction for developing a simple and powerful methodology for real-time imaging of single cellular protein secretion.

Chapter 10, "Novel Biosensing Strategies for the *in Vivo* Detection of microRNA", describes the principles and designs of these detection technologies and discusses their advantages as well as their shortcomings, providing guidelines for the further development of more sensitive and selective miRNA sensing strategies in vivo.

Chapter 11, "Electrochemical Response of Cells Using Bioactive Plant Isolates", probes the electrochemical response of model cells using bioactive compounds captured in bio-zeolites or membrane mimetics. The voltage and current fluctuations emanating from studies establish a correlation between cell death and membrane depolarization.

Dr. Luis Jesús Villarreal Gómez and Dr. Ana Leticia Iglesias
Facultad de Ciencias de la Ingeniería y Tecnología,
Universidad Autónoma de Baja California,
Tijuana, Baja California, México

References

[1] Mehrotra P. Biosensors and their applications - A review. J Oral Biol Craniofacial Res [Internet]. 2016;6(2):153-9. Available from: http://dx.doi.org/10.1016/j.jobcr.2015.12.002

[2] Vigneshvar S, Sudhakumari CC, Senthilkumaran B, Prakash H. Recent advances in biosensor technology for potential applications - an overview. Front Bioeng Biotechnol. 2016;4(FEB):1-9.

[3] Holzinger M, Goff A Le, Cosnier S. Nanomaterials for biosensing applications: A review. Front Chem. 2014;2(AUG):1-10.

[4] Kim J, Campbell AS, de Ávila BE-F, Wang J. Wearable biosensors for healthcare monitoring. Nat Biotechnol [Internet]. 2019;37(4):389-406. Available from: https://doi.org/10.1038/s41587-019-0045-y

[5] Botkin ND, Turova VL. Mathematical models of a biosensor. Appl Math Model. 2004;28(6):573-89.

[6] Singh S, Kumar V, Dhanjal DS, Datta S, Prasad R, Singh J. Biological Biosensors for Monitoring and Diagnosis. 2020;317-35.

Section 1

Nanomaterials in Biosensing

Chapter 1

Nanomaterial-Enhanced Receptor Technology for Silicon On-Chip Biosensing Application

Timothy Anton Okhai, Azeez O. Idris, Usisipho Feleni and Lukas W. Snyman

Abstract

Nanomaterials integration in biosensors designs are known to enhance sensing and signaling capabilities by exhibiting remarkably high surface area enhancement and intrinsic reactivity owing to their distinctive optical, chemical, electrical and catalytic properties. We present the synthesis and characterization of silver nanoparticles (AgNPs), and their immobilization on a silicon on-chip biosensor platform to enhance sensing capability for prostate specific antigen (PSA) - cancer biomarkers. Several techniques, including UV-Visible (UV-Vis) absorption spectrum, Fourier transforms infrared spectroscopy (FTIR), high resolution transmission electron microscopy (HRTEM), scanning electron microscopy (SEM) and field emission scanning electron microscopy (FESEM) were used for characterizing the AgNPs. The biochemical sensor consists of AgNPs immobilized on the receptor layer of a silicon avalanche mode light emitting device (Si AM LED) which enables on-chip optical detection biological analytes. A bio-interaction layer etched from the chip interacts with the evanescent field of a micro dimensioned waveguide. An array of detectors below the receptor cavity selectively monitor reflected light in the UV, visible, infrared and far infrared wavelength regions. AgNPs used as an immobilization layer in the receptor layer enhances selective absorption analytes, causing a change in detection signal as a function of propagation wavelength as light is dispersed. The analytes could range from gases to cancer biomarkers like prostate specific antigen.

Keywords: silicon avalanche mode LED, silver nanoparticles, biochemical sensors, optical sensor, nanomaterials, receptor technology

1. Introduction

Biosensors and lab-on-chip (LOC) devices have become a subject of growing professional interest world-wide. This is evident in the growing number of scientific publications, and the astronomical growth in the world market for biosensors and lab-on-chip devices over the past ten years. This has been possible, on a large part, due to rapid improvements in sensing techniques, innovation and growth in the development of new biomaterials such as conducting polymers, copolymers and sol-gels, multiplexing capabilities that promote versatility in new generation sensor devices, the possibility of integration on standard silicon integrated circuit chip, and miniaturization possibilities down to micro- and nano-dimensions. Recently, researchers have been successful in developing light emitting devices that can be realized in standard silicon integrated circuitry, and have also proposed diverse applications for these in the future [1–5]. The main advantage of these devices may be the ease of integration into mainstream silicon manufacturing technology such as complementary metal oxide silicon (CMOS) and radio frequency (RF) bipolar technologies. Through recent research, light emission from silicon devices has been achieved in various reverse-biased p-n avalanche structures. This development has now been nomenclated as "silicon light-emitting diodes that operate in the reverse avalanche mode" (Si AMLEDs) [6–10]. If the detailed dispersion characteristics observed per solid angle for a particular device is known, it can enable the design of novel and futuristic on-chip electro-optic applications. Examples of such applications could include wavelength multiplexers for on-chip communication, diverse futuristic on-chip micro- and nano-dimensioned gas sensors and even on-chip biosensors [11–14]. In this chapter, a two-junction micro-dimension p + −np + Silicon Avalanche-based Light Emitting Device (Av Si LED) has been analyzed in terms of radiation geometrical dispersion characteristics, and with particular interest in the different wavelengths of light (colors) being emitted at different emission angles from the surface of the device. It is worthy of note that the detailed dispersion characteristics will be a function of the device structure, the number of transparent over layers with each having different optical refractive index, and even the final topography or curvature of the various surface layers.

2. Light emitting characteristics from silicon AMLEDs

Light emitting devices (LEDs) have become a subject of growing research interest in recent times. A series of LEDs have been realized in standard Complementary Metal Oxide Silicon (CMOS) technology by Kramer et al., [15] and Snyman et al. in [15–19]. These structures emit light through phonon-assisted intra-band and inter-band recombination phenomena [20–22]. Subsequent devices were developed by Du Plessis et al., which showed increased light emission when additional carriers are injected into avalanching Si n + p light emitting junctions [23, 24]. Further work by Xu et al. led to the realization of a series of CMOS integrated LED devices with third terminal gated control [8]. Subsequently, the temperature, carrier density, and electric field encountered in Silicon Avalanche Mode Light Emitting Devices (Si AMLEDs) were analyzed by Duttal and Steeneken et al. They also suggested operation of gated Si LED operating in the forward-biased mode and emitting in the 1100 nm region [12]. A major advantage with these devices is the realization of high modulation speeds ranging into the GHz due to the reverse bias configuration of Si AMLEDs [25, 26]. Potential applications of these devices can be found in hybrid optical RF systems, on-chip micro-photonic systems, and CMOS-based optical interconnect. In a recent work by Xu and Snyman, they demonstrated enhanced emission intensities of 0.1 to about 200 nW/μm^2 from Si AMLEDs in the 650–750 nm emission regime by using enhanced impurity scattering and extended E-field profiling in the device [27, 28].

We present in this chapter a specific p + np + graded junction type Si AMLED device (**Figure 1(a)**) that was realized in a 0.35 micron Si bipolar process with a high frequency RF application capability. This process enabled an "elongated pillar" structure to be etched out on a broad silicon semi-insulating p-substrate. These structures could hence effectively confine the lateral carrier diffusion and

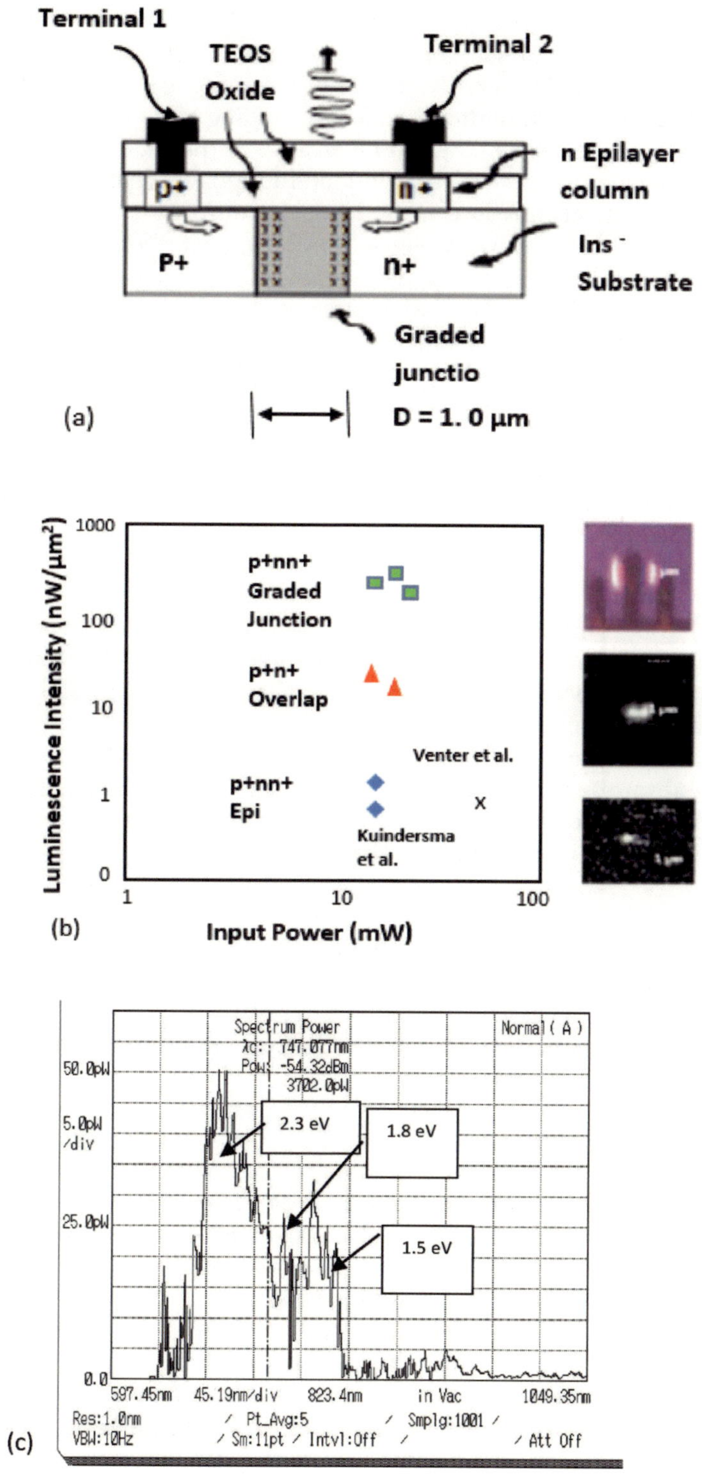

Figure 1.
Device design (schematic), considerations of a p + nn + Si avalanche mode LED in RF bipolar integrated circuitry [27] (a) lateral cross-section of the device. (b) Device optical performance characteristics as compared with other previous devices [27]. (c) Spectral characteristics of the emitted optical radiation (for below 570 nm consult Ref. [17]). Inserts show optical emission micrographs of the LEDs taken at normal angles to the surface of the device.

maximize the diffusing carrier density in the device. The device used n + and p + regions in the substrate region of the silicon, and positioned a distance 1 micron apart from each other. Subsequently, up to 1 micron graded doping profiles were formed at the edges of these regions, while overlapping of dopants occurred in the center region of the device [27]. For illustrative purposes, device design and performance characteristics relative to previous designs are again presented in **Figure 1(b)**. The optical emissions from the device were measured with an Anritso MS9710B Spectrum Analyzer with a lensed-probe optical fiber. The device and the lensed probe were electronically micro manipulated to within 0.1 mm of the light-emitting device. The total emission intensities with cross-sectional conduction areas of about 1 micron square as indicated at the surface of the device was measured to be in the order of 200 nW per μm^2. **Figure 1(c)** depicts the main spectral components as observed for these types of devices. Clear peaks and prominent peaks of 2.8 eV, 2.3 eV, 1.8 eV, and 1.5 eV were observed in the spectrographic measurements for the devices and are shown in the spectrum when converting the nm emissions to corresponding eV emissions [19, 27]. Overall, the spectrum represent a broad spectrum from 450 nm to about 850 nm with main characteristic peaks at 450 nm (2.8 eV) (blueish), 550 nm (2.0 eV) (greenish), 600 nm (2.3 eV) (reddish), and at 750 to 850 nm (1.5 and 1.8 eV) (infrared). To form the on-chip biosensor, a bio-interaction layer etched from the Si AMLED chip interacts with the evanescent field of a micro dimensioned waveguide. An array of detectors below the receptor cavity selectively monitor reflected light in the UV, visible, infrared and far-infrared wavelength regions.

AgNPs used as immobilization layer in the receptor layer enhances sensitivity and selective absorption of antigens and biomarkers, like the prostate specific antigen (a biomarker for prostate cancer), causing a change in detection signal as a function of propagation wavelength as light is dispersed.

3. Transducers and transduction mechanisms in biosensors

Integrated biosensors can be categorized in several ways, one of which is their transduction mechanism. Below is a brief description of some of the main transducers used in biosensor mechanisms:

3.1 Transduction mechanisms

Electrochemical or Electroanalytical transducers: These types of transducers exploit analyte capturing to change the electrochemical characteristics of electrode-electrolyte systems. Hassibi, and Lee [29] described one of the first reports of a CMOS electrochemical biosensor array chip capable of performing impedance spectroscopy, amperometric analysis, and cyclic-voltammetry techniques. The Electrical performance of this CMOS multi-functional chip is comparable to state-of-the–art electrochemical measurement instruments currently used in molecular biology. Prior efforts in this area are limited only to ISFET [30] and conduction-based sensor arrays [31] in CMOS compatible processes.

Mechanical transducers: Mechanical transducers in biosensors are systems in which an electromechanical parameter of the system (e.g., mass of a cantilever) is changed by the additional mass of the captured analytes. Mechanical transducers cannot be fabricated using standard CMOS processes. This is largely because CMOS processes, unlike many MEMs processes, offer no component or device, which can move in response to mechanical motion [32, 33].

Thermal transducers: They are used to measure the temperature change during biological thermal reactions to detect the total number of molecules involved in the reaction [34].

Acoustic transducers: Acoustic transducers are based on the principle of using acoustic waves to develop biosensing devices. Acoustic waves can be used to analyze biochemical reactions in different fluid (liquid and gas) environments because they have the ability to travel through them easily. Different mechanisms can be employed to either generate or receive acoustic waves, including piezoelectric, magnetostrictive, optical and thermal techniques. The surface or the acoustic biosensor can be functionalized using standard methods, and the binding of the target analyte will induce a change in the acoustic wave. By measuring and subsequently analyzing this variation in the resonant frequency, it is possible to determine the correlation between the acoustic signal and the interaction of the molecule. One important advantage of acoustic transducers is the ability to operate using wireless excitation. This makes it extremely important for sensing in difficult-to-reach or hazardous environmental conditions. Additionally, the compatibility with integrated circuit technology permits a high efficiency in the fabrication process. The main drawback of this technique is the fact that any little vibration induced in the system can produce artifacts that will require complex algorithms to differentiate from the true biosensing signals [35].

Optical transducers: Optical biosensors can easily fulfill the requirement for high sensitivity, fast response and the potential for real-time measurements. They also lend themselves to optical measurements through different techniques like emission, absorption, fluorescence, refractometry, or polarimetry. Optical biosensors based on evanescent wave detection have unique properties such as extremely high sensitivity for direct, real-time measurement of biomolecular interactions in label-free schemes. The advantages of optical sensing are significantly improved when this approach is used within an integrated optics context. Integrated optics technology allows the integration of passive and active optical components (including fibers, emitters, detectors, waveguides, and related devices) onto the same substrate, allowing the flexible development of miniaturized compact sensing devices, with the additional possibility to fabricate multiple sensors on a single chip. The integration offers additional advantages such as miniaturization, robustness, reliability, potential for mass production with consequent reduction of production costs, low energy consumption, and simplicity in the alignment of the individual optical elements [36].

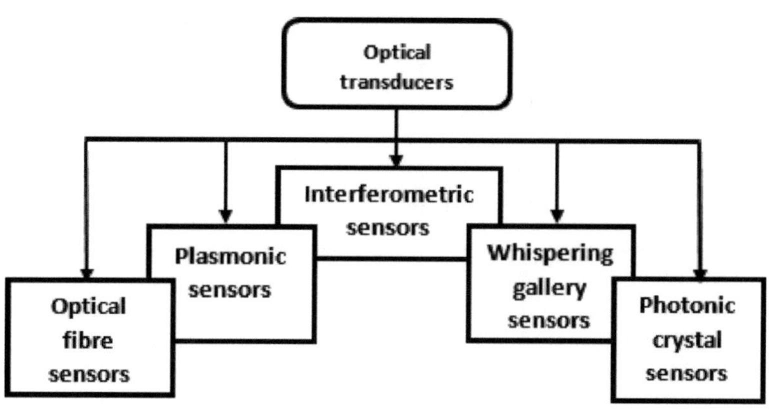

Figure 2.
Categories of optical transducers used for biosensor applications.

Independent of the transduction method used in integrated biosensors, one challenge is always to adequately immobilize capturing probes on the surface to create the capturing spot. Our design addresses this challenge by etching a receptor cavity through the silicon substrate, and by using AgNPs as immobilization layer in the receptor layer to enhance selective absorption of the target analyte.

3.2 Optical transducers categories

Optical transducers can be further categorized into the different categories shown in **Figure 2** above.

4. Waveguide structures

In waveguide structures, light is guided in the plane of the thin film, facilitating the integration of such a sensor, along with source and detector components, into a single integrated chip device [37]. This is a significant advantage in the development of on-chip micro- and nano-optical biosensors. Secondly, for porous silicon waveguides, the active sensing layer is the top porous layer, eliminating the infiltration difficulties that can plague Bragg mirrors, rugate filters, and micro-cavities, where biomolecules must filter through many layers of both high and low porosity. As a result of both advantages mentioned above, waveguide sensors display electric field confinement, sharp resonance peaks, and a thin sensing layer, all qualities that facilitate a fast response and a high sensitivity detection of molecules.

4.1 Optical waveguide biosensors

Various modalities have been developed for optical waveguide biosensor applications. They include grating-coupled waveguide sensors, interferometric waveguide sensors, photonic crystal waveguide sensors and resonant optical microcavity sensors, among others. **Figure 3** below provides examples for each of the optical waveguide options mentioned.

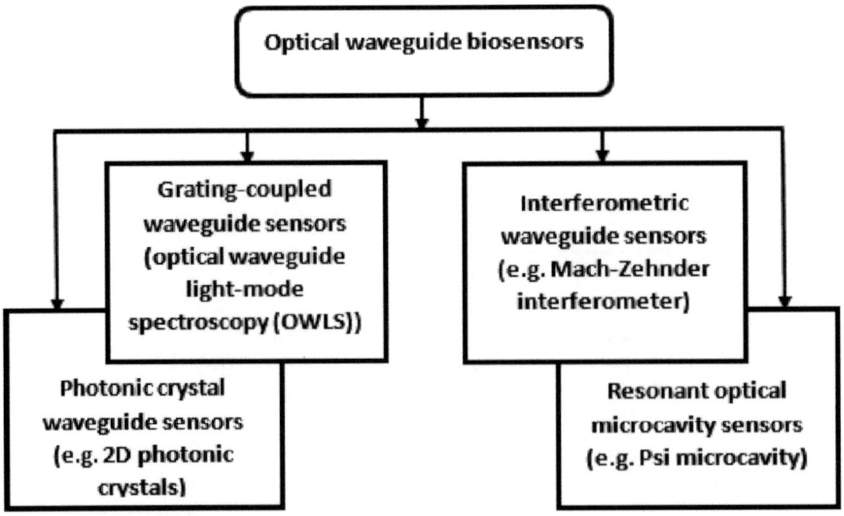

Figure 3.
Optical waveguide biosensor modalities and examples of their applications.

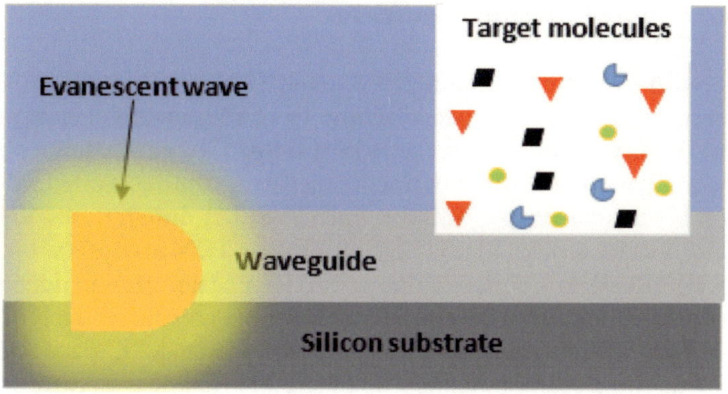

Figure 4.
Schematic representation of an optical biosensor based on evanescent wave interaction. Due to interaction of the light with the target molecules (analytes) within the cavity in the interaction area, the optical wave undergoes a change in its propagation constant due to the variation in the effective refractive index.

4.2 Receptor layer in waveguide and evanescent field

The difference in refractive index between the core and cladding of an optical waveguide exist. Thus, light is guided via the core with a higher refractive index on account of total internal reflection, which generates an evanescent optical field that decays exponentially from the sensor surface, as in **Figure 4**. Biomolecular binding events modulate the refractive index contrast and thus attenuate the propagation of light through the waveguide. By monitoring the coupling and/or propagation properties of light through an appropriately modified waveguide, it is possible to construct sensors responsive to the target biomolecular analytes of interest, as shown in **Figure 4**.

5. Synthesis and characterization of nanomaterials

Silver nanoparticles were, characterized and applied in the receptor layer to enhance the sensitivity of the biosensor. The synthesis method and materials, and the characterization procedures and results are discussed in the following sections.

5.1 Synthesis procedure and materials

Silver nanoparticles were prepared by chemical reduction method, using silver nitrate ($AgNO_3$) as the silver precursor. The preparation procedure of silver nanoparticles is adopted from Muzamil et al., [38] with minor modification. All reagents were of analytical grade and used without any further purification. The reagents include Silver nitrate ($AgNO_3$, ≥99%), Trisodium citrate ($Na_3C_6H_5O_7$, 1%), Polyethylene glycol ($C_2nH_4n + 2On + 1$, ≥99%), and Sodium hydroxide (NaOH, ≥99%), and were all purchased from Sigma Aldrich. The experiment was conducted at room temperature (23°C) unless otherwise stated. To synthesize silver nanoparticles, 50 ml of 1 mM silver nitrate solution and 5 ml of polyethylene glycol were taken and heated till boiling on a magnetic stirrer. When the solution started to boil, 1% trisodium citrate solution of 4 ml was quickly added with constant stirring. A few minutes later, the solution turned into yellow color, hinting the formation of silver nanoparticles. The pH of the nanoparticles was kept at 7.6 by adding NaOH. Afterward, it was cooled to room temperature and stored at 4°C before use.

5.2 Characterization of silver nanoparticles

The prepared AgNPs were characterized using SEM, FESEM, HRTEM, SAXS, FTIR Spectroscopy, and UV–Vis spectroscopy. The SEM images of samples were obtained from JEOL Scanning Microscope JSM-6400. The surface morphology and elemental analysis of the silver nanoparticles were studies using JSM-7800F Field Emission Electron Scanning Microscope (FESEM), integrated with energy-dispersive x-ray spectroscopy (EDS). High resolution TEM analysis was carried out using Hitachi H-800 electron microscope at 200 kV acceleration to determine the size distribution and elemental composition of samples respectively. Small angle x-ray scattering (SAXS) spectroscopy was performed with SAXSpace Spectrometer from Anton-Paar, Graz, Austria, using a solid sample. The X-ray scattering spectra were plotted with a SAXdrive software. GIFT software was used to Fourier transform the scattering data to obtain the pair distance distribution function (PDDF) and size distribution spectra. The functional groups of the nanomaterials were done on a Perkin Elmer FTIR spectrometer Frontier (Spectrum 100 spectrometer) in the range

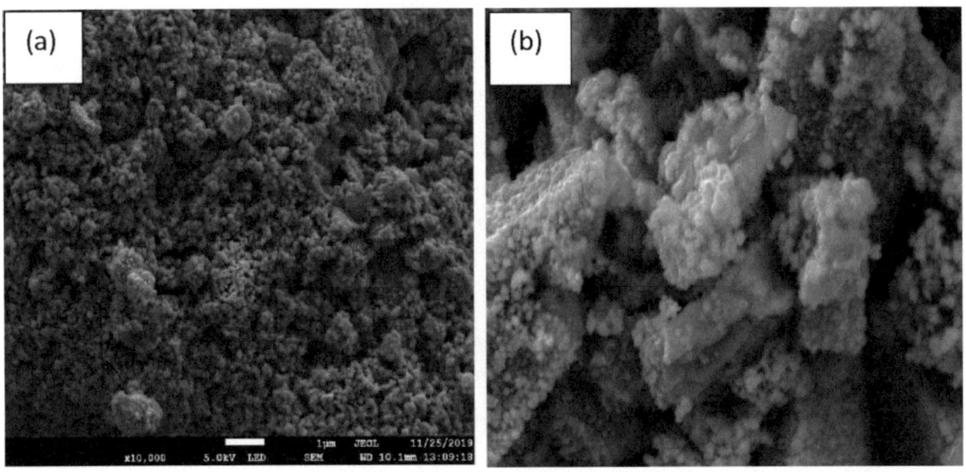

Figure 5.
Electro-micrograph image of (a) SEM analysis, and (b) FESEM analysis at a magnification of x10,000.

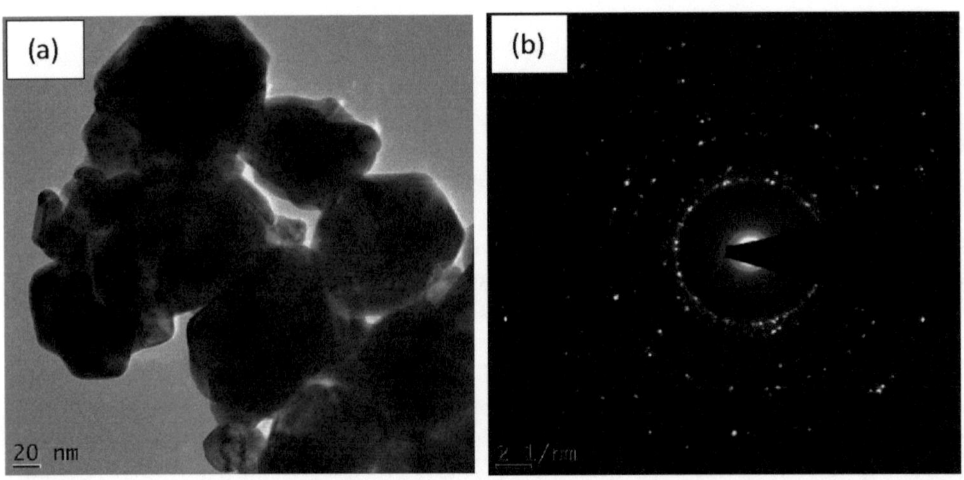

Figure 6.
(a) HRTEM electro-micrograph at 20 nm scale view and (b) SAED pattern of AgNPs.

of 400–4000 cm^{-1} using the KBr pellet method. UV-vis spectra were acquired over the range of 200–800 nm using PerkinElma Lambda 650S UV/Visible Spectrometer. To produce graphs and curves that are clear enough for reporting, Origin 8.0 software was used to plots the data obtained from the characterization equipment.

5.3 Results and discussion

Scanning electron microscope (SEM) and FESEM were used for topographical imaging of the nanoparticles, and to investigate the size, shape, impurities &

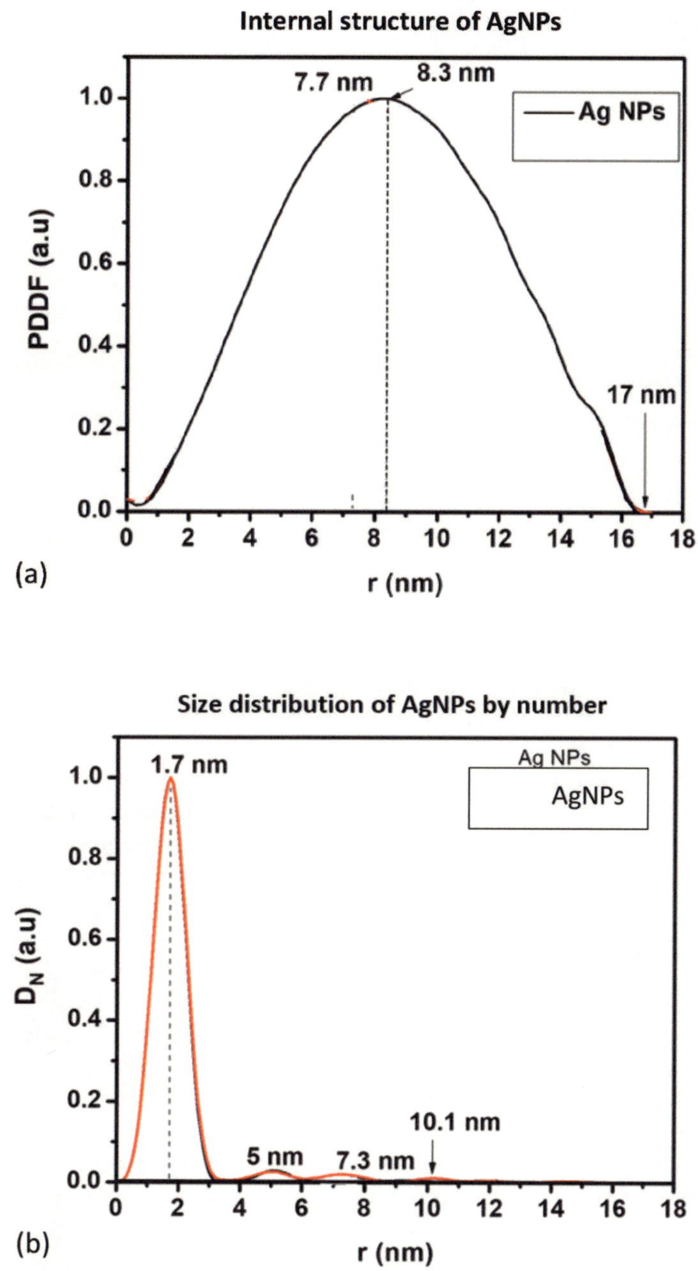

Figure 7.
(a) SAXS analysis showing (a) internal structure of AgNPs (b) size distribution by number.

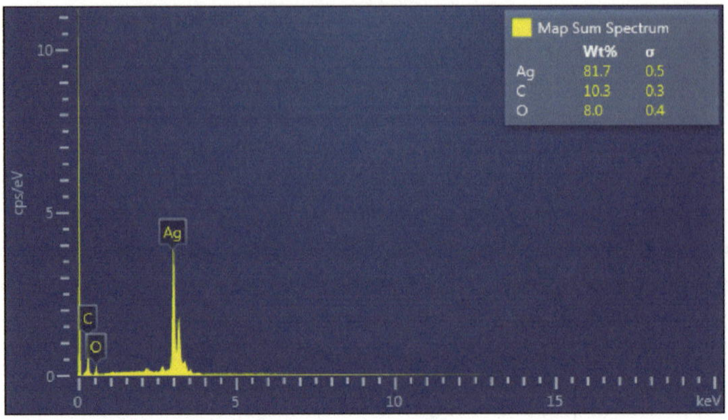

Figure 8.
EDS spectrum confirming the presence of silver, carbon and oxygen.

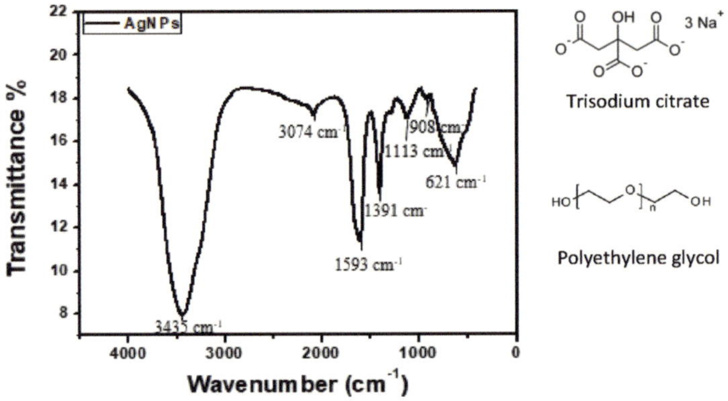

Figure 9.
FTIR graph showing prominent peaks representing the unique fingerprint of AgNPs that was synthesized.

stabilization of the particles, as shown in **Figure 5(a)** and **(b)**. The SEM image of the AgNPs shown in **Figure 5(a)** reveals a globular-shaped morphology, which was further confirmed by the FESEM image in **Figure 5(b)**. The FESEM confirmed the globular-cluster shaped morphology of the silver nanoparticles.

Interestingly, the HRTEM image in **Figure 6(a)** showed that the AgNPs are spherical at nano-range with spherically shaped internal structures. This is supported by the selected area diffraction structure (SAED) image in **Figure 6(b)**. HRTEM results also complement the SAXS results, which show that most of the particles are spherical or cuboidal in shape.

The SAXS analysis in **Figure 7** was used to investigate the internal structure of the nanoparticle, and it revealed that the AgNPs show lattice fringes, which confirms that the particles are crystalline. In addition, they exhibited a quarzi-spherically shaped internal structure as expected. **Figure 7(a)** shows the internal structure of the AgNPs, while **Figure 7(b)** shows their size distribution by number.

The elemental composition of the AgNPs was evaluated by energy dispersion x-ray spectroscopy (EDS) to find out the purity of the nanomaterials. From the layered images and the EDS spectrum analysis, we confirm the presence of silver, carbon and oxygen, as shown in **Figure 8**. The presence of carbon was due to the carbon tape used for coating the nanomaterial before the analysis.

The morphology is consistent with the expectation for silver nanoparticles, and we functionalized our silver with polyethylene glycol. The sizes (width and diameter) for the AgNPs could not be clearly determined due to agglomeration of the particles. In the FTIR analysis represented by the graph in **Figure 9**, prominent peaks were observed for different stretches of bonds. The peak at 3435 cm^{-1}, representing N-H stretch, 3074 cm^{-1} assigned to C-H stretching vibrations, and 1593 cm^{-1} corresponding to stretching vibration of C=O bond. The peak at 1391 cm^{-1} corresponds to C-C and C-N stretching, while 1113 cm^{-1} assigned to –C = bond, and 908 cm^{-1} and 621 cm^{-1} are for C-H out-of-plane bend and CH bending vibrations, respectively. These peaks are comparable to [39].

UV Visible spectroscopy is one of the most important techniques which can confirm that the prepared material are nanoparticles [40]. **Figure 10** shows the plot of absorption spectrum obtained from the UV-Vis spectroscopic analysis of the AgNPs over a range of 200 to 800 nm. The exact peaks occurred at 310 and 400, which is indicative of the peak of silver nanoparticles [41, 42]. The bandgap from the Tauc plot in **Figure 10(b)** for the synthesized AgNPs is 3.26 eV, which implies that the nanomaterials will absorb in the UV-Vis range.

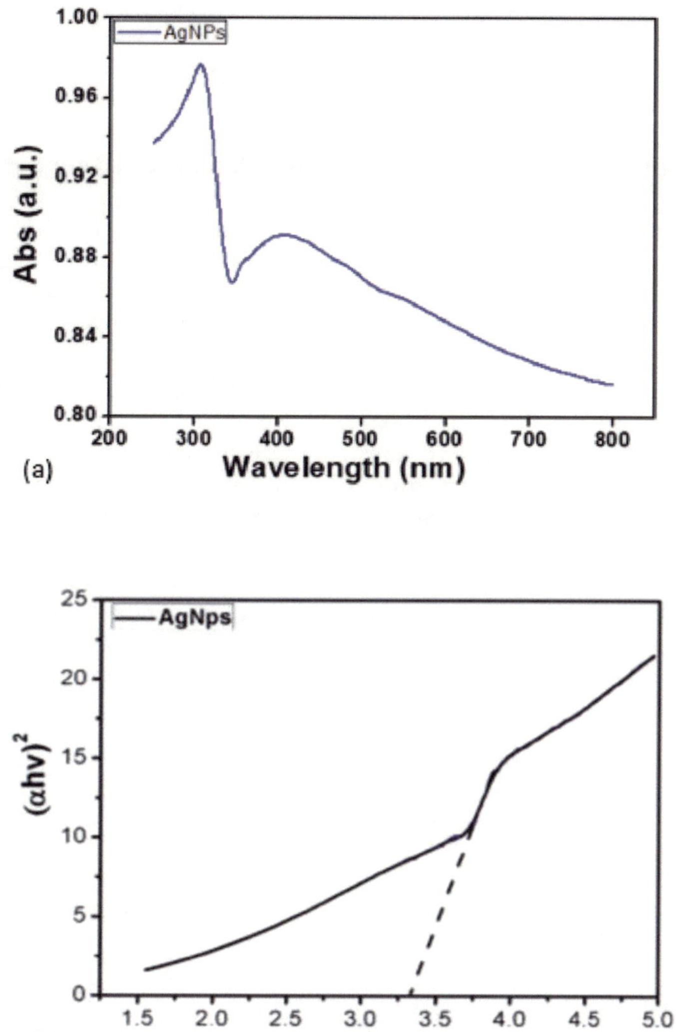

Figure 10.
UV-Vis results for AgNPs showing (a) the absorption spectrum, and (b) the bandgap from Tauc plot.

6. Design, simulations and potential applications

We present in this section the design, simulation results and potential futuristic on-chip applications of our device.

6.1 Software simulation and design

To model how the evanescent waves would couple with bio-species in a cavity etched in the nitrite layer as light waves travel through the waveguide, we performed optical simulations using RSoft BeamProp optical simulation software. As represented in **Figure 11**, light emitted from the optical source travels through the waveguide. As the resultant evanescent wave travels through the cavity etched deep into the nitride layer, it is exposed to specific analyte material trapped within the cavity. In this design, a multimode wave travels through high refractive index bridge waveguide and interacts with material within the etched cavity in the nitride layer. The interaction, in this case, would be primarily a function of the specific refractive index of the analyte inside that cavity, since the multimode light traveling in the waveguide will interact and be diverted into the absorbed analyte. The unique fingerprints of each material within the cavity then produces a change in signal that is recognizable by the detector, as in **Figure 11(a)**.

6.2 Applications in futuristic micro- and nano-dimensioned devices

Applications already proposed and demonstrated for Si Av LEDs include micro displays [44, 45] and Lab-on-chip systems [46, 47]. Analyses of test results from our device open up exciting possibilities for potential applications for the derived technology in futuristic integrated on-chip optoelectronic and biosensor applications.

These applications can be achieved through (1) placements of specific designed optical sources with specific directional and dispersive emission characteristics; (2) design and placement of micro wavelength dispersive coupling into micro dimensioned on-chip optical waveguides, and (3) design and placement of broadband wavelength emitters for diverse on-chip electro-optic applications. Other possible applications include (4) realization of various on-chip nano- and micro-dimensioned sensors that can detect a variety of parameters, ranging from standard physical parameters to a range of derived bio-parameters through the

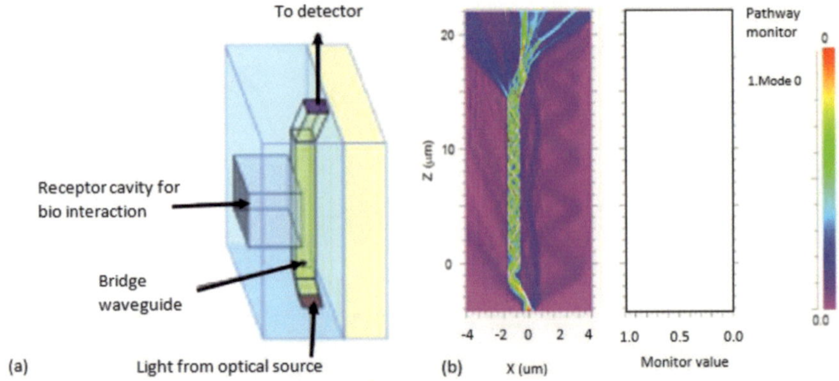

Figure 11.
Bridge waveguide design realization with RSoft BeamProp optical simulation software: (a) design of bridge waveguide device [43], (b) optical simulation run for the bridge waveguide.

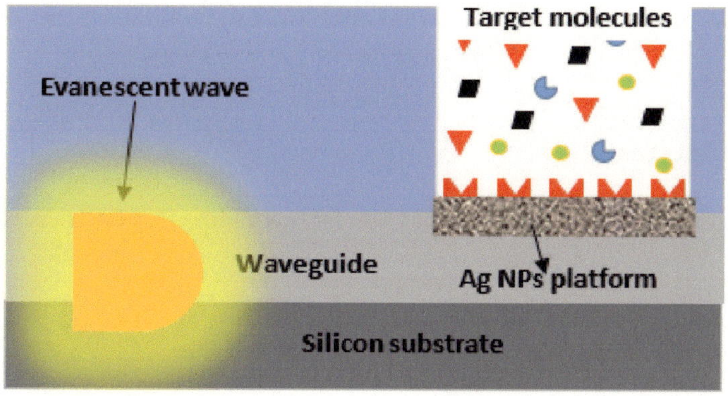

Figure 12.
Application of optical biosensor based on evanescent wave interaction and nanomaterial enhancement for increased sensitivity and selectivity of target analytes in the within the cavity in the interaction area.

use of waveguide optics and intermediate evanescent-based waveguide receptor layers. An attractive feature of these applications is the micro-positioning of the optical source itself through micro- and nano-lithographic technology, the design of waveguides and wavelength dispersers using the same technology, and the design of micro-electronic processing technology in close proximity to the optical source and detectors to process and transfer derived information to adjacent on-chip processing circuitry. **Figure 12** demonstrates a typical application where the AgNPs synthesized are deployed in the etched cavity within the nitrite layer to form a highly sensitive platform for selective detection of analytes like prostate specific antigen, which is a biomarker for prostate cancer cells.

7. Conclusions

The current designs and simulations as demonstrated in this chapter indicate that it would be possible to develop simple to advanced micro and even nano sensors directly on silicon chip, by means of Si AMLEDs and standard silicon integrated circuitry processing. The design of various on-chip nano-and micro-dimensioned sensors that can detect a variety of parameters using waveguide optics and intermediate evanescent- and waveguide-based receptor layers seems possible. The major advantage of such biosensors would be the micro-dimensioning and the integration of such sensors directly on the chip, in conjunction with adjacent on-chip optical processing circuitry. Sensitivity and selectivity of such biosensor devices can be enhanced by creating a layer of nanomaterials in the receptor cavity. Since monolayers of analytes can be detected through the diversion of waveguide traveling radiation into absorbed species with different refractive indices, or through the coupling of species with the evanescent electrical fields of waveguides, the sensors could be made extremely sensitive.

Acknowledgements

This work was supported in part by the National Research Foundation's Rated Researcher Incentive Funding (IFR2011033100025 Grant), Key International Collaboration Grant (KIC 69798), and the Department of Higher Education and Training (DHET) Grant, administered by the Tshwane University of Technology, South Africa. The iNanoWS Laboratory at UNISA, South Africa, is specially thanked for supporting the experimental analyses and facilitating the nanomaterials analysis and characterization work as presented in this chapter.

Conflict of interest

"The authors declare no conflict of interest." or delete this entire section.

Author details

Timothy Anton Okhai[1,3*], Azeez O. Idris[2], Usisipho Feleni[2] and Lukas W. Snyman[2,3]

1 Clinical Engineering Cluster Group, Department of Electrical Engineering, Tshwane University of Technology, Pretoria, South Africa

2 Institute for Nanotechnology and Water Sustainability (iNanoWS), College of Science, Engineering and Technology, University of South Africa, Florida, South Africa

3 Department of Electrical Engineering, College of Science, Engineering and Technology, University of South Africa, Florida, South Africa

*Address all correspondence to: timokhai@yahoo.co.uk

References

[1] Fitzgerald EA, and Kimerling LC. Silicon-based micro-photonics 627 and integrated optoelectronics. MRS Bull: 1998. vol. 23, no. 4, pp. 39-47.

[2] Wada K. Electronics and photonics convergence on Si CMOS platform. In: Proceedings of SPIE. 2004; 5357, p. 16-24.

[3] Alfano RR. The ultimate white light. Sci. Amer. 2006;295: 86-93.

[4] Soref R. The Past, Present, and Future of Silicon Photonics. Selected Topics in Quantum Electronics. IEEE Journal of. 2006;12:1678-1687.

[5] Soref R. Silicon photonics technology: past, present and future. In: Kubby JA, and Jabbour GE. Editors. Optoelectronic Integration on Silicon II. Proceedings of SPIE; 2008.p.5730.

[6] Snyman LW, Ogudo KD, and Foty D. Development of a 0.75 micron wavelength CMOS optical communication system. In: Proceedings of SPIE; 2011; 7943.p. 79430K-1–79430K-12.

[7] Snyman LW. Integrating Micro-Photonic Systems and MOEMS into Standard Silicon CMOS Integrated Circuitry. In: Predeep P, editor. Optoelectronics – Devices and Applications. Croatia; IntechOpen; 2011. p. 23-50. DOI: 10.5772/18810/978-953-51-4921-7.ch2

[8] Xu K, Snyman LW, Polleux J-L, Chen H, and Li G. Silicon Light-Emitting Device with Application in the Micro-opto-electro-mechanical Systems. International Journal of Materials, Mechanics and Manufacturing. 2015; 3; 4; pp282-286. ISSN: 1793-8198

[9] Xu K, Ogudo KA, Polleux J-L, Viana C, Ma Z, Li Z, Yu Q, Li G, and Snyman LW. Light-emitting Devices in Si CMOS and RF Bipolar Integrated Circuits. 2016; 2; 1550-2716. DOI: 10.1080/15502724.2015.1134333

[10] Newman R. Visible light from a silicon p-n junction. Phys. Rev. 1955; 100; 2. 700-704.

[11] Ghynoweth WG, and McKay KG. Photon emission from avalanche breakdown in silicon. Physical Rev. 1956; 102;369-376.

[12] Dutta S, Steeneken PG, Agarwal V, Schmitz J, Annema A-J, Hueting RJE. The Avalanche-Mode Superjunction LED. IEEE Transactions on Electron Devices. 2017; 64; 1612-1618.

[13] Okhai TA, Snyman LW, Polleux J-L. Wavelength dispersion characteristics of integrated Silicon Avalanche LEDs – Potential applications in futuristic on-chip micro-and nano-bio-sensors. In: Proceedings of the SPIE Fourth Conference on Sensors, MEMS and Electro-Optic Systems (SMEOS '17), September 2016; Skukuza, South Africa; SPIE 2017. 10036. p. 1003604-1003604-22.

[14] Hassibi AA, Plummer ID, and Griffin PB. Design requirements for integrated biosensor arrays. Progress in Biomedical Optics and Imaging. In: Proceedings of SPIE; 2017. 5699; 57. p. 403-413. DOI: 10.1117/12.591300

[15] Kramer J, Seitz P, Steigmeier EF, Auderset H, and Delley B. Light-emitting devices in Industrial CMOS technology. Sensors and Actuators. 1993. A37-38. p 527-533.

[16] Bude J, Sano N, and Yoshii A. Hot carrier luminescence in silicon.Phys. Rev. B. 1992; 45: 11. p. 5848-5856.

[17] Akil N, Houstma VE, LeMinth P, Holleman J, Zieren V,

DeMooij D, Woerlee PH, van den Berg A, and Wallinga H. Modelling of light-emission spectra measured on silicon nanometer-scale diode antifuses. Journal of Applied Physics. 2000; 88; 4. p. 1916-1922.

[18] Moll JL and Van Overstraeten R. Charge multiplication in silicon p-n junctions. Solid-State Electron. 1963: 6; 2. p. 147-157.

[19] Snyman LW, du Plessis M, Seevinck E, and Aharoni H. An efficient, low voltage, high frequency silicon CMOS light emitting device and electro-optical interface. IEEE Electron Device Letters. 1999; 20;12. p. 614-617.

[20] Agah A, Hassibi I, Plummer D, and Griffin PB. Design requirements for integrated biosensor arrays. Progress in Biomedical Optics and Imaging. In: Proceedings of SPIE. 2005; 5699: 57. p. 403-413. DOI: 10.1117/12.591300

[21] Lechuga LM. Optical biosensors. In: Gorton L. Biosensors and Modern Biospecific Analytical Techniques. vol. 44 of Comprehensive Analytical Chemistry Series. Editor. Amsterdam: Elsevier Science BV; 2005; 44. p. 209-250.

[22] Healthcare in the palm of your hand. [Internet]. 2019. Available from: hppt://qualcommtricorderxprize.org. [Accessed: 28/12/2019].

[23] Snyman LW, Aharoni H, du Plessis M, Marais JFK, Van Niekerk D, and Biber A. Planar light emitting electro-optical interfaces in standard silicon complementary metal oxide semiconductor integrated circuitry. Opt. Eng. 2002; 41. p. 3230-3240.

[24] Booth N. and Smith AS. Infrared Detectors. New York and Boston. Goodwin House Publishers. 1997; p. 241-248.

[25] Davis AR, Bush C, Harvey JC and Foley MF. Fresnel lenses in rear projection displays. In: SID Int. Symp. Digest Tech. 2001; 32. p. 934-937.

[26] Van Derlofske JF. Computer modeling of LED light pipe systems for uniform display illumination. In: Proceedings of SPIE. 2001; 4445: p. 119-129.

[27] Snyman LW, Xu K, Polleux J-L, Ogudo KA. and Viana C. Higher Intensity SiAvLEDs in an RF Bipolar Process Through Carrier Energy and Carrier Momentum Engineering. IEEE Journal of Quantum Electronics. 2015; 51; 7. P. 3200110-3200125. DOI: 10.1109/JQE.2015.2427036. (ISSN: 0018-9197).

[28] Snyman LW, Polleux J-L, Ogudo KA, and Du Plessis M. Stimulating 600 – 650nm Wavelength Optical Emission in Monolithically Integrated Silicon LEDs through controlled Injection-Avalanche and Carrier Density Balancing Technology. IEEE Journal of Quantum Electronics. 2017; 53: 5. P. 1-9. DOI: 10.1109/JQE.2017.2736254) (ISSN 0018-9197).

[29] Hassibi A, Lee TH. A programmable Electrochemical Biosensor Array in 0.18 μm. In: International Solid State Conference. 2005. Session 30, Displays and Biosensors,30.7

[30] Wong HS, and White MH. A CMOS integrated ISFET-operational Amplifier Chemical Sensor Employing Differential Sensing. IEEE Trans. on Electron devices. 1989; 36. P. 479-498.

[31] Schienle M, et al,. A fully Electronic DNA sensor with 128 positions and In-Pixel A/D Conversion. ISSCC Dig. Tech. Papers. 2004; p. 220-221.

[32] Savran CA, Burg TP, Fritz J, and Manalis SR. Microfabricated mechanical biosensor with inherently differential readout. Appl. Phys. Lett. 2003; 83: 8. p. 1659.

[33] Voiculescu I, Zaghloul ME, McGill RA, Houser EJ, and Fedder GK.

Electrostatically actuated resonant microcantilever beam in CMOS technology for the detection of chemical weapons. IEEE Sensors J. 2005; 5: 4. p. 641-647.

[34] Ramanathan K, and Danielsson B. Principles and applications of thermal biosensors. Biosens. Bioelectron. 2001; 16: 6. p. 417-423.

[35] Lechuga LM. Optical biosensors. In: Gorton L, editor. Biosensors and Modern Biospecific Analytical Techniques. Vol 44 of Comprehensive Analytical Chemistry Series. Amsterdam: Elsevier Science BV; 2005; p. 209-250.

[36] Zinoviev K, Carascosa LG, Rio JSD, Sepulveda B, Dominguez C. and Lechuga LM. Silicon photonic biosennsors for lab-on-a-chip applications. Advances in Optical Technologies. 2008; 383927. DOI: 10.1155/2008/383927.

[37] Ogudo KA, Snyman LW, Polleux J-L, Viana C, Tegegne Z, and Schmieder D. Towards 10-40 GHz on-chip micro-optical links with all integrated Si Av LED optical sources, Si N based waveguides and Si-Ge detector technology. In: Proceedings of SPIE. 2014; 8991. p. 899108.

[38] Muzamil M, Khalid N, Aziz MD and Abbas SA. Synthesis of silver nanoparticles by silver salt reduction and its characterization. Materials Science and Engineering. 2014; 60. P. 012034. DOI: 10.1088/1757-899X/60/1/012034

[39] Devara J, Kumari P, Aarti C, and Renganathan A. Synthesis and characterization of Silver nanoparticles using cannon ball leaves and their cytotoxic activity against MCF-7 line. Nanocomposites. 2013; 598328. DOI: 101155/2013/598328

[40] Mahadevan S, Vijayakumar S, Arulmozhi P. Green synthesis of silver nano particles from Atalantia monophylla (L) Correa leaf extract, their antimicrobial activity and sensing capability of H2O2. Microbial Pathogenesis. 2017; 113. p. 445-450. DOI: 10.1016/j.micpath.2017.11.029

[41] Salari S, Esmaeilzadeh Bahabadi S, Samzadeh-Kermani A, Yosefzaei F. In-vitro Evaluation of Antioxidant and Antibacterial Potential of GreenSynthesized Silver Nanoparticles Using *Prosopis farcta* Fruit Extract. Iranian Journal of Pharm. Res. 2019; 18: 1. p. 430-455. [Internet]. Available from: https://www.ncbi.nlm.nih.gov/pmc/articles/PMC6487442/

[42] Nilavukkarasi M, Vijayakumar S, Prathip Kumar S. Biological synthesis and characterization of silver nanoparticles with *Capparis zeylanica* L. leaf extract for potent antimicrobial and anti proliferation efficiency. Materials Science for Energy Technologies. 2020; 3. p. 371-376. DOI: 10.1016/j.mset.2020.02.008

[43] Xu K, Chen Y, Okhai TA, and Snyman LW. Micro optical sensors based on avalanching silicon light-emitting devices monolithically integrated on chips. Optical Materials Express. 2019; 9. p. 3985-3997.

[44] Venter PJ, Du Plessis M, Bogalecki AW, Goosen ME and Rademeyer P. An 8 × 64 pixel dot matrix microdisplay in 0.35 micron CMOS technology. Optical Engineering. 2012; 51: 014003. Du Plessis et al.: Spectral Characteristics of hot electron electroluminescence. 577

[45] Chen AR, Akinwande AI, and Lee H-S. CMOS-based microdisplay with calibrated backplane. IEEE J. Solid-State Circuits. 2005. P. 40:2746-2755.

[46] Rebohle L, Gebel T, Yankov RA, Trautmann T, Skorupa W, Sun J, Gauglitz G, and Frank R. Microarrays of silicon-based light emitters for

novel biosensor and lab-on-a-chip applications. Opt. Mater. 2005; 27. P. 1055-1058.

[47] Misiakos K, Petrou PS, Kakabakos SE, Vlahopoulou ME, Tserepi A, Gogolides E, and Ruf HH. Monolithic silicon optoelectronic transducers and elastomeric fluidic modules for bio-spotting and bio-assay experiments. Microelectron. Eng. 2006; 83: p. 1605-1608.

Chapter 2

Nucleic Acids for Electrochemical Biosensor Technology

Zihni Onur Uygun, Hilmiye Deniz Ertuğrul Uygun and Ferhan Girgin Sağin

Abstract

Biosensor technology has developed extremely rapidly in recent years. This technology brings along precise measurements as well as specific measurements. Thanks to its ability to be miniaturized and be easily accessible to the end user, it is one-step ahead of other similar methods. The selectivity of biological molecules and the sensitivity of electrochemical methods enable the continuous evolvement of these new technologies. In this chapter, the use of nucleic acids as both recognition agents and target molecules, the way they are used in biosensor technology and their electrical properties are explained in detail with examples. Aptamers, which are synthetic nucleic acids, and their use in electrochemical biosensor systems with different electrochemical and immobilization methods have been compared extensively.

Keywords: biosensor, DNA, RNA, aptamer, electrochemistry, sensor, nanomaterials, impedance, differential pulse voltammetry, cyclic voltammetry, DNA tetrahedron, mediator

1. Introduction

Biosensor technology is a promising field where many outputs are continuously produced thanks to physicochemical techniques and biological materials developed every day. In this technology, a biological molecule interacts with the analyte on the biosensor and this generates a physicochemical signal which is detected by the transducer. Biosensor systems are divided into two classes in terms of biological molecules used, either catalytic-based which transforms the analyte or affinity-based which binds the analyte directly [1]. In terms of physicochemical signal transmitter, it can be designed as electrochemical, optic or piezoelectric. Systems that are combined within also continue to be open to development today. For example, both electrochemistry and optical measurements can be made in spectro-electrochemical techniques. Among these techniques, electrochemical systems [2], which are produced at low-costs without being interfered by the properties of the analyte solution, are used mostly.

The most important element of the biosensor is the biorecognition agent which shows the affinity for the analyte. These agents are of biological origin and are biomolecules with specific substrates such as proteins [3], enzymes [4], nucleic acids [5], antibodies [6], cells [7], cell surface channels. Biosensors can be designed by immobilizing these biomolecules on a suitable signal transmitter based on the working principle. When selecting the biorecognition agent, the specimen containing the analyte to be measured and the characteristics of the reaction that will take place should be considered. It is desired that the biorecognition agent has a maximum activity and that it has a low degree of denaturation.

The living organism's structural and functional strategy is hidden in its genes. The gene structure is based on the bases that form nucleic acids, which are divided into two main groups according to their functions, are deoxyribonucleic acid (DNA) and ribonucleic acids (RNA) [8]. DNA carries the genetic information in the double helix structure that includes adenine (A), guanine (G), cytosine (C) and thymine (T) bases. RNA has two main differences when compared to DNA, which are the inclusion of uracil (U) instead of T and the single stranded nucleic acid structure different from DNA. DNA's double helix structure is formed with hydrogen bonds between the DNA bases of the complementary chains. In the same chain, ester bases between the 5 'OH group on the pentose sugar of a nucleotide and the 3' OH group of the other nucleotide sugar form the single chain structure (**Figure 1**).

Thereby, U, A, G, C and T can be ordered in countless combinations to form genetic sequences. These sequences are copied and then transcribed in the ribosomes to take part in the synthesis of peptides and proteins by encoding one amino acid corresponding to all three bases.

Although they have different structures in different living organisms, the basic function of base sequences does not change. Erwin Chargaff showed that A-T and G-C base pairs in DNA sequences are mutually paired with hydrogen bond [9]. The important point here is that the hydrogen bonds formed between DNA helixes directly affect the physical properties of DNA, since there are three hydrogen bonds between G-C, while there are two hydrogen bonds between A-T. If the G-C ratio is high, it requires more energetic power to separate the double helix. This is a considerable structural characteristic for the electrochemical techniques.

On the other hand, RNA is a single chain nucleic acid produced by using DNA sequences. Besides the three main types of RNA in protein encoding (mRNA, tRNA and rRNA), there are also other types of RNAs that serve in post-translational modifications in DNA replication or as regulators. For example, small nuclear RNA (snRNA) involved in RNA cleavage, guide RNA (gRNA) involved in CRISPR-Cas9 system, micro RNA (miRNA), small interfering RNA (siRNA) and viral RNA. These different nucleic acids are worth to identify their function and structure [10].

Today, DNA or RNA analysis can be done quite precisely. Therefore, genetic sequences have a central role in diagnosis and treatment processes and they guide the scientists for development of new techniques. RNA and DNA sequences can be easily illuminated with polymerase chain reactions (PCR) and next-generation sequencing analyzers [11]. Like every method, these methods have limitations. For PCR, it is necessary to use consumables for reproduction and analysis of the nucleic acid sequences. This increases analysis costs and affects the analysis time. The disadvantages of the methods naturally make it inevitable to develop new and efficient methods. Although there are different nucleic acid analysis methods, simple and precise methods are needed. Bioelectronics systems are preferable as they are in the front line with their low cost, fast analysis time, minimum consumable requirement and lower margin of errors. Efficient properties of biological molecules with physicochemical transducer sensitivity increase the preferability. These basic mini analyzers are able to provide fast, low cost and precise analysis, based on the immobilizing biological molecules on a physicochemical transducer. The term biosensor is developed by immobilizing a biomolecule of biological origin that provides the biochemical reaction on a transducer. In terms of classification, it can be divided into different areas according to both the working principle of the biomolecule and the working principle of the transducer.

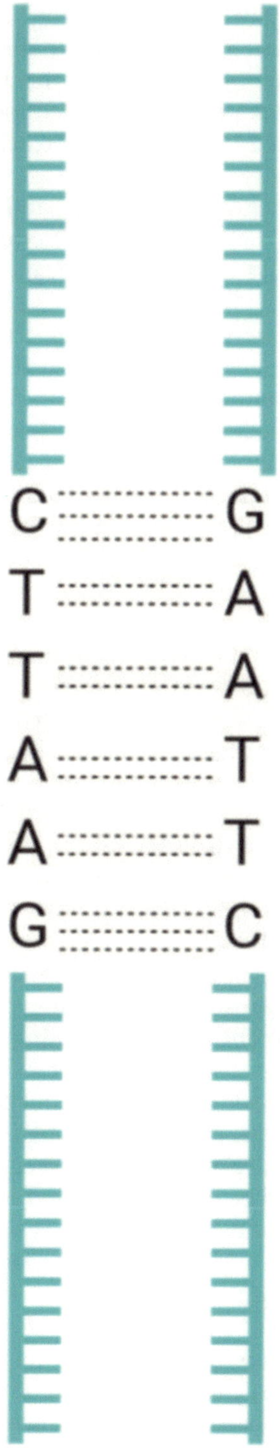

Figure 1.
Representation of the hydrogen bonds between DNA chains.

In electrochemical nucleic acid biosensor systems, the electrical signal occurs because of the interaction between the biorecognition agent and the analyte. As a result of the biochemical reaction, if an electron is formed, amperometric measurement can be performed. If a molecule is formed it can be detected by potentiometric or direct affinity-based binding can be measured as impedimetric/capacitive. When there is no molecule being exposed, only affinity-based biosensor systems can be designed amperometrically. In this design, when the interaction between biomolecules occurs, a secondary molecule (label) can generate an electrochemical signal. Measurements can be performed through the electrochemical activity of the label used here. Electrical conductivity is an extremely important parameter, especially in biosensor systems. Nucleic acids, on the other hand, can be considered as ideal transistors, because of their structure, they show conductive nanocable characteristics and are very efficient in use in electrochemical biosensors in order to be found in many different conformations. The DNA helix has between 3.4-angstrom base pairs, and the aromatic ring structure facilitates electron flow. This structure, that is the closeness between the bases, is similar to the Z-directional space of graphite and provides conductivity. Moreover, the π electrons on DNA also help electrical conductivity [10]. They help electrochemical conductivity due to structural variability.

On the other hand, beside the electroactivity of DNA, the electrochemical measurement method is important in the design of nucleic acid biosensors. Some electroactive secondary molecules can be used for the electrochemical detection. Mediators, which are frequently used in biosensor systems, can also be used to measure molecules that interact with DNA. Mediator is an intermediary molecule that facilitates electron exchange in an electrochemical reaction and lowers the reduction/oxidation potential of the detection system and also has regeneration potential [1]. The most important feature of a mediator is that it can signal in a low and narrow potential ranges. This feature increases the sensitivity of the biosensor since signaling of other electroactive species can be prevented in lower potentials.

Electroactive species can be determined using techniques such as differential pulse voltammetry (DPV) and cyclic voltammetry (CV) in studies that require the measurement of electroactive species, and the measurement of the amount of DNA through the reduction or oxidation of these species. The basic principle of the measurements is the presence of electroactive species on DNA (guanine base) or the formation of signals by binding some mediators or indicators to DNA. Indicators such as ruthenium complexes, ferrocene and methylene blue are often used for nucleic acid based biosensors. Measurement can be performed by chemically marking the DNA or RNA at the end or forming a complex with DNA helix. Measuring current generated by electroactive species in these electrochemical techniques is extremely important, but can also limit the effectiveness of measurement systems. In other electrochemical measurement systems where mediators are not used, different electrochemical techniques that can measure nucleic acid binding or conformational changes may be used. These methods are performed in redox probe solutions to characterize electrode surface. Here, CV is capable of measuring physical changes on the surface with the help of a redox probe. When the sensitivity of CV in affinity based non-electroactive detections is insufficient, electrochemical impedance spectroscopy (EIS) or capacitance (C) measurement can also be used in affinity-based nucleic acid biosensors. These two methods are really sensitive methods to detect biomolecules, charge transfers and mass transfers with reaction kinetics and also are affected by electrode surface charges [12]. Therefore, nucleic acid length, base composition, and conformational changes after target molecule binding had to be considered before study design. Moreover, the negatively charged redox probe usage reduces the interference of the redox probe interaction between nucleic acid in the measurement.

Another advantage of nucleic acids is that there is no denaturation or loss of activity like proteins. The most important point to consider here is to take measures to reduce the effectiveness of DNase and RNase enzymes that break down nucleic acids. Some examples of methods that can be used when designing a biosensor system with nucleic acids are given in the following pages.

2. Nucleic acids as biorecognition receptors and target

With 5 different base sequences on nucleic acids, the potential for an almost unlimited sequence is theoretically available. Their use as both a biorecognition agent and a target molecule to be analyzed is among its advantages. By its ability to form a complementary structure even within itself, it shows the feature of an analyte-biorecognition agent.

2.1 DNA and RNA usage in biosensor technology

In studies where DNA is used as a biorecognition agent, biosensor systems can be designed by measuring molecules that interact directly or indirectly with DNA. Especially in genetic analysis, DNA determinations have been performed based on complementary base pairings (**Figure 2**).

Chen et al. [13] developed a DNA biosensor whose signal was increased in triplicate for the determination of transgenic soybeans. Signal enhancement was performed as rolling circle amplification (RCA). In the biosensor system Chronocoulometry was used to detect DNAs via electrode surface charges. Firstly, Fe_3O_4@Au magnetic nanoparticles were produced and the electrode was modified with SH modified DNAs to capture the target DNA sequence. After this immobilization on carbon electrode and incubated by dropping target DNA, complementary DNA forms a double structure with the target DNA. Afterwards, the double helix was cut and removed with ExoIII and 4 single-stranded ssDNA with a gold nanoparticle cube in the center was added to the free cutted ends, and binding was achieved with the help of Phi29 DNA polymerase and T4. $[Ru(NH_3)_6]^{3+}$, which forms a complex with anionic phosphates, is used as a complex mediator specifically bound on this quaternary structure. The amount of DNA was determined chronocoulometrically over the electrochemical signals generated by the ruthenium complex. A linear calibration curve was obtained between 10^{-16} and 10^{-7} M, and LOD was calculated as 4.5×10^{-17} M. Target DNA analysis took 2 hours. By the help of this complex DNA analysis, the authors managed to develop an ultra-sensitive system. Sensitivity is increased with the DNA immobilization steps used here. However, since the study requires a repetitive enzyme treatment, it seems costly and time consuming in developmental process.

Nucleic acid biosensors can also be developed by using enzymes used in DNA analysis. In recent years, studies using the CRISPR-Cas9 system are used in biotechnological studies as a genetic editing molecule. Uygun et al. [14] developed an impedimetric graphene oxide electrode modified with CRISPR-dCas9 for the determination of the target circulating tumor DNA molecules containing the PIK3CA exon 9 mutation, which is used as a biomarker in breast cancer and is referred to as a liquid biopsy biomarker. In this study, deactivated Cas9 (dCas9) proteins without exonuclease activity, were used as biorecognition receptor by modifying them with a sgRNA that would recognize the target ctDNA sequence. Graphene oxide electrodes were modified with dCas9 and sgRNA, consequently. In this way, the modification for ctDNA analysis is completed. The short analysis time (40 seconds) needed was a great advantage. The impedimetric measurement method with a 1.92 nM LOD in the range of 2–20 nM ctDNA concentration has been developed.

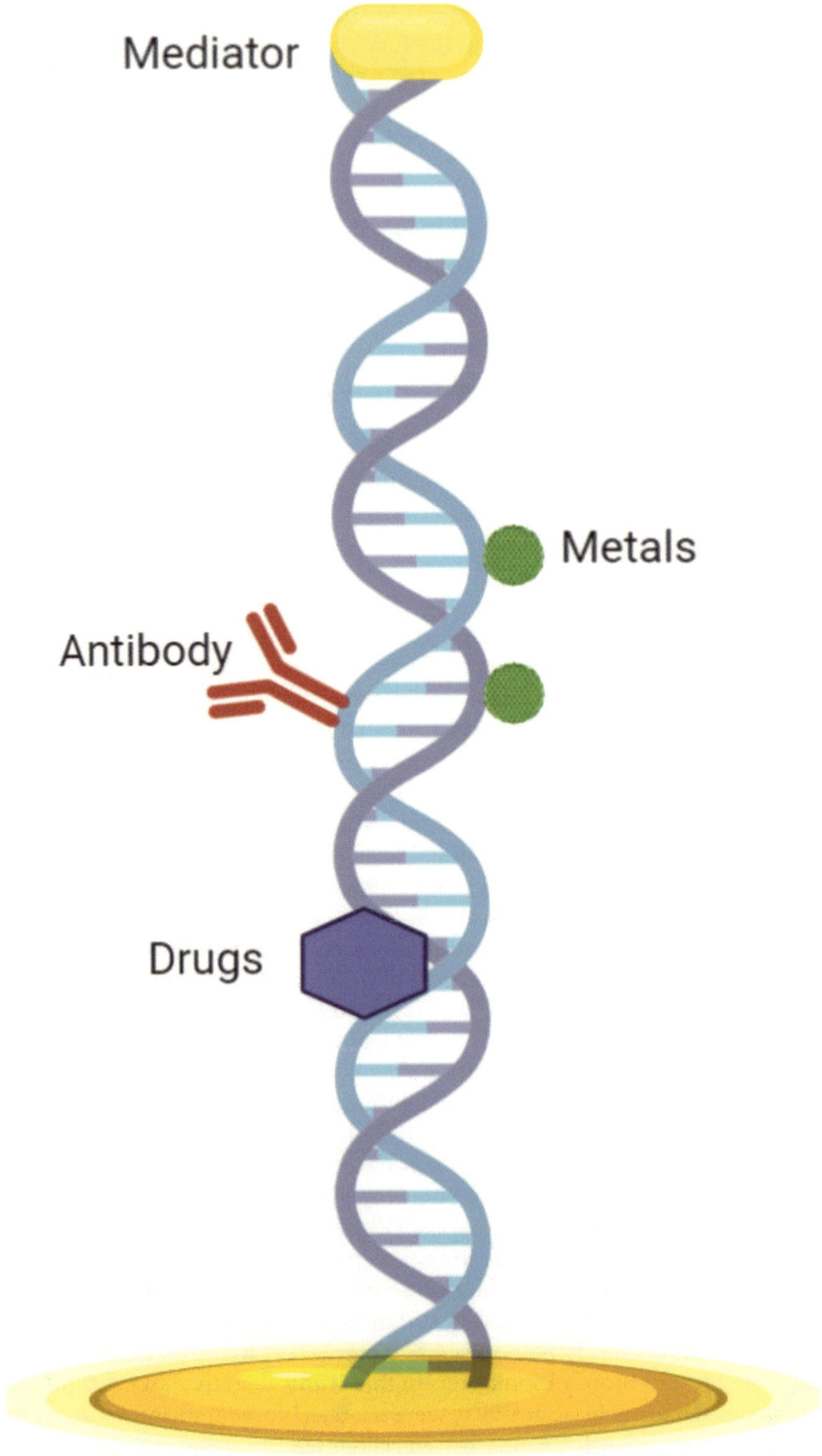

Figure 2.
Schematic representation of the DNA as biorecognition receptor.

Because of the charges on the DNA, analysis of cations, where the bases show selectivity, can be detected. In another biosensor study, due to its negatively charged structure, the ability of chelating properties of DNAs for metal ions is used. Zhang et al. [15] used DNA molecules for the determination of mercury ions. DNA probes modified with the DNA sulfur group formed a self-assembly monolayer on the gold electrode. Afterwards, the electrode modified with the reporter DNA, which has a gold nanoparticle in the center, was measured by binding mercury ions. Both impedance and CV were used in the study. The linear measuring range was set as 1–200 nM and the LOD was calculated as 0.05 nM. By this study, thanks to the use of DNA molecules, the mercury molecule was determined with a relative standard deviation of 3% within real samples.

To observe the complementary base pairing and post translational modifications, secondary conjugates such as antibody or enzyme can be used in the DNA based biosensor studies. Huang et al. [16] developed a biosensor to determine DNA methylation levels. In this study, the methylation level was determined with the help of a bioconjugate modified by a secondary antibody. This conjugate is formed on graphene oxide layers that target CpG and have horseradish peroxidase (HRP)-labeled anti-5-methylcytosine antibodies. The signal generated by HRP is directly proportional to the presence of methyl groups, and DPV was used in this enzymatic reaction-based study. Hydroquinone as a mediator, i.e. electron transmitter, also reduced the reaction voltage and made it more selective. Then, the measurement was carried out on the complex of the bioconjugate with cytosine containing methyl groups. While the biosensor reaches 1 fM LOD value, it can measure in the linear range between 1 fM and 10 nM. The preparation process of the biosensor took approximately 5 hours. In this study, since DNA methylation is performed by measuring the enzyme activity on the bioconjugate, the measurement efficiency is based on the performance of the antibody, enzyme and the mediator.

Jahandari et al. [17] developed a biosensor modified with gold nanoparticles for DNA-based Temodal (anticancer drug) determination. They also modified dsDNA molecules electrochemically on the gold nanoparticles deposited on the pencil graphite electrode. The binding of the Temodal to the DNA on the biosensor was measured by DPV. Here, the main measurement is not the Temodal measurement directly. As the intercalator agent binds to the DNA, the reduction potential of the guanine base on the DNA decreases due to the amount of Temodal that is bound to DNA. Temodal performed intercalation by the interaction of the minor groove on the DNA. In this system with a maximum measurement time of 8 minutes, a maximum recovery deviation of 5% was observed in real samples. Linearly, it showed 1 nM LOD with measurement performance between 5 nM and 45 μM. The performance and sensitivity of this study are directly proportional to the presence of guanine bases. The base ratio on DNA is important in the design of such studies.

Ebrahimi et al. [18] determined cadmium ions using ethyl green (EG) on a simple DNA-based biosensor system. EG can be used as a hybridization indicator in DNA studies. Cadmium is known as a toxic heavy metal and this heavy metal measurement is especially important for biological samples. Cadmium destabilizes the double helix by forming a bond through the N7 atom of the guanine base on DNA. Similarly, in this study, measurement was performed using differential pulse voltammetry signals of EG. The signal generated by DPV is the oxidation signal that occurs as the result of the release of EG by destabilizing double helix. In other words, EG among the DNA helix is released as the result of the binding of cadmium to DNA, and it forms a destabilized DNA signal with cadmium. Measurement of cadmium ions showed 0.3 pM LOD with a linear measurement between 1 pM and 1 nM and between 10 nM and 1 μM. The limitation of the study is the accumulation performance of EG on DNA. The degree of this accumulation determines the sensitivity. It is difficult to determine the low amounts of cadmium in drinking water with a relative standard deviation of 8%.

In biosensors developed with DNA, the properties of DNA hybrids can be used. Yang et al. [19] have developed an electrochemical biosensor for the determination of MCF-7 cells, which are breast cancer cells. In this biosensor, DNA molecules were used for modification. The system provided linear measurement between 100 and 1 million cells in 1 mL and the LOD was found to be 80 cells/mL. The biosensor system was developed as a sandwich-type and the signal was made more sensitive with nanomaterials on antibodies labeled with DNA. With the 3D nanomaterials used in the design of the system, the modification steps are quite highly complex and difficult in terms of workload. In the study, the electrode was first modified with 3D-graphenes and then was modified with gold nanocages with antibody on the carbon nanotubes and immobilized on the electrode. DNA fragments labeled with a secondary antibody bonded on MCF-7 bound on these antibodies, and the measurement was performed with DPV. Here, MCF-7 measurement was performed by DNA hybridization, that is, by measuring the degree of binding of the complement bound to the ssDNA labeled with the last bound antibody.

Saeedfar et al. [20] developed a biosensor using multi-walled carbon nanotubes modified with gold nanoparticles to determine the sex of Arowana fish. The process of determining the sex of the Arowana fish before maturation is quite difficult. Arowana is an ancient and very expensive fish. This biosensor was developed as it is a very advantageous approach for the fish farming industry to distinguish the gender of the fish in time. For this, a hybridization-based approach has been adopted. Carbon nanotubes were used as a hybridization agent by complexing with ruthenium (III) chloride hex ammoniate in this study. DNA determination was performed between 10^{-21} M and 10^{-9} M and 1.55×10^{-21} M was the lowest detection limit.

Apart from DNA and proteins used in DNA determination, uncharged DNA variant known as Peptide Nucleic Acid (PNA) is also used. Unlike DNA, instead of a phosphate backbone, this molecule contains a backbone made of neutral amino acids. PNA of this nature can be used as potential probes for both DNA and RNA determination. The advantage of PNA is that it provides a great advantage in reducing the determination time. Tian et al. [21] used graphene field-effected transistors in their PNA-modified electrochemical biosensor study. In the DNA analysis study by measuring the gate voltage, it reached the level of 0.1 aM LOD and performed between 0.1 aM and 1 pM.

Due to their structural features, RNA biosensors can also be used in biosensor development, just like DNA biosensors. The structural differences of RNA with DNA were mentioned above. Apart from their metabolic functions, RNA and DNA are similar except for the difference in oxidation in ribose sugar. Studies have also been carried out which DNA and RNA can be used together in biosensor studies, especially using complementary DNAs for RNA analysis. In this section, RNA-based biosensors and types of studies are summarized.

Luo et al. [22] have developed an electrochemical DNA biosensor for exosomal miRNA analysis. The study was generally modified by adding a DNA probe modified with methylene blue (MB) over amino groups after the lysine amino acid was electrochemically coated on the glassy carbon electrode. Complementary to this probe, a ferrocene-modified secondary probe is attached. The biosensor was prepared for sample measurement by exosome extraction that releases miRNA to hybridize them to complementary chain and detected by labeled with Ferrocene (Fc). The variation of the Fc signal with the MB folded on itself indicates the miRNA and probe measurement, consequently. It shows performance at 2.3 fM level LOD and linear measurement range between 10 and 70 fM.

As a result, DNA and RNA have been used both as a recognition agent and as a target molecule with successful results. In some of these studies, the determination was carried out by measuring a secondary molecule on the basis of DNA hybridization. Besides, DNA analysis with the use of Cas proteins and DNA analysis with PNA were performed by using different methods and extremely low detection limits were reached.

2.2 Aptamers as synthetic biorecognition receptors

Aptamers have caught a very rapid trend after their discovery. These artificial nucleic acids are produced by the systematic evolution of ligands by exponential enrichment (SELEX) method [5]. By being artificially produced, they show affinity for a wide range of target molecules. They achieve this affinity with easy physical changes. Aptamer sequences designed in the correct sequence for the target molecule work by binding to the target site by undergoing conformational change when the target molecule approaches. The conformational change can be measured by using a label or surface resistance, shown in **Figures 3** and **4**, respectively.

Ohno et al. [23] developed a label-free immunosensor-based aptamer-modified graphene FET. The researchers, who modified the G-FET with IgE aptamers, determined IgG by measuring the gate voltage on the FET. With a protein concentration measurement between 0.29 and 340 nM, a LOD value of 0.29 nM was reached. 47 nM isotherm value was observed as the Kd value. Since nonspecific binding of different proteins except this molecule was not observed.

In another study, Chen et al., [24] developed an aptamer-based biosensor for the electrochemical determination of Human epidermal growth factor (HER2). Differential pulse voltammetry was chosen as a measurement technique. In the study, after modifying the gold nanorod nanomaterials with palladium, they formed a bioconjugate for analysis by modifying it with an aptamer containing SH group and horse radish peroxidase (HRP). Later, they modified the gold electrode with DNA tetrahedrons. DNA tetrahedron is a nanoscale structure designed by using the complementary base pairing reactions of nucleic acids. They modified the single-stranded DNA aptamer from one corner of the DNA tetrahedron structure.

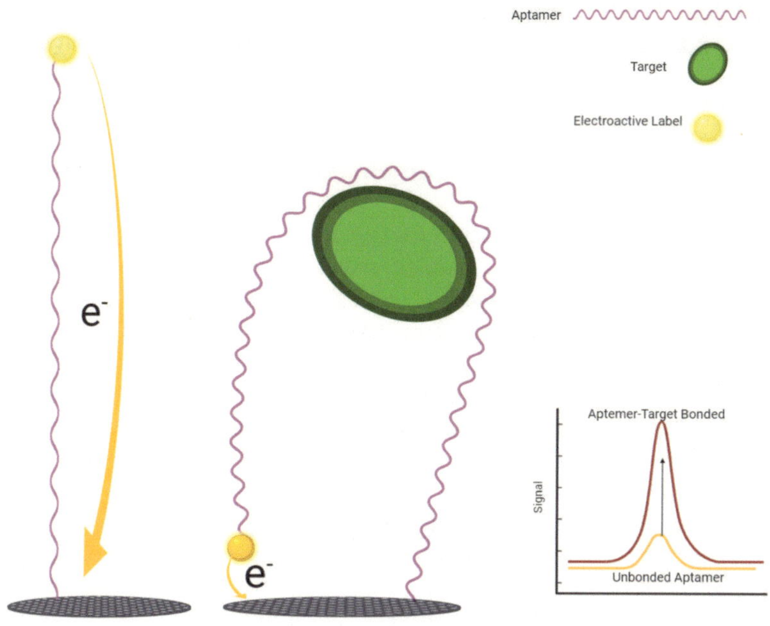

Figure 3.
Labeled-aptamer based electrochemical biosensor technology.

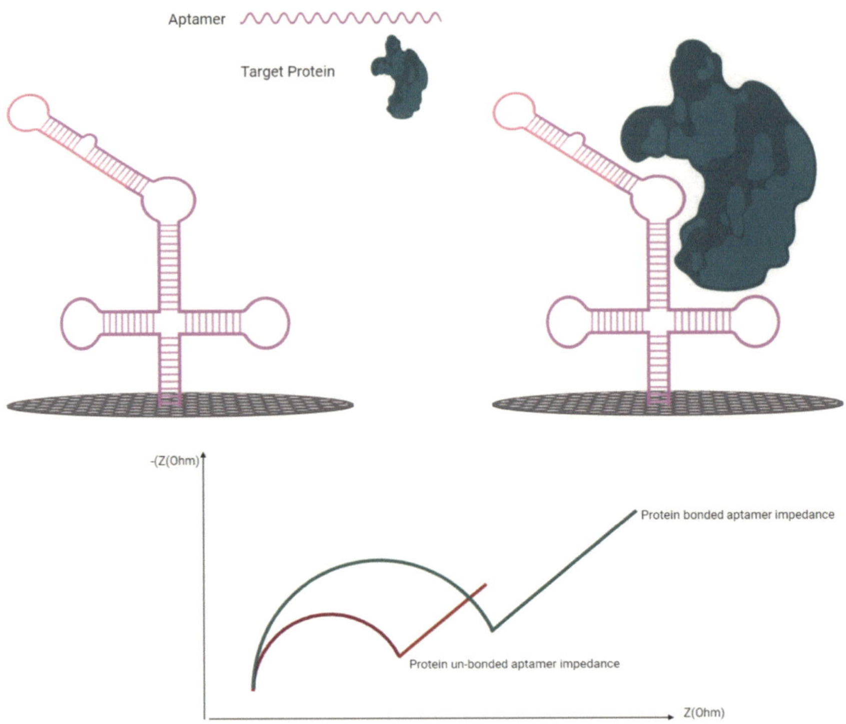

Figure 4.
Schematic representation of the impedimetric aptamer biosensor.

DNA tetrahedron is preferred because of its mechanical structural rigidity and high affinity (5000 times higher for ssDNA aptamer). The DNA was dropped onto the tetrahedron-aptamer modified gold electrode, aptamer's unbound ends were modified with BSA. After HER2 molecules were captured by the aptamer on the electrode, the bioconjugate was added on this modification and the biosensor was constructed???. HER2 measurement was performed indirectly through the conversion of HRP to hydrogen peroxide and the measurement of hydroquinone (mediator) added to the environment. In this study, researchers used the DNA tetrahedron structure and aptamer composite, thus HER2 recognition capacity was increased with this modification. The biosensor, with a working range of 10–200 ng/mL, provided the opportunity to make the analysis in 60 minutes. LOD was found to be 0.15 ng/mL.

Apart from large proteins, aptamer molecules are also used to identify small molecules. Aptamer molecules are particularly useful for the determination of molecules which are extremely difficult and demanding to identify easily. Swensen et al. [25] conducted real-time cocaine measurement in their biosensor study. This determination was carried out in approximately one minute. The microfluidic chip has been modified with cocaine-specific aptamers for cocaine binding. One end of the aptamer is modified with methylene blue. The sample, injected into the microfluidic chamber, was added to the fetal bovine serum with a flow, and the measurement was performed by binding to the aptamer. Rapid measurement is important for the rapid determination of this drug, which has a half-life of 60–90 minutes in serum. Besides the speed advantage, this system has a 20 pM LOD with a linear detection range of 10–2000 μM.

Apart from organic molecules, aptamer-based biosensors have also been developed for the determination of ions. Radi et al. [26] developed a biosensor system for the aptamer-based potassium determination. The gold electrode was made ready for potassium ion measurement after being modified with aptamers with SH at one end and Fc at the other. The biosensor had a measurement limit between 0.1 and 1 mM and reached a value of 0.015 LOD by using electrochemical impedance spectroscopy.

Besides the principle of binding aptamer molecules to a molecule, a bifunctional aptamer-based biosensor for determination of adenosine and lysozyme was developed by Deng et al. [27]. In their study, they performed the determination of adenosine and lysozyme on DNA/DNA duplex. The gold electrode was first modified by a probe with SH group (adenosine selective) and then a secondary probe (lysozyme selective) attached to this probe, and the modification was completed with a DNA loaded nanomaterial with a central gold nanoparticle. Finally, ruthenium complexes were added as electroactive species on this structure. After the primary probe captures adenosine with adenosine binding, the gold nanoparticle structure together with the secondary probe is separated from the biosensor. With lysozyme binding, the secondary structure is separated from the main structure by binding lysozyme. All these bonding and separation reactions were followed by the electrochemical activity of ruthenium complexes. Electrochemical measurement

Electrochemical method	Biorecognition receptor	Target	Linear range	LOD	Reference
Coul	Phi29 DNA polymerase and T4	Transgenic soybeans DNA	10^{-16} and 10^{-7} M	4.5×10^{-17} M	[6]
EIS	CRISP-dCas9	PIK3CA	2–20 nM	1.92 nM	[7]
CV	DNA	Hg^{2+}	1–200 nM	0.05 nM	[8]
DPV	DNA-(HRP)-labeled IgG	DNA Methylation	1 fM–10 nM	1 fM	[9]
DPV	AuNPSs-DNA	Temodal	5 nM–45 μM	1 nM	[10]
DPV	DNA-ethyl green	Cd^{2+}	1 pM–1 nM	0.3 pM	[11]
DPV	DNA-antibody-graphene	MCF-7 Cells	10^2–10^6 cells/mL	80 cells/mL	[12]
DPV	DNA-ruthenium	Arowana fish gender (DNA)	10^{-21}–10^{-9} M	1.55×10^{-21} M	[13]
G-FET	DNA	PNA	0.1 aM–1 pM	0.1 aM	[14]
DPV	DNA-MB, DNA-Fc	Exosomal miRNA	10–70 fM	2.3 fM	[15]
G-FET	IgG aptamer	IgG	0.29–340 nM	0.29 nM	[17]
DPV	DNA tetrahedron – aptamer	HER2	10–200 ng/mL	0.15 ng/mL	[18]
AC voltammetry	Cocaine aptamer	Cocaine	10–2000 μM	20 pM	[19]
EIS	5′-ferrocene(Fc)–DNA–SH-3′	K^+	0.1–1 mM	0.015 mM	[20]
CV	Adenosine-lysozyme aptamers	Lysozyme Adenosine	10–60 μg/mL 0.02–40 nM	0.01 μg/mL 0.02 nM	[21]

DPV: differential pulse voltammetry, EIS: electrochemical impedance spectroscopy, CV: cyclic voltammetry, Coul: coulometry, fc: ferrocene, PIK3CA: phosphatidylinositol-4,5-bisphosphate 3-kinase catalytic subunit alpha, AuNPs: gold nanoparticles, G-FET: graphene field effect transistor, MB: methylene blue, HER2: human epidermal growth factor, AC: alternative current.

Table 1.
Comparison of the nucleic acid based biosensors.

was carried out by CV. Lysozyme and adenosine bifunctional biosensor reached the LOD limits of 0.01 μg/mL and 0.02 nM, respectively. Measurements were made between 0.02 and 40 nM for adenosine and 10–60 μg/mL for lysozyme.

With aptamer nucleic acids, target biomolecules can be easily identified. Although aptamer molecules work similarly to antibodies, they can easily be modified with a secondary biomolecule. Molecules that do not have denaturation problems unlike proteins can be very useful in the development of biosensors, especially in the development of electrochemical biosensors. Electrochemical activation of electroactive species or direct aptamer binding to the target molecule can be measured impedimetrically. As a result, aptamer systems are suitable for affinity-based sensor development in biosensors (**Table 1**).

3. Conclusion

Biosensors are low cost analyzers with high potential to be miniaturized. They also provide short measurement time. Thanks to the numerous combinations of biorecognition receptor and transducers, biosensor systems can easily be adapted for the measurement of any kind of analyte. The biological activity of the biorecognition agent on the transducer is the critical element in a biosensor. Biomolecules with low probability of denaturation, adaptable to all kinds of measurements and strong electrical components should be selected for biosensor development. Nucleic acids meet the needs of biosensors at this point. They are advantageous biomolecules that can interact from metal ions to large proteins thanks to their multiple negative charges. Nucleic acids also have the potential to facilitate the determination of organic molecules, such as drugs and pesticides, which can enter between nucleic acid chains thanks to the electroactive guanine base in their structure. They can be used as simple biorecognition agents, similar to an unlimited antibody-antigen interaction, with the potential to be designed to synthetically show affinity for the target molecule. Another important feature of nucleic acids is the potential of their end portions to be modified by secondary signal transmitters without causing any deactivation. Apart from being both a biorecognition agent and an analyte molecule, their immobilization capacity also increases their usage and advantages. In conclusion, the fact that they can be used as a material which provides stability and ease of modification for analysis in biosensor systems puts nucleic acids one step further among other biorecognition agents.

Acknowledgements

We are grateful to thank The Scientific and Technological Research Council Of Turkey (TÜBİTAK) for the supports for giving the idea to write this chapter by awarded our TÜBİTAK-1001 217S353 project.

Conflict of interest

The authors declare no conflict of interest.

Author details

Zihni Onur Uygun[1*], Hilmiye Deniz Ertuğrul Uygun[2,3] and Ferhan Girgin Sağin[1]

1 Department of Medical Biochemistry, Faculty of Medicine, Ege University, İzmir, Turkey

2 Center for Production and Application of Electronic Materials, Dokuz Eylül University, İzmir, Turkey

3 Nanoscience and Nanoengineering Division, Institute of Natural Sciences, Dokuz Eylül University, İzmir, Turkey

*Address all correspondence to: onur_uygun@hotmail.com

References

[1] A.P.F. Turner, Biosensors: Fundamentals and Applications, Oxford University Press, 1987.

[2] X. Zhang, H. Ju, J. Wang, Electrochemical Sensors, Biosensors and Their Biomedical Applications, 2008. doi:10.1017/CBO9781107415324.004.

[3] E. Povedano, V. Ruiz-Valdepeñas Montiel, M. Gamella, V. Serafín, M. Pedrero, L. Moranova, M. Bartosik, J.J. Montoya, P. Yáñez-Sedeño, S. Campuzano, J.M. Pingarrón, A novel zinc finger protein–based amperometric biosensor for miRNA determination, Analytical and Bioanalytical Chemistry. (2019). doi:10.1007/s00216-019-02219-w.

[4] S. Hashemzadeh, Y. Omidi, H. Rafii-Tabar, Amperometric lactate nanobiosensor based on reduced graphene oxide, carbon nanotube and gold nanoparticle nanocomposite, Mikrochimica Acta. (n.d.). doi:10.1007/s00604-019-3791-0.

[5] S. Tombelli, M. Minunni, M. Mascini, Analytical applications of aptamers, Biosensors and Bioelectronics. 20 (2005) 2424-2434. doi:10.1016/j.bios.2004.11.006.

[6] Z.O. Uygun, Ç. Şahin, M. Yılmaz, Y. Akçay, A. Akdemir, F. Sağın, Fullerene-PAMAM(G5) composite modified impedimetric biosensor to detect Fetuin-A in real blood samples, Analytical Biochemistry. 542 (2018) 11-15. doi:10.1016/J.AB.2017.11.007.

[7] F. Vajhadin, S. Ahadian, J. Travas-Sejdic, J. Lee, M. Mazloum-Ardakani, J. Salvador, G.E. Aninwene, P. Bandaru, W. Sun, A. Khademhossieni, Electrochemical cytosensors for detection of breast cancer cells, Biosensors and Bioelectronics. (n.d.). doi:10.1016/j.bios.2019.111984.

[8] G. Michal, D. Schomburg, eds., Biochemical Pathways, John Wiley and Sons Inc., Hoboken, New Jersey, 2012.

[9] D. Elson, E. Chargaff, On the desoxyribonucleic acid content of sea urchin gametes, Experientia. 8 (1952) 143-145. doi:10.1007/BF02170221.

[10] M. Mozneb, E. Mirtaheri, A.O. Sanabria, C. Li, Bioelectronic properties of DNA, protein, cells and their applications for diagnostic medical devices, Biosensors and Bioelectronics. (2020) 112441. doi:10.1016/j.bios.2020.112441.

[11] F. Rothé, J.-F. Laes, D. Lambrechts, D. Smeets, D. Vincent, M. Maetens, D. Fumagalli, S. Michiels, S. Drisis, C. Moerman, J.-P. Detiffe, D. Larsimont, A. Awada, M. Piccart, C. Sotiriou, M. Ignatiadis, Plasma circulating tumor DNA as an alternative to metastatic biopsies for mutational analysis in breast cancer., Annals of Oncology : Official Journal of the European Society for Medical Oncology. 25 (2014) 1959-65. doi:10.1093/annonc/mdu288.

[12] H.D. Ertuğrul, Z.O. Uygun, Impedimetric Biosensors for Label-Free and Enzymless Detection, Intech. i (2016) 13. doi:http://dx.doi.org/10.5772/57353.

[13] D. Chen, M. Zhang, M. Ma, H. Hai, J. Li, Y. Shan, A novel electrochemical DNA biosensor for transgenic soybean detection based on triple signal amplification, Analytica Chimica Acta. 1078 (2019) 24-31. doi:10.1016/j.aca.2019.05.074.

[14] Z.O. Uygun, L. Yeniay, G. Sağın, Ferhan, CRISPR-dCas9 powered impedimetric biosensor for label-free detection of circulating tumor DNAs, Analytica Chimica Acta. 1121 (2020) 35-41. doi:10.1016/j.aca.2020.04.009.

[15] Y. Zhang, C. Zhang, R. Ma, X. Du, W. Dong, Y. Chen, Q. Chen, An ultra-sensitive Au nanoparticles functionalized DNA biosensor for electrochemical sensing of mercury ions, Materials Science and Engineering C. 75 (2017) 175-181. doi:10.1016/j.msec.2017.02.058.

[16] J. Huang, S. Zhang, F. Mo, S. Su, X. Chen, Y. Li, L. Fang, H. Huang, J. Deng, H. Liu, X. Yang, J. Zheng, An electrochemical DNA biosensor analytic technique for identifying DNA methylation specific sites and quantify DNA methylation level, Biosensors and Bioelectronics. 127 (2019) 155-160. doi:10.1016/j.bios.2018.12.022.

[17] S. Jahandari, M.A. Taher, H. Karimi-Maleh, A. Khodadadi, E. Faghih-Mirzaei, A powerful DNA-based voltammetric biosensor modified with Au nanoparticles, for the determination of Temodal; an electrochemical and docking investigation, Journal of Electroanalytical Chemistry. 840 (2019) 313-318. doi:10.1016/j.jelechem.2019.03.049.

[18] M. Ebrahimi, J.B. Raoof, R. Ojani, Design of an electrochemical DNA-based biosensor for selective determination of cadmium ions using a DNA hybridization indicator, International Journal of Biological Macromolecules. 108 (2018) 1237-1241. doi:10.1016/j.ijbiomac.2017.11.023.

[19] Y. Yang, Y. Fu, H. Su, L. Mao, M. Chen, Sensitive detection of MCF-7 human breast cancer cells by using a novel DNA-labeled sandwich electrochemical biosensor, Biosensors and Bioelectronics. 122 (2018) 175-182. doi:10.1016/j.bios.2018.09.062.

[20] K. Saeedfar, L.Y. Heng, C.P. Chiang, A DNA biosensor based on gold nanoparticle decorated on carboxylated multi-walled carbon nanotubes for gender determination of Arowana fish, Bioelectrochemistry. 118 (2017) 106-113. doi:10.1016/j.bioelechem.2017.07.012.

[21] M. Tian, M. Qiao, C. Shen, F. Meng, L.A. Frank, V. V. Krasitskaya, T. Wang, X. Zhang, R. Song, Y. Li, J. Liu, S. Xu, J. Wang, Highly-sensitive graphene field effect transistor biosensor using PNA and DNA probes for RNA detection, Applied Surface Science. 527 (2020). doi:10.1016/j.apsusc.2020.146839.

[22] L. Luo, L. Wang, L. Zeng, Y. Wang, Y. Weng, Y. Liao, T. Chen, Y. Xia, J. Zhang, J. Chen, A ratiometric electrochemical DNA biosensor for detection of exosomal MicroRNA, Talanta. 207 (2020) 120298. doi:10.1016/j.talanta.2019.120298.

[23] Y. Ohno, K. Maehashi, K. Matsumoto, Label-free biosensors based on aptamer-modified graphene field-effect transistors, Journal of the American Chemical Society. 132 (2010) 18012-18013. doi:10.1021/ja108127r.

[24] D. Chen, D. Wang, X. Hu, G. Long, Y. Zhang, L. Zhou, A DNA nanostructured biosensor for electrochemical analysis of HER2 using bioconjugate of GNR@Pd SSs—Apt—HRP, Sensors and Actuators, B: Chemical. 296 (2019). doi:10.1016/j.snb.2019.126650.

[25] J.S. Swensen, Y. Xiao, B.S. Ferguson, A.A. Lubin, R.Y. Lai, A.J. Heeger, K.W. Plaxco, H.T. Soh, Continuous, real-time monitoring of cocaine in undiluted blood serum via a microfluidic, electrochemical aptamer-based sensor, Journal of the American Chemical Society. 131 (2009) 4262-4266. doi:10.1021/ja806531z.

[26] A.E. Radi, C.K. O'Sullivan, Aptamer conformational switch as sensitive electrochemical biosensor for potassium ion recognition, Chemical Communications. (2006) 3432-3434. doi:10.1039/b606804a.

[27] C. Deng, J. Chen, L. Nie, Z. Nie, *S. Yao*, Sensitive bifunctional aptamer-based electrochemical biosensor for small molecules and protein, Analytical Chemistry. 81 (2009) 9972-9978. doi:10.1021/ac901727z.

Section 2

Wearable Biosensors

Chapter 3

Theranostic Microneedle Devices: Innovative Biosensing and Transdermal Drugs Administration

Principia Dardano, Mario Battisti, Selene De Martino, Ilaria Rea, Bruno Miranda, Luigi Nicolais and Luca De Stefano

Abstract

Biosensing systems based on microneedles can overcome the stratum corneum of the skin, i. e. the outer natural barrier of the human body, without any pain and detect the target analytes directly in the interstitial fluid. Moreover, microneedle-based devices (MNDs) can combine diagnostic sensing and therapeutic administration of drugs in one single tool. From this point of view, more than a painless door to the human body, a MND represents the a perfect example of theranostic instrument, since a single device could quantify the real value of a relevant biomolecule, such as glucose, and accurately deliver a drug, the insulin, if needed. MNDs could be integrated on printed circuit boards, flexible electronics and microfluidic channels, thus allowing a continuous monitoring of the physiological parameters with very low invasiveness, together with sustained and localized administration of drugs. MNDs can be designed for very specific applications, from the detection of skin cancer to the monitoring of metabolic pathways. Moreover, several fabrication approaches have been introduced, from laboratories to large-scale production. Finally MNDs can be properly functionalized to enhance analytical performances.

Keywords: microneedles, theranostics, biosensing, microfabrication, drug delivery

1. Introduction

A new type of biomedical devices was born when technologies and facilities for Micro and Nano Electro Mechanical Systems (MEMS and NEMS) fabrication have met medical and biological issues. These new kinds of biomedical devices are able to easily control physical and chemical parameters at a very small scale, down to nanomolar concentrations and nanometric sizes [1–3]. Moreover, the integration of such a device in wearable and/or mobile systems gave them popularity among commercial devices. In this technological frame, Microneedles based devices (MNDs) were born. Their height is sufficiently large to overcome the outer natural barrier of the human body, the stratum corneum of the skin, but not enough to reach the nerves, resulting in a lack of pain [4]. Usually, MN height is ranging from 10 to

1000 μm, depending on the application and how deep in the epidermis is the specific target analyte. Then, MNs based devices act as an interface between the body of the patient and a biomedical device, whose applications can range from fluid extraction for ex-situ analysis to drug and gene delivery, from *in situ* diagnostic tools to targeted cell therapy [1–4]. Material, length, shape of the body and the tip of the MNs drastically vary depending on the application [2, 3] and the fabrication technology, according to new needs and challenges. Biosensing systems based on MNs have to overcome the stratum corneum without pain and to detect the target

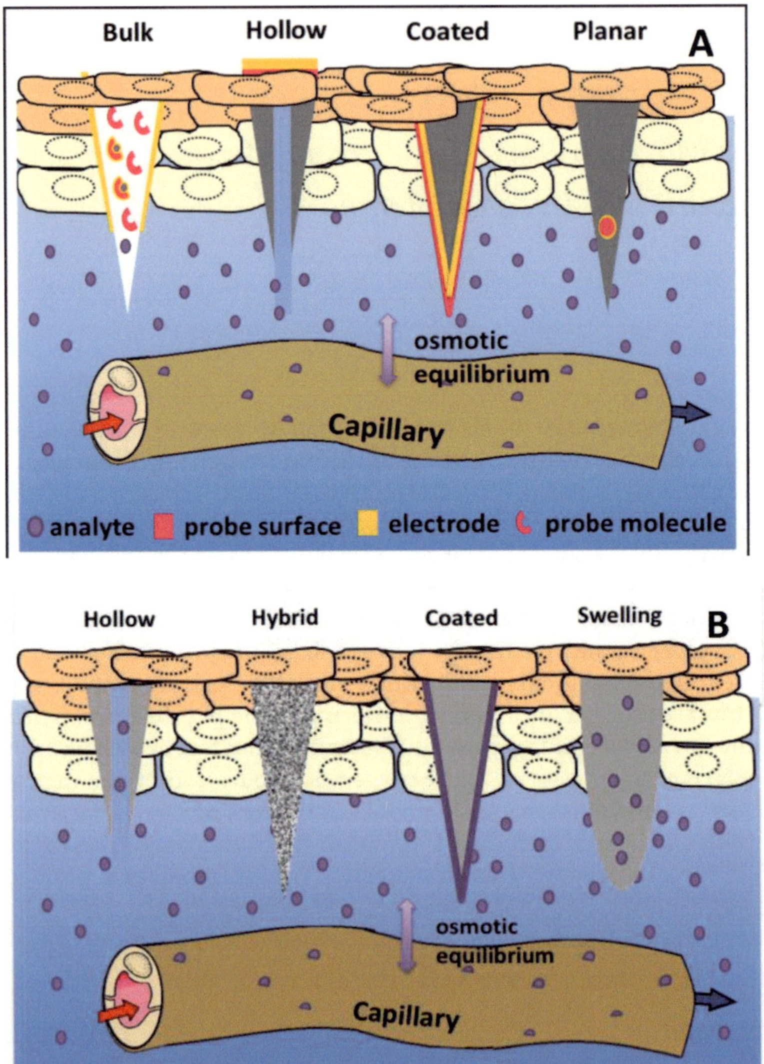

Figure 1.
(A) Sketch of different MNDs for sensing purposes together with their working conditions into the human skin. Starting from the right, they are characterized by the locus of probe-analyte interaction: Swelling bulk MNs sensors (BMNDs), where probe-analyte interaction is inside the volume of MN; hollow MNs sensors (HMNDs), where a small material sampling of ISF is analyzed on or offline; coated MNs sensors (CMNDs), whose surface is the locus of the interaction between analytes and bioprobes; planar MNs sensors (PMNDs), where the probe–analyte interaction is on a specific zone of a flat MNs surface. (B) some configurations for MNs for drugs delivery: (from left) hollow MNs present a inner cavities to immediately administration of high dose and high MW drugs; soluble and hybrid MNs for fast administration with a high doses and medium MW; coated MNs for fast administration of low doses and any MW; swelling MNs for very slow administration of high doses of smaller molecules. Reproduced with permission of Ref. [8].

analytes directly in the interstitial fluid. In those cases, more than a strategy could be used: the functionalization of the surface of MNs with a specific probe, realizing a coated MND [5], the trapping of probe molecules into a swelling material [6] or the extraction of fluids and the analysis into a microfluidic system [7] are only some examples. In **Figure 1A** a sketch of different MNDs for sensing purposes is shown.

Moreover, microneedle-based devices (MNDs) can combine diagnostic sensing and therapeutic administration of drugs in one single tool. From this point of view, more than a painless door to the human body, a MND represents the a perfect example of theranostic instrument, since a single device could quantify the real value of a relevant biomolecule, such as glucose, and accurately deliver a drug, the insulin, if needed. MNDs are particularly interesting as simple drug administration tools, too. In fact, the transdermal route for drug administration is a very fascinating way, not only for the very low invasiveness and the easiness of self-administration, but also for the absence of first pass metabolism. However, the intercellular lipid matrix of the epidermis consists of ceramides, free fatty acids, and cholesterol, a complex mixture of neutral lipids arranged as bilayers with hydrophobic chains facing each other (lipophilic bimolecular leaflet) [9]. Transdermal delivery works only for lipophilic uncharged drugs with low MW (<500 Da), which need low dose and continuous delivery. Moreover, components, formulations and drugs must be non-irritating and non-sensitizing. MNs can be used with both lipophilic and hydrophilic formulations, both charged and uncharged drugs, both small and oversized molecules.

For all these cases, MN configurations are illustrated in **Figure 1B**, where the possibility to use solving or hybrid soluble/insoluble MNs are considered.

MNDs could be integrated on printed circuit boards, flexible electronics and microfluidic channels, thus allowing a continuous monitoring of the physiological parameters with very low invasiveness, together with sustained and localized administration of drugs. MNDs can be designed for very specific applications, from the detection of skin cancer to the monitoring of metabolic pathways.

2. Microneedles array fabrication

Technologies, skills and facilities for Micro and Nano Electro Mechanical Systems (MEMS and NEMS) fabrication are the key elements for the development of new biomedical devices [1–3, 10]. Fabrication methods for Microneedles (MNs) strongly depend on the MNs shape, tip model, length, density of the MNs matrix, and the material of which they are made of.

Moreover, structural characteristics of the MNs matrix in turn depend on the specific application considered [11]. In fact, MNDs are exploited in fluid extraction [12] and *in-situ* diagnosis of diseases [13], in drug and gene delivery strategies [1, 11], in cell therapy [3] and so on.

At first, Silicon and silicon-based nanostructured materials, such as porous silicon, were largely employed in MNDs fabrication due to the well-established functionalization chemistry protocols and fabrication techniques, extenseively used in microelectronics, which simplified the integration into more complex systems [14]. However, silicon revealed to be a non-biocompatible material, due to its fragility and to the local inflammations (silicosis) it could provoke; for this reason its use has been limited in cell applications [15].

To overcome limitations on the use of silicon, polymers have been extensively proposed as alternative materials in many applications. Poly Dimethyl Siloxane

(PDMS) is one of the most used materials in microfluidics to design biomedical devices, due to its well-known biological compatibility [16]. Usually, PDMS is employed as mold to fabricate MNDs by replica molding (see **Figure 2**). In case of PDMS molding, the fabrication involves the following steps: female PDMS mold fabrication by means of standard photolithography or laser drilling; patterned MNs in PDMS mold filling with liquid polymers in vacuum conditions; curing of the polymers by temperature and/or UV exposure; mold removal; eventually, an additional curing step [16]. Biodegradable polymers have been largely employed in MNDs for drugs delivery application [20–24], but the biodegradability is not required for biosensing.

A direct method for MNDs fabrication is the so-called drawing lithography [19]. Drawing lithography is a fabrication method, which does not need light irradiation and a mask, since it is based on the use of a thermosetting polymer directly drawn from a 2D solid surface (see **Figure 2**). In drawing lithography, commercial photoresist is usually spin coated or drop casted onto the substrate and cooled down. Drills are fixed in an array on a PDMS frame and used as pillars contacted with the photoresist. Conical-shaped bridges between the substrate and the pillars appear when their relative distance is increased by drawing (elongation). The bridges are cured to generate a rigid structure. Finally, the separation of the bridges produces the desired MND.

However, drawing method lacks in flexibility and the curing at high temperature of the polymers encapsulating biopharmaceutical molecules can cause their denaturation or inactivation. In fact, MNDs encapsulating drugs or bio-probes must be fabricated in a controlled environment to preserve the biological activity.

The increasing demand for simple methods that preserve the biological activity by utilizing the natural properties of polymers has conducted to the idea of centrifugal lithography [17]. In [17], centrifugal lithography was used for the fabrication of MNDs in a single centrifugation, by exploiting the self-shaping properties

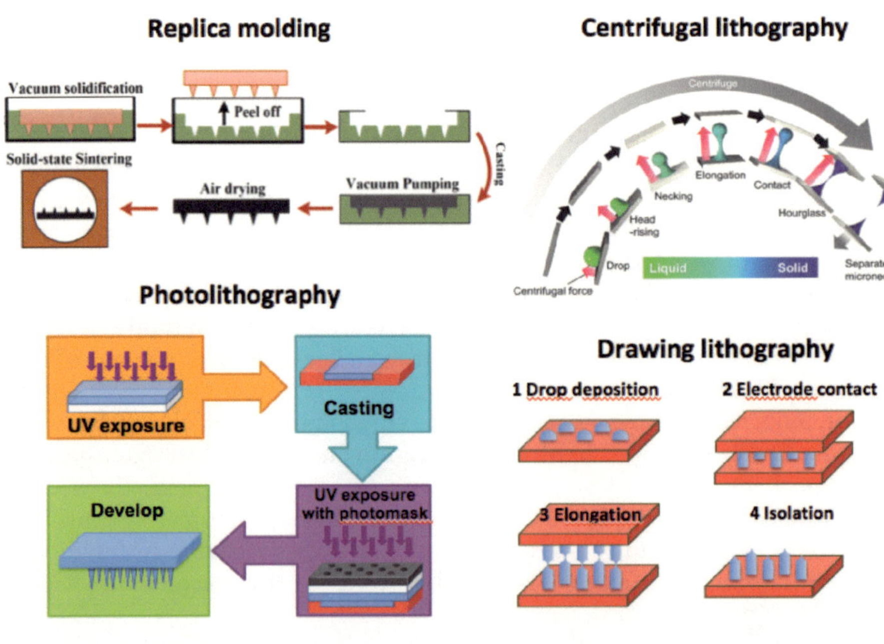

Figure 2.
Main fabrication strategies for MNs fabrication. Replica molding [16] centrifugal lithography [17] photolithography [18] drawing lithography [19].

of hyaluronic acid (HA). Briefly, fabrication involves the following steps: HA drops encapsulating drugs molecules are casted onto the substrate; centrifugal force is applied under refrigerated conditions (4°C) to the droplets in order to shape in hourglass microstructures; finally, the mirroring shapes are separated to form MNs. Also in the case of HA, drug delivery is successfully obtained, but biosensing is unavailable due to its biodegradability.

On the other hand, hydrogel polymers are very attractive materials for MNDs and, generally, for biomedical devices, since a hydrated gel provides near physiological conditions. These gels are excellent encapsulation matrices for biological probes, such as enzymes and peptides [18, 20, 25, 26]. Moreover, the standard photolithographic processes can be employed to fabricate micrometric devices based on polymeric hydrogels [materials] (**Figure 2**). In [6, 18, 27, 28], authors proposed procedures of standard direct photolithography, where a mixture of Poly(ethylene glycol) diacrylate (PEGDA) and a commercial photoinitiator were used as an ordinary photoresist, without any etching step being required. In fact, PEGDA is a biocompatible polymer that solidifies at room temperature in presence of a photoinitiator after exposure to ultraviolet (UV) light for few seconds. In case of photolithographic process, the fabrication involves the following steps: the liquid photosensitive polymeric mixture is casted onto a UV-transparent substrate and exposed to ultraviolet radiation, in order to fabricate the MNDs base; a vessel is fulfilled with a second quantity of liquid mixture and the MNDs base is put on; a second exposure through a mask, whose pattern is an array of holes, is applied; finally the structure is developed by simply washing in deionized water. The PEGDA mixture can be customized to encapsulate a variety of drugs or sensing probes as biological molecules or inorganic nanoparticles [29–31].

Comparing the fabrication methods, all produced MNs have demonstrated high quality in indentation proof and a good grade of reproducibility, with some critical issues during the mold removal step in replica molding method.

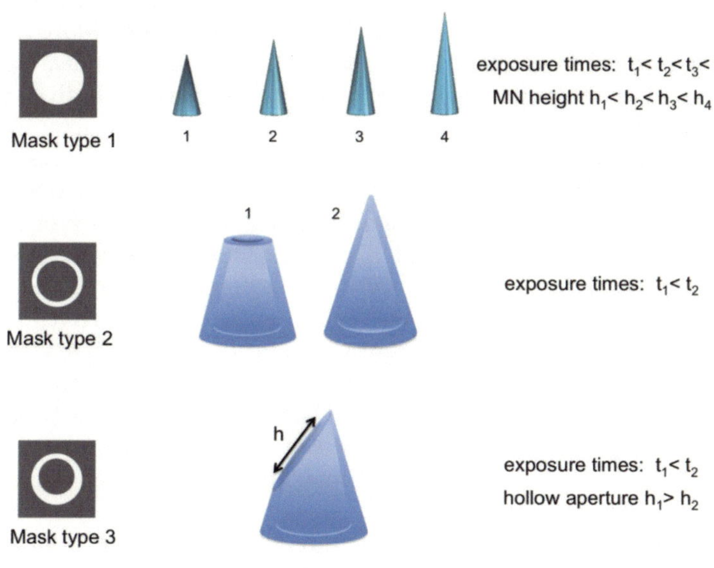

Figure 3.
The photolithographic methods offer a wide range of solutions for MNDs. Changing time exposure and/or photolithographic mask several configurations and arrays of MNs for both therapeutics and biosensing can be fabricated. From above: Mask type 1 (simple circle) enables MNs with several heights depending on time exposure; mask type 2 (ring) enables hollow MNs with height and closure depending on time exposure; mask type 3 (mismatched concentric ring) enables in one only exposure hollow MNs with a lateral oblique aperture, which is smaller as the exposure time increases.

Finally, we highlight that the photolithographic approach allows the fabrication of MNDs for a wide range of applications. In fact, this process allows the design of a wide range of MN types with different shape, length and tip, simply by adjusting the exposure parameters or shape photolithographic masks [18, 28]. In **Figure 3**, the whole range of possibilities enabled by photolithographic method are summarized: mask type 1 (simple circle) enables MNs with several heights depending on time exposure; mask type 2 (ring) enables hollow MNs with height and closure depending on time exposure; mask type 3 (mismatched concentric ring) enables in a single exposure the fabrication of hollow MNs with a lateral oblique aperture as in hypodermic syringes. Also in this case, lateral aperture is smaller as the exposure time increases.

3. Drug delivery patches

MNs represent actually a flexible technological platform, which enables innovative diagnostic solutions and breakthrough therapeutic issues in biomedicine [1–3]. First, finding a painless alternative to hypodermic injections has driven researchers to the development of MNDs. In fact, belonephobia, which is the unreasonable fear of needles, affects up to 10% of the population and has implications for treatment and follow up, especially in the pediatric patients [32]. In reverse, the sensation caused by MNs has proved to be statistically indistinguishable from a smooth surface and the pain caused by a hypodermic needle has been perceived substantially more than MNs [4]. Moreover, as previously stated, the transdermal route for drug administration is a very fascinating way, not only for the very low invasiveness and the easiness of self-administration, but also for the absence of first pass metabolism. However, the intercellular lipid matrix of the epidermis consists of ceramides, free fatty acids, and cholesterol, a complex mixture of neutral lipids arranged as bilayers with hydrophobic chains facing each other (lipophilic bimolecular leaflet) [9]. Transdermal delivery works only for lipophilic uncharged drugs with low MW (<500 Da), which need low dose and continuous delivery. Moreover, components, formulations and drugs must be non-irritating and non-sensitizing. MNs can be used with both lipophilic and hydrophilic formulations, both charged and uncharged drugs, both small and oversized molecules. In fact, currently, interesting MNDs are involved in clinical trials both for some topical applications, as analgesic compounds, anti-inflammatory or anesthetic drugs, and for some traditional systemic drugs, such as anticancer drugs, vaccines, insulin or hormones [33].

Among the topical applications, MNDs can replace very invasive methods for warts therapy, such as electrocautery and cryotherapy. A MND developed by Ryu et al. for warts treatment resulted to be innovative and effective [34]. In this study, quite 40 patients with wart lesions were enrolled and referred less pain than cryotherapy, as well as more tolerability with respect to electrocautery. Other skin diseases have been treated by means of MNDs, as melasma in [35], where authors fabricated biocompatible polymeric MNs based on methacrylic acid and polyvinyl pyrrolidone (PVP) to locally administer tranexamic acid, an innovative molecule that inhibits excessive melanin production by acting on melanocytes.

Acne vulgaris is another common inflammatory skin disease, affecting both physiologically and psychologically on patients. Barrier properties of skin strongly limit the usual antibiotic drug creams used to cure acne, but the use of MNs can overcome this limits, by using a reactive oxygen species–responsive [36]. In some *in-vivo* studies, MNDs for anti-acne therapy demonstrated bioresponsivity and efficiency to prevent bacterial growth. Finally, among the local administration taking advantage of MNs, the treatment of cornea diseases must be quoted. In particular, using dissolving polymeric microneedles to deliver besifloxacin to the cornea, a significant improvement in besifloxacin deposition and permeation were proven after only 5 minutes of application [37].

On the other hand, also administration of systemic drugs by means of MNDs showed good results in effectiveness, safe and economic efficiency as disposal devices. A wide range of molecules has been proven to be compatible with MNDs and each category of drug showed specific advantages compared to the use of oral or hypodermic administration.

First of all, vaccine delivery is probably the most involved health issue in MN technology, due to the large number of people involved each year. Nguyen and Park recently reviewed MNDs enrolled in human studies and reported the progress of MNDs in the clinical trials [38]. Finally, the use of MNs in therapy for clinical vaccine was recognized as very important, but further tests are recommended.

When MNDs is used to deliver vaccines based on DNA, some studies show that the gene expression is improved with respect to the results of conventional hypodermic injection. Consequently, the use of MNs to administrate DNA based vaccine results in an improvement of the immune responses [38, 39]. In [39], Authors hypothesized that the improvement of the immune response by delivering DNA vaccine by means of MNs could be due to the enhancement of the protein expression of the encoded gene.

Another important issue of vaccine administration improved by MNDs is the stability of the active ingredients into dissolving or swellable MNs. Encapsulation of inactivated polio vaccine (IPV) into dissolving MNs gains a better thermal stability with respect to that of the conventional liquid formulation of IPV [40]. The greater thermostability of the MN patches can generally enable a mass distribution with less constrains on cold chain storage resulting in a great reduction of costs, since global vaccination strategies require large immunization coverage. Moreover, new MNDs have been proposed as an alternative solution to the standard needle injections, for the advantage of self-vaccination.

Further studies have been done to elucidate the interactions between polymers and vaccines, as in the case of hydrogel based MNs and dissolving MNs. In these cases, the antigen ovalbumin was used as a model protein interaction with polymers and the consequences on the immune response [40, 41].

Hollow MNs have the advantage of overcoming the skin barrier imposed by the stratum corneum and delivering bigger molecules, such as macromolecules or nanoparticle systems, in the fastest possible way. Polymeric nanoparticles encapsulating the model antigen ovalbumin have been intradermal delivered by means of hollow MNDs by Niu et al., reporting that this kind of delivery is a promising approach to improve the effectiveness of vaccine formulations [42]. Among the dissolving devices, MNs based on hyaluronic acid (HA) resulted a promising encapsulation method of high content of antigen molecules in intradermal vaccination [43].

Also anticancer drugs belong to an important field of application of MNDs: two research groups have investigated on DOX administration by means of MNs in [44] and in [45]. Nguyen et al. found *in vitro* studies that Polyvinyl Alcohol (PVA) MNs enhance the transdermal delivery of DOX. In an *in vivo* antitumor study of Hao et al., a near-infrared responsive PEGylated gold nanorod (GNR-PEG) and DOX-loaded dissolvable HA-based microneedle (GNR-PEG&DOX@HA MN) has been developed against cancer of epidermis. In the study, mice treated with GNR-PEG&DOX@HA MNs taken remarkable advantage in antitumor efficacy in only one treatment, such that all mice have been cured without recurrence.

Moreover, lipophilic drugs found a lot of benefits from the use of MNs: poorly soluble drugs were encapsulated and easily administrated by MNDs, as in the case of the widely used specific 5-HT3 receptor antagonist, namely granisetron, that prevents nausea and vomiting during emetogenic chemotherapy in cancer patients [46]. *In vivo* results in [46] proved the evidence of controlled release systemic delivery.

An innovative pharmaceutical solution involving a MND in the field of HIV treatment has been proposed by Yavuz et al. in [47]. Also in this case, the self-injection route of administration represents the key issue for care improvement, since it limited the risks of contamination of the personnel involved in therapy and guaranteed a painless delivery for the patients via patches of microneedles.

New drugs and innovative therapies have been put in place with the help of MNDs. In particular, polymeric MNs have been widely exploited for their porous nature, which is expressed both by soluble MNs and by simply biocompatible ones. In [48, 49], anti-obesity substances have been successfully administered. These substances modified the metabolic process by increasing the energy consumed and

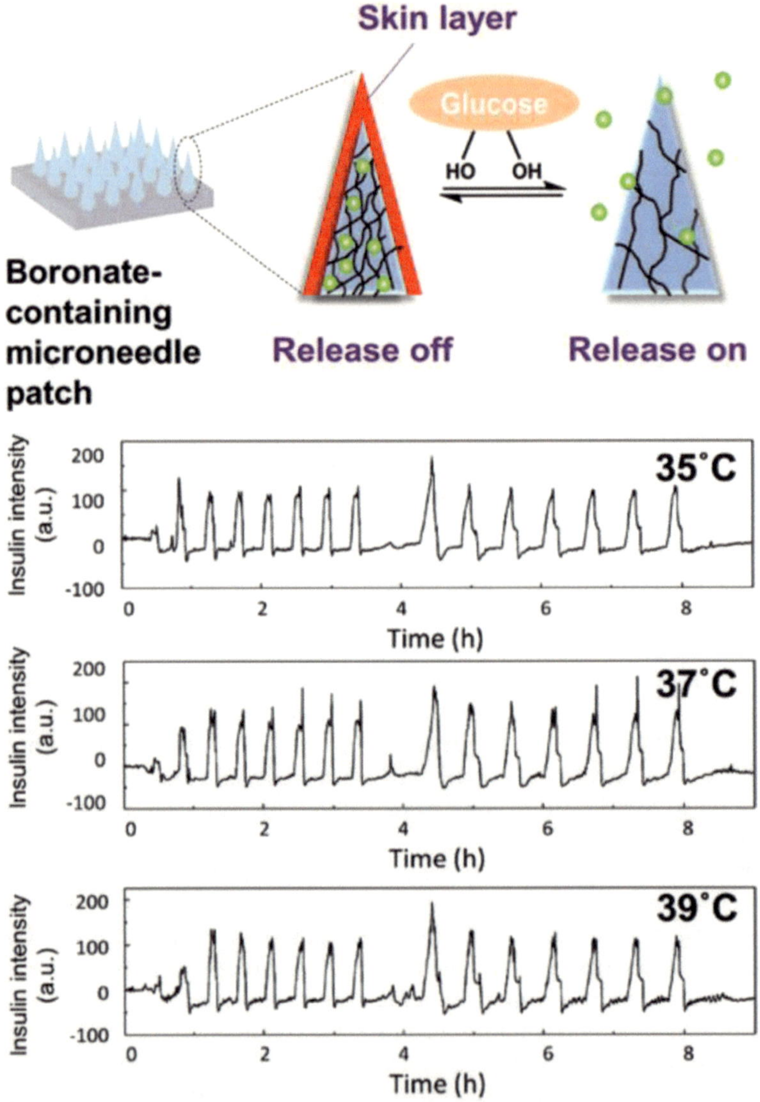

Figure 4.
Adapted with permission from ACS Appl. Polym. Mater. 2020, 2, 7, 2781–2790. Copyright (2020) American Chemical Society. Sketch of device and in vitro *FITC-labeled insulin release at various temperatures, pH 7.4.*

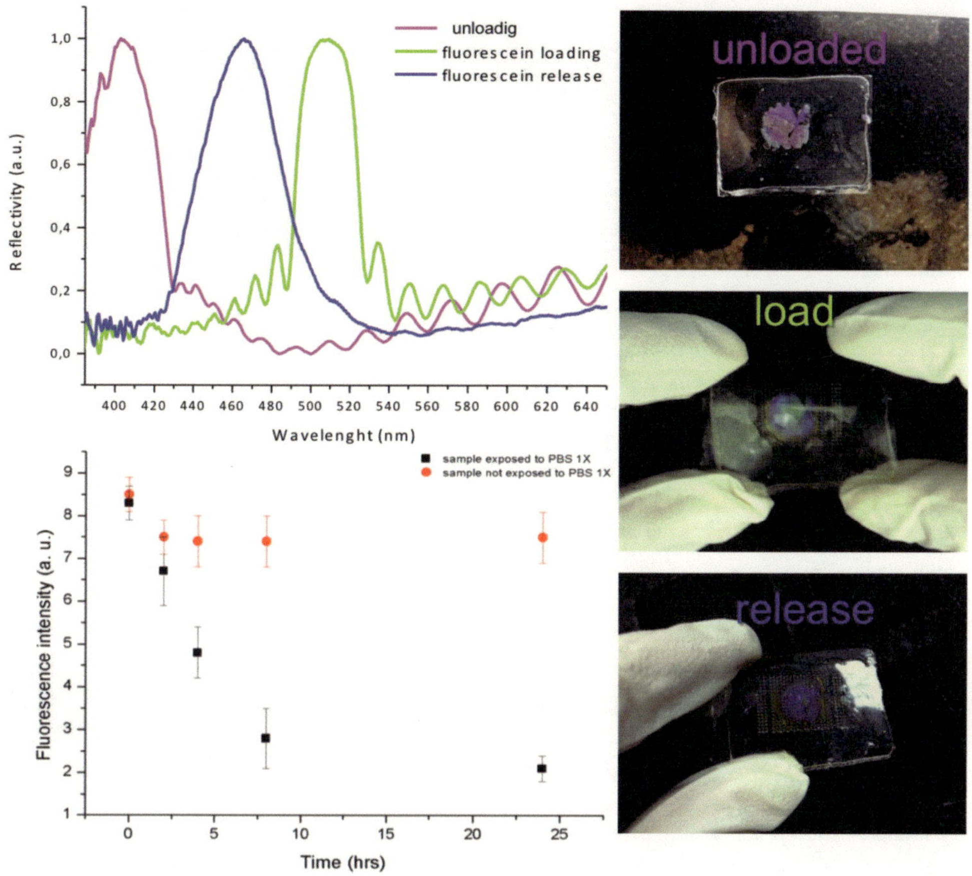

Figure 5.
The optical integrated MND presented in [6] have got a naked-eye monitor made up with a psi membrane to follow the release of a drug loaded in.

transforming the white fat that stores calories into brown fat that burns calories [48]. While in [49], gelatin MNDs were used to induce lipolysis and suppress adipocyte lipogenesis in fatty rats.

Particular attention has to be paid on insulin delivery, since diabetes is one of the most common diseases, not only in elder patients, but also in obesity-affected patients.

Avoiding use of enzymes, a polymeric MND has been developed for on-demand insulin delivery by Chen et al. [50]. Continuous and acute glycemic control was realized with a long-acting, safe, stable, economically efficient and on-demand insulin delivery by MND, without depending on patient compliance. Thus, this technology opens to next generation of diabetes therapies.

In the same field, the treatment of individuals with type II diabetes mellitus has been successfully obtained with metformin HCl, the most widely used drug for this disease, delivered by means of hydrogel MNs [51].

In [52], authors proposed a temperature-independent MND for glucose-responsive insulin release. The rapid and sustained regulation is enabled through a "skin layer" of Phenylboronic acid (PBA), formed on the surface of MNs. PBA is a synthetic hydrogel with reversible binding capability with glucose. Compared to other glucose-responsive MNDs based on nanoparticles or glucose oxidase, the proposed patch overcomes the safety concerns and provides a good sustainability for large-scale production. In **Figure 4**, a sketch of the proposed glucose-responsive

MN type	Disease	Experiments	Refs.
Swelling	Acne vulgaris	*In vivo* (mouse)	[36]
Swelling	Diabetes	*In vitro*	[50]
Swelling	Diabetes	*In vivo* (mouse)	[51]
Swelling	Immunity (vaccines)	*In vitro*	[40]
Swelling	Nausea and vomiting	*In vivo*	[46]
Swelling	Keloid scar	*Ex vivo*	[53]
Swelling/hybrid	—	*in vitro*	[6]
Hollow	Immunity (vaccines)	—	[42]
Dissolving	Melasma	*In vivo* (mouse)	[35]
Dissolving	Ocular infection	*Ex vivo* (cornea)	[37]
Dissolving	Cancer	*In vitro*	[44]
Dissolving	Cancer	*In vivo* (mouse)	[45, 54]
Dissolving	Immunity (vaccines)	*In vivo* (mouse)	[41, 43]
Dissolving	Obesity	*In vivo* (mouse)	[48, 49]
Dissolving	Vitamin K deficiency	*In vitro*	[55]
Coated	Warts	*In vivo* (human)	[34]
Coated	Immunity (vaccines)	*In vivo* (mouse)	[39]
hybrid	Diabetes	*In vivo* (mouse)	[52]

Table 1.
Main studies on therapeutic delivery with MNDs. Adapted from [56].

insulin dispensing MND is presented together with main results in on-demand insulin release at physiological temperature.

Finally, we cite the engage of MNDs in effective administration of small peptides, vitamin K and mRNA administered, both *in vitro* and *in vivo* studies [53–56].

In **Table 1**, main studies on therapeutic delivery with MNDs are summarized. Another important issue is the integration of MNs in optical, microelectronic or microfluidic devices. In [6], authors present the proof-of-concept of an optical integrated MNDs based on polymeric MNs and porous silicon (PSi) for transdermal drug delivery (**Figure 5**). Since its surface can be chemically modified, PSi is one of the most popular porous material used in drug administration [57]. Moreover, PSi structures have a tunable refractive index that depends on their porosity [58]. The MND presented in [6] is based on PEGDA hydrogel MNs and includes a PSi free-standing membrane with a Bragg mirror optical structure, i.e. an optical structure that reflects a specific wavelength (color) in the visible spectrum. Furthermore, the Psi membrane not only acts as a drug/biomolecules reservoir, but also it can be used to optically monitor the released drug, since the reflected wavelength changes with the emptying of pores (**Figure 5**). In [6], the integrated-chip optical device guarantees the optimum disposable MND, which can be self-administrated and self-wasted, once the drug has been all delivered by only looking at the color variation at naked-eye.

4. Biosensing with microneedles

Human interstitial fluid (ISF) is on average between 9 and 13.5 L [59, 60]. Fluid moves from the lymphatic vasculature into the interstitium, among the endothelial walls of cells, then to the blood plasma, and finally returns to the lymphatic vasculature. Analytes enter into the ISF through three paths: first, by transcellular path, through the capillaries; secondly, by paracellular path, through the cell walls; finally, by vesicular path, from the cells to the ISF [61, 62]. ISF moves within a network of glycosaminoglycans, elastin, and collagen and transports electrolytes and metabolites to muscle cells, bone cells, cartilage, tissues, organs and so on [60, 63].

Dermal ISF is localized in the extracellular spaces between the vasculature, connective tissues and the cells. A lot of research efforts have been done to develop extraction methods of ISF in order to obtain an analytical composition and understand the relationship between plasma and ISF. **Table 2** summarizes the main ISF constituents, measured concentrations, and typical concentration ranges for healthy people [63].

Since its location just under human skin (the largest human organ) and its relationship with the vasculature system, analysis of ISF has received interest for the realization of new wearable devices.

On the other hand, new diagnostic methods can sensitively, rapidly and accurately detect, analyze and monitor relevant diseases of social interest, and can lead to an effective management of healthcare. Biomarkers and biosensors research receive, then, a constantly increasing thrust.

Despite the transduction method used, innovation in standard sensing technologies is continuously pursued. Although several optical techniques, such as fluorescence, surface plasmon resonance and surface enhanced Raman spectroscopy have been exploited, electrochemical methods, based either on voltammetry or impedance spectroscopy, have been demonstrated to quantify analytes in ISF with high sensitivity and easily integration into a MND [8].

Standard electrochemical sensors are realized confining bioprobes onto an electrode surface directly immersed in a solution, as the ISF. A key issue in the innovation of electrochemical devices is the design of the so-called working electrode, that can increase the performance of the whole biosensor. The development of electrochemical engineered biosensors has been recently the focus of many research groups, which provided several fabrication strategies [64].

Electrochemical sensors based on MNs can analytically monitor biomarkers, drug release, metabolites, electrolytes and other chemical species present in dermal ISF and involved in biological functions. Recently, in [65] authors gave a proteomic characterization of the dermal ISF, extracted by means of a hollow MND. In this work, 407 proteins have been found and quantified [65]. Moreover, less than 1% of these proteins have been identified only into the ISF, confirming that the ISF is strictly connected to both plasma and serum. Then, the MNDs can be minimally

ISF constituent	Measured concentration	Typical concentration ranges
Glucose	4–8 mM	4.5–8 mM
Cortisol	24–40 nM	Morning: 1–50 nM Afternoon: 27–42 nM
Lactate	1.17 ± 0.23 mM	1–2 mM
Lipids	1.5 ± 0.3 μM	Not reported
Na+	141 mM	135–150 mM
K+	4.4 mM	3.8–4.9 mM
Cl–	110 mM	99–117 mM

Table 2.
Main ISF constituents, measured concentrations and typical concentration ranges for healthy people [63].

invasive alternative devices to blood-derived fluids sensors with potential for real-time monitoring applications. In addition, in [66] an extremely small quantity (<1 nL) of the ISF was extracted by means of a hollow MN to measure drug concentrations and the typically painful blood drawn was avoided. In [66], the inner cavity of a hollow MN was derivatized to bind vancomycin. Optical absorbance is used as off-line transducer method, after extracting ISF with an integrated optofluidic device. The optofluidic MND detected the vancomycin in a sample volume of 0.6 nL with a limit of detection (LoD) of less than 100 nM.

Before being widely adopted into clinical practice, MNDs used as biosensors have to pursuit some general issues: a low cost fabrication; continuous monitoring and/or long-lasting working time; the possibly of integration in MEMS; the protection of the bioprobe, critical in enzyme-based detection; a good electrical conductivity (EC) for electrochemical sensing [67]. Moreover, the biofouling at the tissue–device interface must be avoided to successfully realize a wearable MND sensor [68]. According to Da Silva et al., currently, wearable sensors are still not yet ready for commercial develop, but within a few years MNDs biosensors will conquer the market [69].

In the field of MNDs for diagnostics, as well as for therapy, the approach can drastically vary with shapes and materials; **Figure 1A** shows a sketch of different MNDs for sensing purposes together with their working conditions into the human skin. Starting from the right, **Figure 6** reports: swelling bulk MNs sensors (BMNDs), whose diagnostic approach includes a volume effect in the probe-analyte interaction that will be considered separately; hollow MNs sensors (HMNDs), where a small material sampling of ISF is analyzed on or offline [70–72]; coated MNs sensors (CMNDs), whose surface is the locus of the interaction between analytes and bioprobes [73–81]; planar MNs sensors (PMNDs), where the probe–analyte interaction is on a specific zone of a flat MNs surface [82].

The bulk volume of solid MNs (BMNDs) is often exploited in electrochemical biosensing. Usually, hydrogels and swelling polymers are employed in the fabrication of BMN. Examples are polyethylene glycol diacrylate (PEGDA), polyvinyl pyrrolidone (PVP), polyvinyl alcohol, poly(acrylic acid), poly-l-lactide,

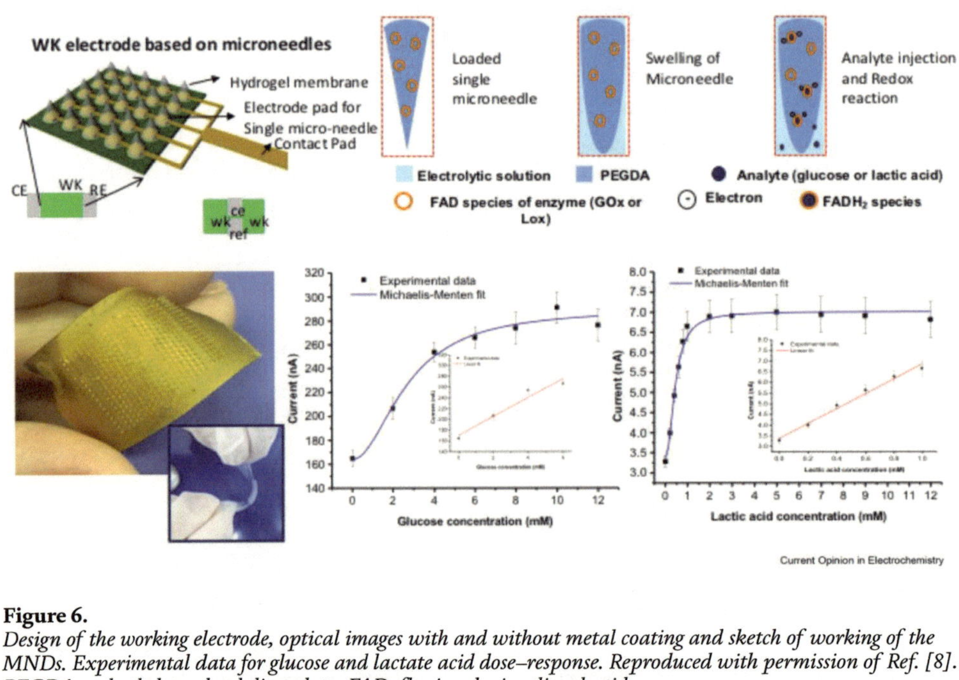

Figure 6.
Design of the working electrode, optical images with and without metal coating and sketch of working of the MNDs. Experimental data for glucose and lactate acid dose–response. Reproduced with permission of Ref. [8]. PEGDA, polyethylene glycol diacrylate; FAD, flavin adenine dinucleotide.

poly(lactide-coglycolide acid) and poly-N-isopropylacrylamide [83, 84]. These types of polymers can be processed by several fabrication techniques, such as replica molding, photolithography, drawing lithography and more [85]. Usually, probes and enhancers of transduction mechanisms are directly embedded in the porous polymer matrix during the fabrication. This environment protects probes without avoiding interaction between target analytes and bioprobes.

Caliò et al. trapped enzymes with vinyl-ferrocene mediator into a polymeric matrix of PEGDA in order to detect glucose and lactate exploiting the volume effect of the hydrogel matrix [27]. After being in contact with the ISF, the PEGDA matrix swells and the analytes solved into ISF enter the volume of the MNs, where a large number of probe molecules (enzymes) can be stored. The redox reaction takes place inside the volume and is transmitted to the electrode. The fabrication of the electrochemical MN biosensor only required a single further step (metal coating) in addition to the direct photolithographic process. The hybrid device traps GOx and LOX enzymes to enable the electrochemical detection of glucose and lactic acid, respectively, in physiological solution. The sensing MND showed a linear response from 0 to 4 mM for glucose, and from 0 to 1 mM for lactic acid (**Figure 6**) and a LoD of about 1 μM was found for both cases. **Figure 6** shows design of the MN based working electrode, optical images with and without metal coating and a sketch of the working principle of the swelling MNDs. Moreover, experimental data for glucose and lactate acid dose–response are reported.

5. Conclusions

Appeared on scene as a painless alternative to syringes, MNDs have conquered the biomedicine. The flexibility of these innovative devices makes these technological platforms really attractive for even new fields of application. Almost all materials can be used in the fabrication of MNDs: noble metals (gold and silver), semiconductors (silicon), plastics (polymers and hydrogels), amorphous materials (ceramics) and artificial nanostructured materials (porous silicon). MNDs have been used for drug delivery, cosmetic industry or biosensing, where the MN microstructures have been used as electrodes for electrochemical transduction. For biosensing systems, pros and cons have been highlighted for each device type in terms of analytical performances such as LoD, detection time, sensitivity and so on. In all the application cases, considerations about the safety of MNDs is due, since MNDs are conceived for being in contact with the human body. Then, inert, biocompatible, or physiologically dissolvable materials have to be engaged for device fabrication, even if they show lower analytical or delivery performances. After the overcoming of the skin natural barrier, MNs are directly in contact with human ISF. Hollow, coated, and swelling MNDs are all used in two ways: sensing of analytes and delivery of drugs; biosensing and administration; therapy and diagnosis.

Conflict of interest

The authors declare no conflict of interest.

Thanks

The Authors would like to thank all the Materias s.r.l. staff for supporting. In particular, Caterina Meglio, Aniello Cammarano, Maria Emilia Mercurio and Maria Grazia Ramaglia, those continuously help our research with their work.

Author details

Principia Dardano[1*], Mario Battisti[2], Selene De Martino[2], Ilaria Rea[1], Bruno Miranda[1,3], Luigi Nicolais[2] and Luca De Stefano[1]

1 Institute of Applied Sciences and Intelligent Systems, National Council of Research, Naples, Italy

2 Materias s.r.l., Naples, Italy

3 "Federico II" Naples University, Naples, Italy

*Address all correspondence to: principia.dardano@cnr.it

References

[1] Henry S., Mcallister, D.V., Allen, M.G., Prausnitz, M.R. Microfabricated microneedles: A novel approach to transdermal drug delivery. J. Pharm. Sci., 1998, 87, 922-925.

[2] Ashraf, M.W., Tayyaba, S., Afzulpurkar, N. Micro electromechanical systems (MEMS) based microfluidic devices for biomedical applications. Int. J. Mol. Sci., 2011, 12, 3648-3704.

[3] Philip R. Miller et al., Multiplexed microneedle-based biosensor array for characterization of metabolic acidosis, Talanta, 2012,Volume 88, 739-742

[4] Kaushik, Shilpa, Hord, Allen H., Denson, Donald D., McAllister, Devin V., Smitra, Sudhasinee, Allen, Mark G., Prausnitz, Mark R., Lack of Pain Associated with Microfabricated Microneedles, Anesthesia and Analgesia, 2001, 92, 502-504, doi: 10.1213/00000539-200102000-00041

[5] Fanmao Liu, Zhihong Lin, Quanchang Jin, Qianni Wu, Chengduan Yang, Hui-Jiuan Chen, Zihan Cao, Di-an Lin, Lingfei Zhou, Tian Hang, Gen He, Yonghang Xu, Wenhao Xia, Jun Tao*, and Xi Xie*, Protection of Nanostructures-Integrated Microneedle Biosensor Using Dissolvable Polymer Coating, ACS Appl. Mater. Interfaces, 2019, 11, 5, 4809-4819 https://doi.org/10.1021/acsami.8b18981

[6] Dardano, A. Caliò, J. Politi, I. Rea, I. Rendina, L. De Stefano, Optically monitored drug delivery patch based on porous silicon and polymermicroneedles, Biomed. Opt. Express, 2016, 7 (5), 1645-1655.

[7] Miller, Philip R., et al. Extraction and biomolecular analysis of dermal interstitial fluid collected with hollow microneedles. Communications Biology, 2018, 1.1, 1-11.

[8] Dardano, P., I. Rea, and L. De Stefano. Microneedles-based electrochemical sensors: New tools for advanced biosensing., Current Opinion in Electrochemistry, 2019, 17, 121-127.

[9] Montagna W., Kligman A.M., Carlisle K.S, Blood Vessels. In: Atlas of Normal Human Skin. Springer, New York, NY, 1992.

[10] Pasut, G., Veronese, F.M. Polymer-drug conjugation, recent achievements and general strategies. Progress Polym. Sci., 2007, 32, 933-961

[11] Valdés-Ramíreza, G., Windmiller, J.R., Claussen, J.C., Martinez, A.G., Kuralay, F., Zhou, M., Zhou, N., Polsky, R., Miller, P.R., Naravan, R., et al. Multiplexed and switchable release of distinct fluids from microneedle platforms via conducting polymer nanoactuators for potential drug delivery. Sens. Actuators B, 2012, 161, 1018-1024.

[12] Mukerjee, E.V., Collins, S.D., Isseroff, R.R., Smith, R.L. Microneedle array for transdermal biological fluid extraction and in situ analysis. Sens. Actuators A Phys., 2004, 114, 267-275.

[13] Donnelly, R.F., Morrow, D.I. J., McCarron, P.A., Woolfson, A.D., Morrissey, A., Juzenas, P., Juzeniene, A., Iani, A., McCarthy, H.O., Moan, J. Microneedle-mediated intradermal delivery of 5-aminolevulinic acid: Potential for enhanced topical photodynamic therapy. J. Controll. Release, 2008, 129, 154-162.

[14] Wilke, N., Mulcahy, A., Ye, S.R., Morrissey, A. Process optimization and characterization of silicon microneedles fabricated by wet etch technology. Microelectron. J., 2005, 36, 650-656.

[15] Hansel, C. S., Crowder, S. W., Cooper, S., Gopal, S., João Pardelha

da Cruz, M., de Oliveira Martins, L.,.. & Bakal, C., 2019, Nanoneedle-mediated stimulation of cell mechanotransduction machinery. ACS nano, 13(3), 2913-2926.

[16] Jiyu Li,Bin Liu,Yingying Zhou,Zhipeng Chen,Lelun Jiang,Wei Yuan,Liang Liang, Fabrication of a Ti porous microneedle array by metal injection molding for transdermal drug delivery, 2017, 12.2, e0172043. https://doi.org/10.1371/journal.pone.0172043

[17] Lee, Kwang, and Hyungil Jung, Drawing lithography for microneedles: a review of fundamentals and biomedical applications, Biomaterials, 2012, 33, 30, 7309-7326.

[18] P. Dardano, A. Caliò, V. Di Palma, M.F. Bevilacqua, A. Di Matteo, L. De Stefano, A photolithographic approach to polymeric microneedles array fabrication, Materials, 2015, 8 (12), 8661-8673.

[19] Yang, Huisuk, et al. Advanced healthcare materials, 2017, 6, 19.

[20] Su, Y., Mainardi, V. L., Wang, H., McCarthy, A., Zhang, Y. S., Chen, S.,.. & Xie, J., Dissolvable Microneedles Coupled with Nanofiber Dressings Eradicate Biofilms via Effectively Delivering a Database-Designed Antimicrobial Peptide. ACS nano, 2020, 14(9), 11775-11786.

[21] Sun, W., Araci, Z., Inayathullah, M., Manickam, S., Zhang, X., Bruce, M.A., Marinkovich, P.M., Lane, A.T.,Milla, C., Rajadas, J., et al. Polyvinylpyrrolidone microneedles enable delivery of intact proteins fordiagnostic and therapeutic applications. Acta Biomater., 2013, 9, 7767-7774.

[22] Kim, M.Y., Jung, B., Park, J.H. Hydrogel swelling as a trigger to release biodegradable polymermicroneedlesin skin. Biomaterials 2012, 33, 668-678.

[23] McGrath, M.G., Vucen, S., Vrdoljak, A., Kelly, A., O'Mahony, C., Crean, A.M., Moore, A. Production of dissolvable microneedles using an atomised spray process: Effect of microneedle composition on skin penetration. Eur. J. Pharm. Biopharm., 2014, 86, 200-211.

[24] Choi, C.K., Lee, K.J., Youn, Y.N., Jang, E.H., Kim, W., Min, B.K., Ryu, W.H. Spatially discrete thermal drawing of biodegradable microneedles for vasculardrug delivery. Eur. J. Pharm. Biopharm., 2013, 83,224-233.

[25] Mellott, M.B., Searcy, K., Pishko, M.V. Release of protein from highly cross-linked hydrogels of poly(ethylene glycol) diacrylate fabricated by UV polymerization. Biomaterials, 2001, 22, 929-941.

[26] Di Matteo, A., Di Palma, V., Bevilacqua, M.F., Cimmino, A. Biosensor. U.S. Patent 13,929,654, 16 January 2014.

[27] A. Calio, P. Dardano, V. D. Palma, M. F. Bevilacqua, A. D. Matteo, H. I. Uele and L. D. Stefano, Polymeric microneedles based enzymatic electrodes for electrochemical biosensing of glucose and lactic acid, Sens. Actuators, B, 2016, 236, 343-349

[28] Luca De Stefano, Principia Dardano, Luigi Nicolais, Hollow microneedle for transdermal delivery of active molecules and/or for the sampling of biological fluids and manufacturing method of such hollow microneedle, World patent WO2019243915A1, 2018

[29] Hahn, M.S. Patterning of PEG-based hydrogels—Engineering spatial complexity. Mater. Matters, 2010, 5, 62-66.

[30] Politi, J., Spadavecchia, J., Iodice, M., de Stefano, L. Oligopeptide-heavy metal interaction monitoring by hybrid

gold nanoparticle based assay. Analyst, 2015, 140, 149-155.

[31] Nada, A.M.A., Dawy, M., Salama, A.H. Dielectric properties and ac-conductivity of cellulose polyethylene glycol blends. Mater. Chem. Phys., 2004, 84, 205-215.

[32] Thurgate, Claire, and Sue Heppell., Needle phobia changing venepuncture practice in ambulatory care., Paediatric nursing, 2005, 17, 9, 15-19.

[33] M. R. Prausnitz and R. Langer, Transdermal drug delivery, Nat. Biotechnol., 2008, 26(11), 1261-1268.

[34] H. R. Ryu, H. R. Jeong, H. S. Seon Woo, J. S. Kim, S. K. Lee, H. J. Kim, J. O. Baek, J. H. Park, J. Y. Roh, Efficacy of a bleomycin microneedle patch for the treatment of warts, Drug Delivery Transl. Res., 2018, 8, 273.

[35] S. A. Machekposhti, M. Soltani, P. Najafizadeh, S. A. Ebrahimi, P. Chen, Biocompatible polymer microneedle for topical/dermal delivery of tranexamic acid, J. Controlled Release, 2017, 261, 87.

[36] Y. Zhang, P. Feng, J. Yu, J. Yang, J. Zhao, J. Wang, Q. Shen, Z. Gu, ROS-Responsive Microneedle Patch for Acne Vulgaris Treatment, Adv. Ther., 2018, 1, 1800035.

[37] S. Bhatnagar, A. Saju, K. D. Cheerla, S. K. Gade, P. Garg, V. V.K. Venuganti, Corneal delivery of besifloxacin using rapidly dissolving polymeric microneedles, Drug Delivery Transl. Res., 2018, 8, 473.

[38] T. T. Nguyen, J. H. Park, Human studies with microneedles for evaluation of their efficacy and safety, Expert Opin. Drug Delivery, 2018, 15, 235.

[39] S. Zhang, S. Zhao, X. Jin, B. Wang, G. Zhao, Hum. Microneedles improve the immunogenicity of DNA vaccines, Gene Ther, 2018, 29, 1004.

[40] C. Kolloru, Y. Gomoaa, M. R. Prausnitz, Development of a thermostable microneedle patch for polio vaccination, Drug Delivery Transl. Res., 2019, 9, 192.

[41] A. J. Courtenay, A. M. Rodgers, M. T. McCrudden, H. O. McCarthy, R. F. Donnelly, Novel hydrogel-forming microneedle array for intradermal vaccination in mice using ovalbumin as a model protein antigen, Mol. Pharmaceutics, 2018, 16, 118.

[42] L. Niu, L. Y. Chu, S. A. Burton, K. J. Hansen, J. Panyam, Intradermal delivery of vaccine nanoparticles using hollow microneedle array generates enhanced and balanced immune response, J. Controlled Release, 2019, 294, 268.

[43] Leone, M., Romeijn, S., Slütter, B., O'Mahony, C., Kersten, G., & Bouwstra, J. A. , Hyaluronan molecular weight: Effects on dissolution time of dissolving microneedles in the skin and on immunogenicity of antigen. European Journal of Pharmaceutical Sciences, 2020, 146, 105269.

[44] Y. Hao, Y. W. Chen, M. Y. Lei, T. Y. Zhang, Y. P. Cao, J. R. Peng, L. J. Chen, Z. Y. Qian, Near-Infrared Responsive PEGylated Gold Nanorod and Doxorubicin Loaded Dissolvable Hyaluronic Acid Microneedles for Human Epidermoid Cancer Therapy, Adv. Ther., 2018, 1, 1800008.

[45] H. X. Nguyen, B. D. Bozorg, Y. Kim, A. Wieber, G. Birk., D. Lubd, A. K. Bang, Poly (vinyl alcohol) microneedles: fabrication, characterization, and application for transdermal drug delivery of doxorubicin, Eur. J. Pharm. Biopharm., 2018, 129, 88-103.

[46] G. Yang, M. He, S. Zhang, M. Wu, Y. Gao, An acryl resin-based swellable microneedles for controlled release intradermal delivery of granisetron, Drug Dev. Ind. Pharm., 2018, 44, 808-816.

[47] B. Yavuz, J. L. Morgan, L. Showalter, K. R. Horng, S. Dandekar, C. Herrera, P. LiWang, D. L. Kaplan, Pharmaceutical approaches to HIV treatment and prevention, Adv. Ther., 2018, 1, 1800054.

[48] A. Than, K. Liang, S. Xu, L. Sun, *H. duan*, F. Xi, C. Xu, P. Chen, Transdermal Delivery of Anti-Obesity Compounds to Subcutaneous Adipose Tissue with Polymeric Microneedle Patches, Small Methods, 2017, 1, 1700269.

[49] S. M. An, K. Y. Seong, S. G. Yim, Y. J. Hwang, S. H. Bae, S. Y. Yang, B. S. An, Intracutaneous delivery of gelatins induces lipolysis and suppresses lipogenesis of adipocytes, Acta Biomater., 2018, 67, 238.

[50] S. Chen, H. Matsumoto, Y. Morooka, M. Tanaka, Y. Miyahara, T. Suganami, A. Matsumoto, Microneedle-Array Patch Fabricated with Enzyme-Free Polymeric Components Capable of On-Demand Insulin Delivery, Adv. Funct. Mater., 2019, 29, 1807369.

[51] E. M. Migdadi, A. J. Courtenay, I. A. Tekko, M. T. McCrudden, M. C. Kearney, E. McAlister, H. O. McCarthy, R. F. Donnelly, Hydrogel-forming microneedles enhance transdermal delivery of metformin hydrochloride, J. Controlled Release, 2018, 285, 142.

[52] Chen, S., Miyazaki, T., Itoh, M., Matsumoto, H., Morooka, Y., Tanaka, M., ... & Matsumoto, A., Temperature-stable Boronate Gel based Microneedle Technology for Self-Regulated Insulin Delivery, ACS Appl. Polym. Mater., 2020, 2, 7, 2781-2790.

[53] S. Liu, D. C. Yeo, C. Wiraja, H. L. Tey, M. Mrksich, C. Xu, Bioeng., Peptide delivery with poly(ethylene glycol) diacrylate microneedles through swelling effect, Transl. Med., 2017, 2, 258.

[54] K. J. Koh, Y. Liu, S. H. Lim, X. J. Loh, L. Kang, C. Y. Lim, K. K.L. Phua, Formulation, characterization and evaluation of mRNA-loaded dissolvable polymeric microneedles (RNApatch), Sci. Rep., 2018, 8, 11842.

[55] A. R.J. Hutton, H. L. Quinn, P. J. McCague, C. Jarrahian, A. Rein Weston, P. S. Coffey, E. Gerth Guyette, D. Zehrung, E. Larrañeta, R. F. Donnelly, Transdermal delivery of vitamin K using dissolving microneedles for the prevention of vitamin K deficiency bleeding, Int. J. Pharm., 2018, 541, 56.

[56] Dardano, P., Battisti, M., Rea, I., Serpico, L., Terracciano, M., Cammarano, A., De Stefano, L, Polymeric microneedle arrays: versatile tools for an innovative approach to drug administration. Advanced Therapeutics, 2019, 2(8), 1900036.

[57] J. R. Henstock, L. T. Canham, and S. I. Anderson, "Silicon: The evolution of its use in biomaterials," Acta Biomater., 2015, 11, 17-26.

[58] L. De Stefano, L. Moretti, I. Rendina, and A. M. Rossi, "Time-resolved sensing of chemical species in porous silicon optical microcavity," Sens. Actuators B Chem., 2004, 100(1-2), 168-172.

[59] J.V.M. Mathew, Physiology, Blood Plasma, StatPearls Publishing, 2020,

[60] K. Aukland, G. Nicolaysen, Interstitial fluid volume: local regulatory mechanisms, Physiol. Rev., 1981, 61 (3), 556-643

[61] J. Heikenfeld, et al., Accessing analytes in biofluids for peripheral biochemical monitoring, Nat. Biotechnol., 2019, 37 (4), 407-419

[62] Madden, J., O'Mahony, C., Thompson, M., O'Riordan, A., & Galvin, P., Biosensing in dermal interstitial fluid using microneedle based electrochemical devices., Sensing

and Bio-Sensing Research, 2020, 100348.

[63] J.H.V. Scallan, R.J. Korthuis, Capillary Fluid Exchange: Regulation, Functions, and Pathology. Chapter 2 The Interstitium Morgan & Claypool Life Sciences, San Rafael (CA), 2010.

[64] Li M, Lv M, Wang L, Fan C, Zuo X, Engineering electrochemical interface for biomolecular sensing., Curr Opin Electrochem, 2019, 14,71-80.

[65] Tran BQ, Miller PR, Taylor RM, Boyd G, Mach PM, Rosenzweig CN, Baca JT, Polsky R, Glaros T, Proteomic characterization of dermal interstitial fluid extracted using a novel microneedleassisted technique. J Proteome Res, 2017, 17,479-485.

[66] Ranamukhaarachchi SA, Padeste C, Dübner M, Häfeli UO, Stoeber B, Cadarso VJ, Integrated hollow microneedleoptofluidic biosensor for therapeutic drug monitoring in subnanoliter volumes. Sci Rep, 2016, 6,29075.

[67] Sharma S, El-Laboudi A, Reddy M, Jugnee N, Sivasubramaniyam S, El Sharkawy M, Georgiou P, Johnston D, Oliver N, Cass AE, A pilot study in humans of microneedle sensor arrays for continuous glucose monitoring. Anal. Methods, 2018, 10, 2088-2095.

[68] Cass AEG, Sharma S, Microneedle enzyme sensor arrays for continuous in vivo monitoring. Methods Enzymol, 2017, 589, 413-427.

[69] Pereira da Silva Neves MM, González-GarcÃ-a MB, Hernández-Santos D, Fanjul-Bolado P, Future trends in the market for electrochemical biosensing. Curr Opin Electrochem, 2018, 10, 107-111.

[70] Mohan AM Vinu, et al., Continuous minimally-invasive alcohol monitoring using microneedle sensor arrays. Biosens Bioelectron, 2017, 91,574-579.

[71] Mishra RK, Mohan AV, Soto F, Chrostowski R, Wang J, A microneedle biosensor for minimally-invasive transdermal detection of nerve agents. Analyst, 2017, 142,918-924.

[72] Ciui B, Martin A, Mishra RK, Brunetti B, Nakagawa T, Dawkins TJ, Lyu M, Cristea C, Sandulescu R, Wang J, Wearable wireless tyrosinase bandage and microneedle sensors, toward melanoma screening. Adv Healthc Mater, 2018, 7, 1701264.

[73] Zhou JX, Tang LN, Yang F, Liang FX, Wang H, Li YT, Zhang GJ, MoS 2/Pt nanocomposite-functionalized microneedle for realtime monitoring of hydrogen peroxide release from living cells. Analyst, 2017, 142,4322-4329.

[74] Tang L, Li Y, Xie H, Shu Q, Yang F, Liu YL, Liang F, Wang H, Huang W, Zhang GJ, A sensitive acupuncture needle microsensor for real-time monitoring of nitric oxide in acupoints of rats. Sci Rep, 2017, 7,6446.

[75] Chinnadayyala SR, Park I, Cho S, Non-enzymatic determination of glucose at near neutral ph values based on the use of nafion and platinum black coated microneedle electrode array. Microchim. Acta, 2018, 185, 250.

[76] Bollella P, Sharma S, Cass AEG, Antiochia R, Microneedlebased biosensor for minimally-invasive lactate detection. Biosens Bioelectron, 2019, 123,152-159.

[77] Parrilla M, Cuartero M, Padrell Sánchez S, Rajabi M, Roxhed N, Niklaus F, Crespo GA, Wearable all-solid-state potentiometric microneedle patch for intradermal potassium detection. Anal Chem, 2018, 91,1578-1586.

[78] Jin Q, Chen HJ, Li X, Huang X, Wu Q, He G, Hang T, Yang C, Jiang Z, Li E, Zhang A, Lin Z, Liu F, Zhang A, Reduced graphene oxide nanohybrid-assembled microneedles as mini-invasive electrodes for real-time transdermal biosensing. Small, 2019, 1804298.

[79] Mehmet S, Dervisevic M, Voelcker NH, Gold microneedles fabricated by casting of gold ink used for urea sensing. Mater Lett, 2019, 243,50-53.

[80] Zuliani C, Ng FS, Alenda A, Eftekhar A, Peters NS, Toumazou C, An array of individually addressable micro-needles for mapping pH distributions. Analyst, 2016, 141,4659-4666.

[81] Harper JC, Brozik SM, Flemming JH, McClain JL, Polsky R, Raj D, Ten Eyck GA, Wheeler DR, Achyuthan KE, Fabrication and testing of a microneedles sensor array for p-cresol detection with potential biofuel applications. ACS Appl Mater Interfaces, 2009, 1,1591-1598.

[82] Ribet F, Stemme G, Roxhed N, Ultra-miniaturization of a planar amperometric sensor targeting continuous intradermal glucose monitoring. Biosens Bioelectron, 2016, 90,1-7.

[83] Ye Y, Yu J, Wen D, Kahkoska AR, Gu Z, Polymeric microneedles for transdermal protein delivery. Adv Drug Deliv Rev, 2018, 127,106.

[84] Xue K, Wang X, Yong PW, Young DJ, Wu Y-L, Li Z, Hydrogels as emerging materials for translational biomedicine. Adv Ther, 2019, 2,1800088.

[85] Gao Y, Hou M, Yang R, Zhang L, Xu Z, Kang Y, Xue P, Highly porous silk fibroin scaffold packed in PEGDA/sucrose microneedles for controllable transdermal drug delivery, Macromol Mater Eng, 2018, 303,1800233.

Chapter 4

Control Strategy for Underactuated Multi-Fingered Robot Hand Movement Using Electromyography Signal with Wearable Myo Armband

Ruthber Rodríguez Serrezuela, Roberto Sagaro Zamora and Enrique Marañón Reyes

Abstract

The main goal of this research is to develop a control strategy for an underactuated robotic hand, based on surface electromyography (sEMG) signal obtained from a wireless Myo gesture armband, to distinguish six, several hand movements. The pattern recognition system is employed to analyze these gestures and consists of three main parts: segmentation, feature extraction, and classification. A series of 150 trials is carried out for each movement and it is established which was most suitable for electromyography signals that can be later used in recognition systems. A backpropagation neural network was used as a classifier. The architecture has a hidden network and six output layers. The number of neurons of the hidden network (20) was determined based on the performance in training progress. The proposed system is tested on datasets extracted from five healthy subjects. A great accuracy (94.94% correct assessment). between the experimentally values and those predicted by the artificial neural network (ANN) was achieved. In addition, kinematic analysis of the proposed underactuated hand has been carried out to verify the motion range of the joints. Simulations and experiments are carried out to verify the effectiveness of the proposed fingers mechanism and the hand prosthesis to generate grasp or postures.

Keywords: underactuated prosthesis, electromyography signal, Myo armband gestures, four-bar mechanism

1. Introduction

Due to its use in majority of activities of daily living (ADL), the human hand is one of the most essential body parts, which enables humans to perform basic daily activities ranging from hand gestures to object manipulation [1]. Amputation results from accidents at work, armed conflicts, diseases, and malformations [2], and it is a severe mental and physical trauma with the loss of both motor and sensory perceptions [3].

High-performance prosthetic hands significantly improve the quality of life for upper limb amputees. Passive prosthetic hands are lightweight, robust, and quiet but can only perform a limited subset of activities. Therefore, researchers have investigated externally powered prosthetic hands for upper limb amputees for more than a century. Regarding the prostheses development, the main contributions are the robotic hand designs such as Vincent hand [4], iLimb hand [5], iLimb Pulse [6], Bebionic hand [7], Bebionic hand v2 [8], Michelangelo hand [9], Metamorphic hand [10], etc. (**Figure 1**). These devices, which emulate with human hand, are characterized by complex systems based on microprocessor technology.

All these myoelectric prostheses harness the EMG signals of residual limb muscles to trigger the function of a robotic prosthetic arm or hand. While these devices have been greatly improved over the past decade, they are still limited due to their number of controllable degrees of freedom, intuitiveness, and reliability. Additional restrictions include weight, limited battery life, cost (there are very expensive due to the amount of actuators, sensors, and the electronics involved), and the user's inability to control multiple degrees of freedom simultaneously and consistently [11]. Therefore, despite numerous advances in the field, rates of user abandonment for upper limb prosthetic systems remain high.

Underactuated robotic prosthesis (URP) is an emerging research direction in the field of robotic medical devices. The control input of the underactuated prostheses is less than the degree of freedom of the system. It has the advantages of

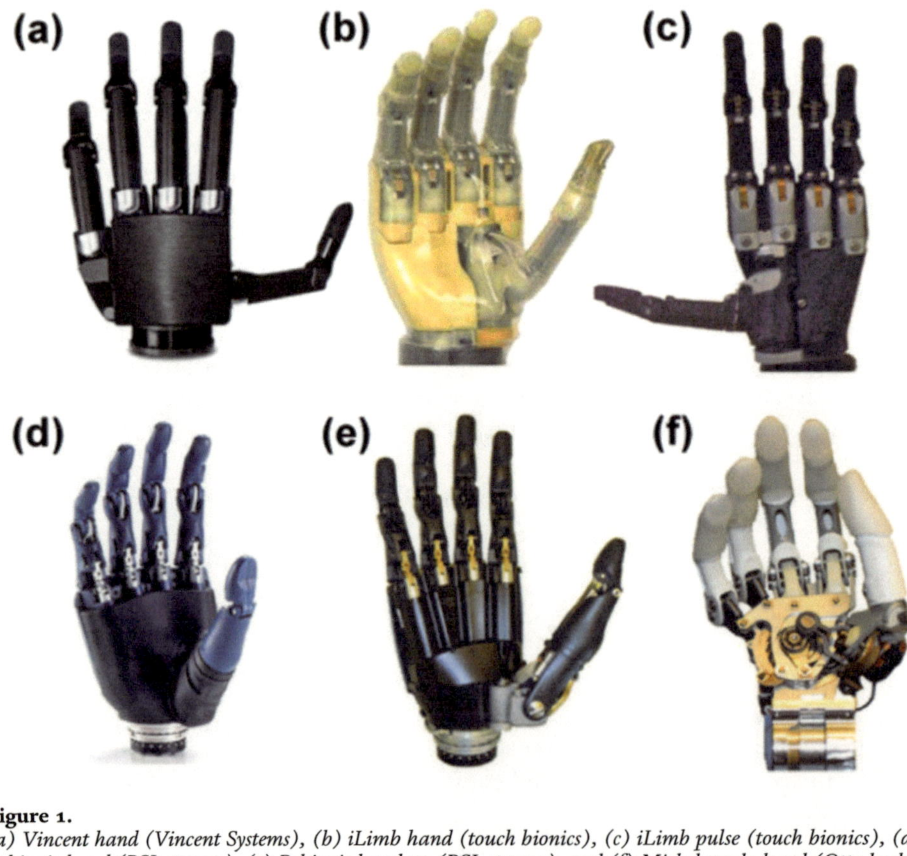

Figure 1.
(a) Vincent hand (Vincent Systems), (b) iLimb hand (touch bionics), (c) iLimb pulse (touch bionics), (d) Bebionic hand (RSL steeper), (e) Bebionic hand v2 (RSL steeper), and (f) Michelangelo hand (Otto bock).

lightweight, low energy consumption, and excellent performance. Compared with full-drive prostheses, URP has fewer drives while maintaining the same DOF, thus reducing mass, volume, and energy consumption. It is ideal for applications where quality, volume, low power consumption, and low cost are desirable.

Natural muscles provide mobility in response to nerve impulses. Electromyography (EMG) measures the electrical activity of muscles in response to a nerve's stimulation. Surface electromyography (SEMG) is a noninvasive method of measurement of the bioelectrical activity of muscles. EMG signals have been used extensively in the identification of user intention to potentially control assistive devices such as smart wheelchairs, exoskeletons, and prosthetic devices [4, 7, 8]. Feature extraction and signals' classification are essential subsystems of this approach.

Pattern recognition-based myoelectric control consists of feature extraction and feature classification of segmented data in signal processing to command to the motor controller. Some signal processing may include feature reduction or feature selection between extraction and classification, depending on the number of features. In general, various features are extracted in time, frequency, and time-frequency to identify the information content of EMG signals [12]. Surface electromyography (sEMG) signals are information bearers that correspond to the hand posture intention. Finite gestures could be identified [13], if considering that the characteristics extracted from each sEMG signal are directly related to the gesture and the number of gestures (including their positions and speeds).

2. Materials and methods

2.1 Data acquisition

Raw sEMG signals were collected with Myo armband placed on forearm's transradial portion as usually performed in common applications. The Myo armband is a wireless wearable technology (**Figure 2**) and has eight medical grade stainless steel EMG sensors. Similar to other surface electrodes, the EMG signals returned by the sensors represent the electric potential of the muscles because of muscle activation. The Myo armband also has a nine-axis inertial measurement unit (IMU) which contains a three-axis gyroscope, three-axis accelerometer, and a three-axis magnetometer [14].

From these units, the orientation and movement of a wearer's arm can be determined through analyzing the spatial data provided. The angular velocity of the armband is provided in a vector format and the accelerometer represents the acceleration the Myo armband is undergoing at a given time. However, the Myo armband is better suited for determining the relative positioning of the arm rather than the absolute position, a consideration to be aware of when applying pattern recognition algorithms. Currently, the Myo armband is able to pull IMU data at sampling rate of 50 Hz. The system is supported on Windows, IOS. MAC and Android and has a Bluetooth 4.0 Smart Wireless connection and a 32-bit ARM Cortex M4 processor with a lithium battery. Signals extracted by Myo armband was processed using Matlab software.

The Myo gesture control armband was used to identify six hand gestures that are the basic ones to achieve the improvement of the grasp: power grasp, palm inward, palm out, open hand, grasp type grasp and hand in rest (**Figure 3**).

Eight datasets were recorded of six hand gestures for five healthy subjects (three males, two females). All subjects did not have any experience in attending this kind of research before. The inclusion criteria adopted in this research were as follows: no evidence in their medical history of peripheral neuropathy, diseases of the

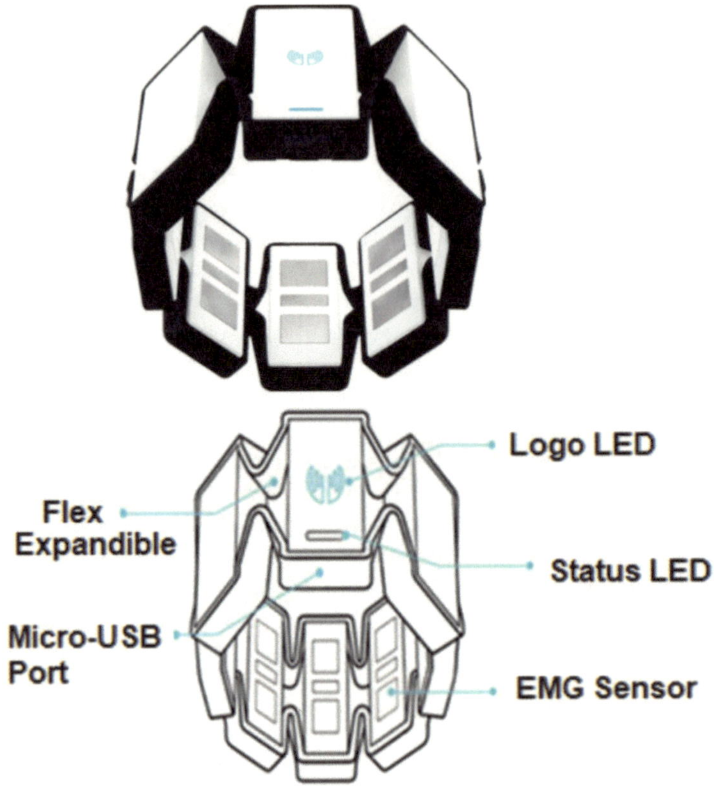

Figure 2.
MYO gesture armband device and its parts, Thalmic Labs.

Power Grasp	Palm inward	Palm out	Open hand	Grasp type clip	Hand in rest
		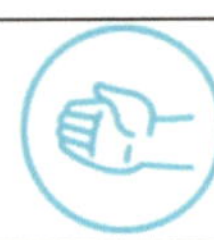	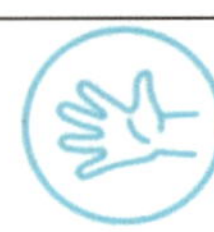	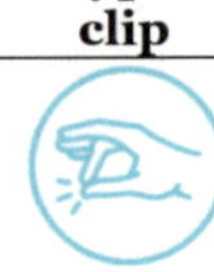	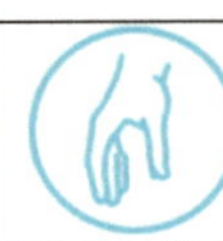

Figure 3.
Hand gestures identify with the MYO device.

central nervous system, and restricted mobility. The EMG signal has a typical amplitude of ±6 mV, and the useful frequency is in the range from 10 to 500 Hz with the greatest amount of concentrated energy up to 150 Hz [15]. According to Calderon et al. [16], the first 400 ms of a muscular activity are enough for the identification of the movement, so the signal was extracted considering this elapsed time as shown in **Figure 4**.

The performed sequence to capture the myoelectric signals is as follows: 200 samples per second were taken for each grasp or hand gesture in an interval of 20 s, it means, there are 4000 samples per sensor. Between each one of the six proposed hand gestures transitions of 5 s were made as was recommended in [15]. The myoelectric signals capture of each sensor was executed at a frequency of 200 Hz [16].

An application for signal processing using a GUI, in the MATLAB® Classification Learner library was developed (**Figure 4**). The GUI shows nine graphs, one for each channel of the myoelectric signals with the Myo armband device and one

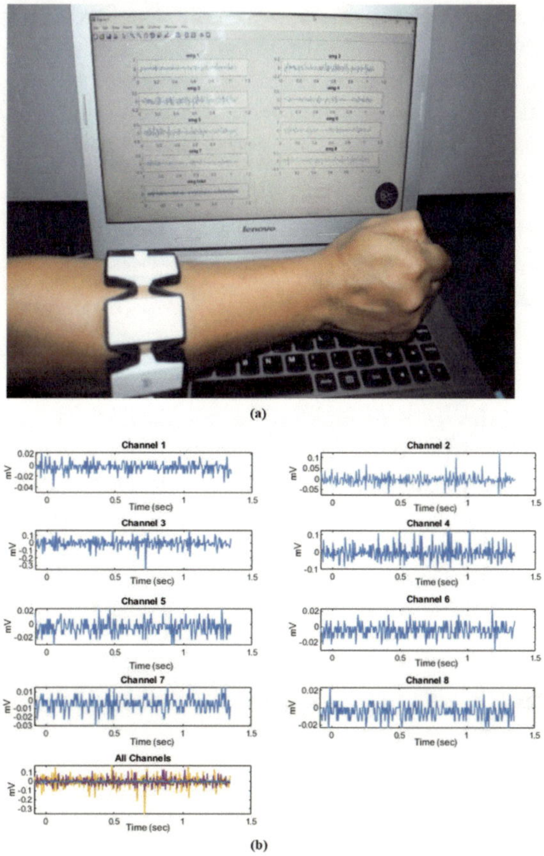

Figure 4.
(a) Acquisition of sEMG signals through the developed application in Matlab. (b) Signals obtained from the eight sensor channels.

where all the signals are displayed. The computed data of these myoelectric signals are stored as matrices format for later offline processing.

2.2 Pattern recognition system

The proposed system for sEMG processing that includes several blocks of preprocessing, segmentation, feature extraction and the neural network development is shown in the flowchart of **Figure 5**.

2.3 Preprocessing

Usually, the collected sEMG signals are normally noisy due to ambient noise, motion artifact, inherent noise in electronics equipment, and inherent instability of the sEMG signal. When using the Myo gesture armband, practically the noise ratio in sEMG signals is low and does not affect the sEMG.

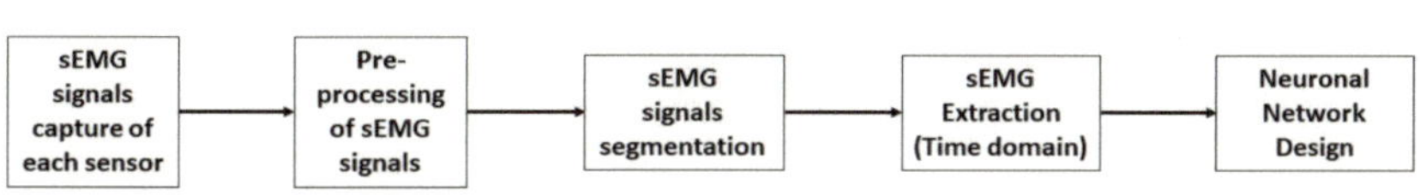

Figure 5.
A flowchart for the proposed extracting sEMG signals.

However, in the preprocessing analyses signals was forced to pass through band pass filters or adaptive filtering to eliminate the undesirable frequency content [17]. The adaptive filter is a system that receives two signals: $x(n)$ and $e(n)$, the latter is called an error signal and becomes from the subtraction of a signal called the desired signal or reference, $r(n)$, and another that is the filter outlet $y(n)$ (see **Figure 6**).

$$e(n) = r(n) - y(n) \tag{1}$$

The filter coefficients are called $w(n)$, which are those that multiply the input $x(n)$ to obtain the output.

$$y(n) = w(n) * x(n) \tag{2}$$

The purpose of the device is to make the error signal to be zero. For this, the system must be configured so that, from the input signal $x(n)$, the output $y(n)$ is generated and it is equal to the signal reference $r(n)$. Each way to minimize that error is an example of implementing adaptive filters. For instance, it could be proposed to minimize the cost function $J = 2 * e(n) * x(n)$, applying the delta rule would obtain the new coefficients such as:

$$w(n+1) = w(n) - \alpha \nabla J \tag{3}$$

where the constant "α" is used to adjust the convergence speed and avoid possible instabilities. Solving, then:

$$w(n+1) = w(n) - 2\alpha * e(n) * x(n) \tag{4}$$

The algorithm implemented for learning an adaptive system could be:

1. Initialize the weights randomly
2. Choose an "α" value
3. Calculate the output y(n)
4. Calculate the error e(n) Eq. (1)
5. Update the weights with the chosen cost function
6. Repeat a certain number of times from point 3

The differences between raw and filtered signals are presented in **Figure 7**.

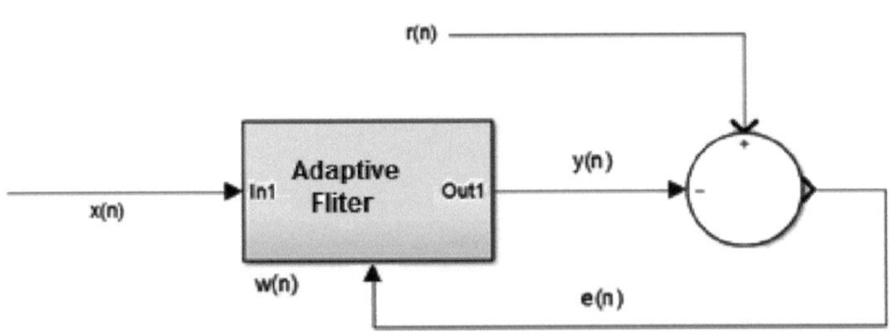

Figure 6.
Flowchart of an adaptive filter.

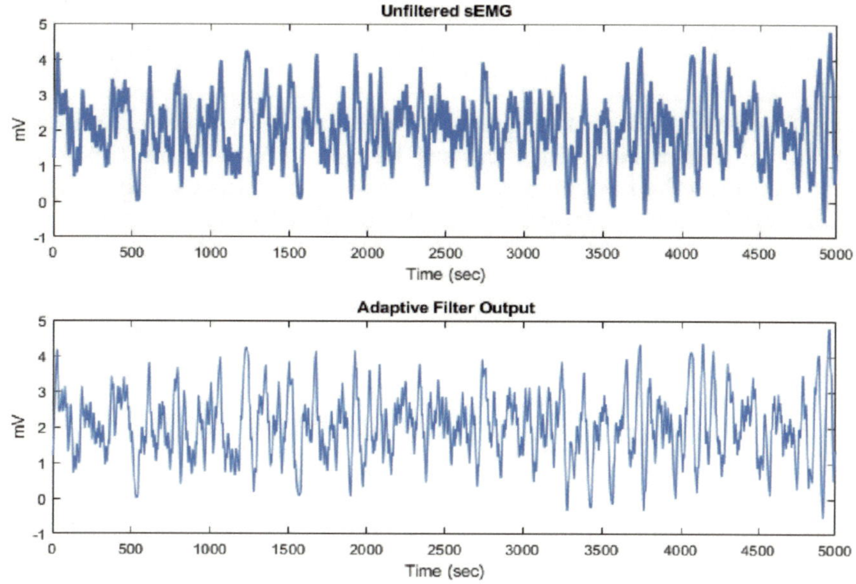

Figure 7.
The difference between raw and filtered signals.

2.4 Segmentation

These are disjoint EMG segmentation and overlapped segmentation. In disjoint segmentation (a), different segments are used which have predefined length and these segments are used for feature extraction. In case of overlapped segmentation (b), a new segment is placed over the present segment with an increment. Thus, the disjoint segmentation deals only with the segment length while the overlapped segmentation deals with segment length and increment. Overlap technique is chosen for segmenting portion of the signal in this research work.

2.5 Feature extraction

The time domain (TD) feature is the feature extracted from EMG signal in time representation [16, 18]. TD features such as mean absolute value (MAV), zero crossing (ZC), Wilson Amplitude (WAMP), variance (VAR), and wavelength (WL) were most popular in EMG pattern recognition due to high processing speed in classification. MAV is defined as the average of total absolute value of EMG signal [6, 14]. It can be calculated as:

1. Mean absolute value: the appreciation of the absolute mean value of the x signal in segment i of N samples is given by equation:

$$\overline{X}_t = \frac{1}{N}\sum_{K=1}^{N} |x_k|, para\ i = 1, \ldots, I-1 \tag{5}$$

2. Wavelength (WL): WL is an improvement of integrated EMG feature and is defined as a cumulative length waveform over the segment. It can be represented as:

$$l = \sum_{K=1}^{N} |x_k - x_{k-1}| \quad (6)$$

3. Zero crossing (ZC): it has frequency related features, which represents counts of how much signal amplitude crosses the zero amplitude over time segment. It is measuring the frequency shift and shows the number of signal sign variations. The mathematical representation of ZC is as follows

$$ZC = \sum_{K=1}^{N} sgn\left([x_k - 0.4][x_{k+1} - 0.4]\right) \quad (7)$$

where

$$sgn\,(x) = \begin{cases} 1\, x > Limit \\ 0\; the\; rest \end{cases}$$

4. Wilson amplitude (WAMP): this is the number of times that the difference between two consecutive amplitudes in a time segment becomes more than threshold. It can be formulated:

$$WAMP = \sum_{K=1}^{N} f(|x_k - x_{k+1}|) \quad (8)$$

5. Variance (VAR): it is used to determine thickness, density of EMG signal power.

$$VAR = \frac{1}{N-1} X_k^2 \quad (9)$$

2.6 Classification

The EMG data taken from muscle myoelectric signals were grouped in a vector to be used as inputs in a creation of a back-propagation neural network as in [19–21], with 20 neurons in the occult layer and 6 outputs. Thirty characteristic vectors were taken for each of the six selected movement patterns (power grasp, inward palm, outward palm, open hand, pincer grasp and rest), which allowed the training of the network.

2.7 Creation of the artificial neural network

Neural networks are created using Matlab software. To train and test the network, the dataset is divided into three sets. Datasets were divided in 60% for training, 20% for testing and 20% for validation. This is the most common method of neural network validation [19, 22, 23]. The true error is calculated directly as the test set error, and bias can be calculated by subtracting the apparent error (training set error) from the test set error.

2.8 CAD design

The five-fingered underactuated prosthetic hand was design using Solidwork 2019 package. This hand has five fingers, driving each one by a DC motor, a worm gear transmission and a four bar mechanisms [24–27] (**Figure 8**). Each finger has three joints. The manufacturing of the hand prostheses was carried out with an

Ultimaker 3 printer for its good performance and excellent print quality of the figures with a thickness, height and amplitude from a design made by a computer. The polylactic acid or polylactide thermoplastic was used as a raw material.

2.9 Control system

The control system was implemented using the prosthetic hand, Arduino UNO microcontroller, laptop computer, and Myo armband. The Arduino has 14 pins that can be configured as input or output which have the advantage of being able to connect any device that is suitable for transmitting or receiving digital signals of 0 and 5 V. It also has analog inputs and outputs. By means of analog inputs, sensor data can be achieved in the form of continuous variations of a voltage. The analog outputs can normally be used to send control signals in the form of pulse width modulation (PWM) signals.

Labview software was used as a graphical development environment platform, ideal for designing systems with a friendly programming language. It allows to structure and perfect professional works of any system. Communication is made through the serial port between the Arduino and Labview. Through the Arduino UNO card using PWMs, the system controls the DC motors to achieve the different positions and grasps previously established.

Tests were carried out for each one of the actuators to be manipulated and it was verified that the position of each finger for the different types of grasps already proposed to be carried out were those established. For the handling of the robotic hand, a checking was made in the LabVIEW interface. To ensure that the time and angles of the servomotors are correct, tests and measurements were carried out to analyze the inverse and direct kinematics of the prototype, which are analyzed in specific details in the following section.

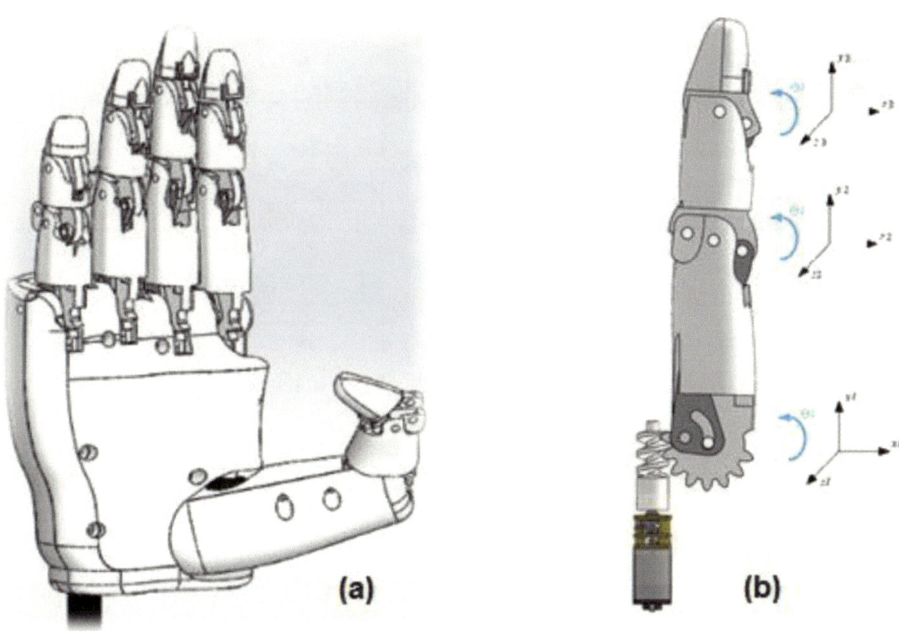

Figure 8.
Design of the anthropomorphic under-performed hand. (a) Proposed prosthetic hand. (b) Underactuated finger.

3. Results and discussion

3.1 Pattern recognition system

Feature extraction was carried out with each posture using the series of time domain, and processing with the Matlab software for six motions or positions of the hand. From **Figure 9**, it can be seen the system behavior trough the developed GUI. Below, eight myoelectric channels are shown. Likewise, at the bottom, on left, real-time motions or types of gestures can be observed.

Figure 10 displays the results of feature extraction, in this case for the power grasp gesture. The less useful features are preferably deleted to decrease the

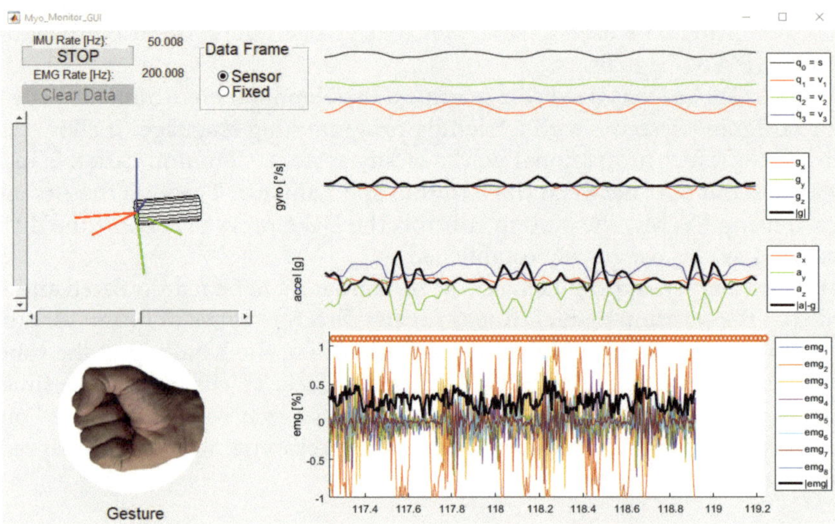

Figure 9.
Feature extraction for the open hand gesture trough GUI.

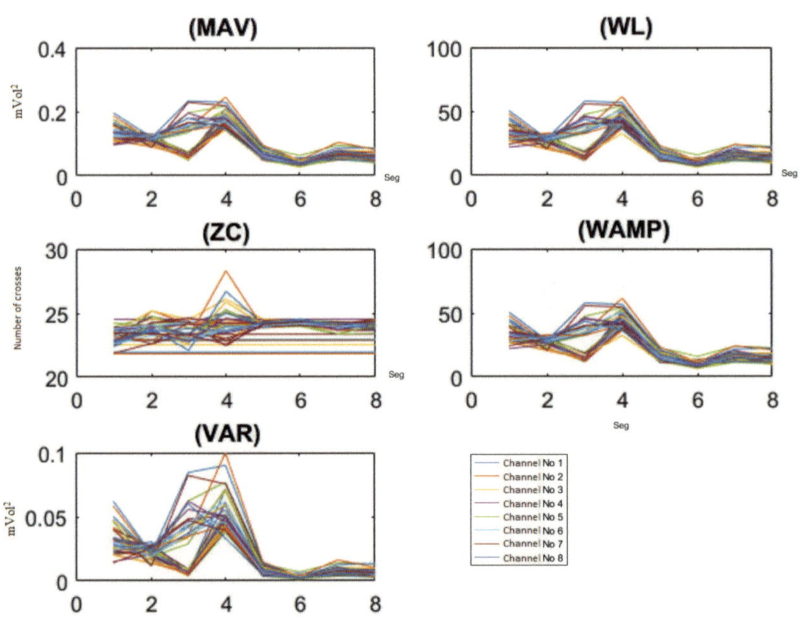

Figure 10.
Feature extraction for the power grasp gesture.

computational time, especially in real-time. It can be observed that characteristic with less accuracy (37.18%) was the Wilson amplitude for the identification of the pronation, and the best one with the better identification (96.45%) was the mean absolute value (MAV) in a 50 mS window.

Figure 11 and **Table 1** explain feature effectiveness gesture hand. From **Figure 11** and **Table 1**, it is concluded that the maximum percentage, 96.55% in this 50 mS window, was obtained with the characteristic of Wilson's Amplitude in the grasp gesture. Similarly, the lowest percentage of 37.18% in this window was also obtained with the same characteristic but in the pronation gesture. Likewise, the AVM in this 50 mS window presents an average of 82.31%, which is higher in all characteristics.

Figure 12 and **Table 2** identify the features effectiveness for 100 mS windows. It is concluded that the maximum percentage, 99.25% in this 100 mS window, was obtained with the characteristic of MAV in the repose gesture. Similarly, the lowest percentage of 42.68% in this window was obtained with the VAR characteristic in the extension gesture. Likewise, the MAV in this 100 mS window presents an average of 85.36%, which is higher in all characteristics.

Figure 13 and **Table 3** identify the features effectiveness for 250 mS windows. It is concluded that the maximum percentage, 99.53% in this window, was obtained with the characteristic of MAV in the repose gesture. Similarly, the lowest percentage of 37.18% in this window was obtained with the Wilson's Amplitude in the grasp gesture. Likewise, the MAV in this window presents an average of 86.06%, which is higher in all characteristics.

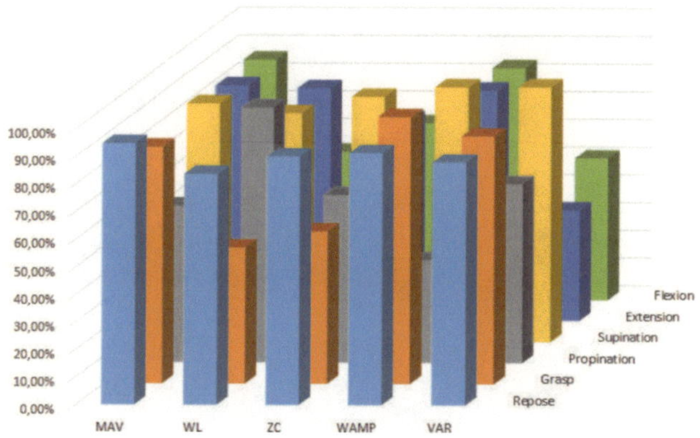

Figure 11.
Features extraction of myoelectric signals for the six gestures at 50 mS window.

			Ventana de 50 mS			
Caracteristica EMG	**Repose**	**Grasp**	**Propination**	**Supination**	**Extension**	**Flexion**
MAV	94.45%	85.54%	56.63%	85.94%	84.79%	86.48%
WL	83.35%	49.25%	92.24%	82.50%	83.87%	53.36%
ZC	89.83%	55.16%	60.61%	88.48%	72.91%	63.72%
WAMP	91.11%	96.51%	37.18%	92.01%	83.17%	83.65%
VAR	87.78%	89.65%	64.72%	92.13%	39.95%	51.22%

Table 1.
Feature records for selected gestures at 50 mS window.

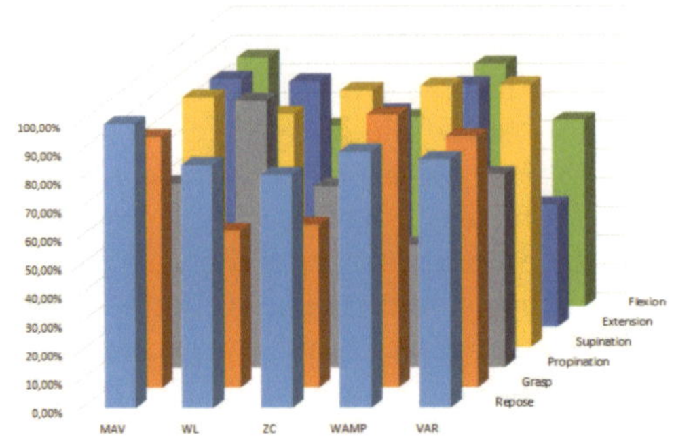

Figure 12.
Features extraction of myoelectric signals for the six gestures at 100 mS window.

Ventana de 100 mS						
Caracteristica EMG	**Repose**	**Grasp**	**Propination**	**Supination**	**Extension**	**Flexion**
MAV	99.25%	87.45%	64.25%	87.37%	86.71%	87.13%
WL	84.67%	54.78%	93.18%	81.56%	85.81%	63.21%
ZC	81.23%	56.89%	63.23%	89.75%	75.36%	66.25%
WAMP	89.34%	95.34%	42.87%	91.34%	84.67%	84.83%
VAR	86.63%	87.58%	67.39%	91.67%	42.68%	65.24%

Table 2.
Feature records for selected gestures at 100 mS window.

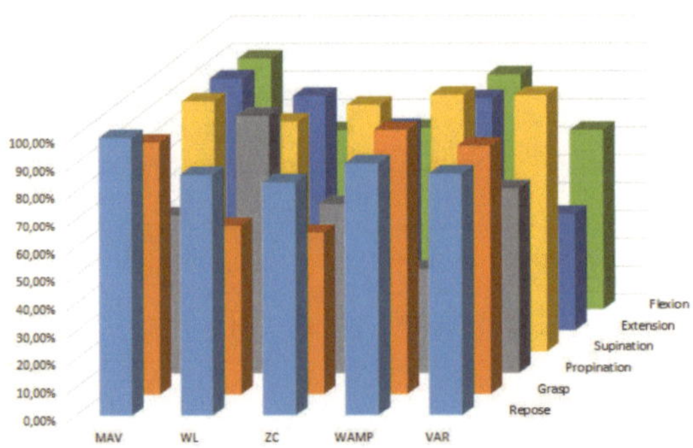

Figure 13.
Features extraction of myoelectric signals for the six gestures at 250 mS window.

From the previous data, it can be concluded that from the probability matrices obtained for each of the characteristics, with the highest accuracy was the time domain features of mean absolute value (MAV). It guarantees the highest probabilities of success were obtained compared to the other characteristics. Similarly, it is conclusive as in [18, 28], that with just one measure such as the MAV, the different movements can be fully identified.

Likewise, such features show a greater percentage of accuracy as the windowing increases in the samples analyzed by the different features in the time domain. These results match others like [15–17].

Ventana de 250 mS						
Caracteristica EMG	**Repose**	**Grasp**	**Propination**	**Supination**	**Extension**	**Flexion**
MAV	99.53%	90.29%	56.63%	89.78%	90.31%	89.84%
WL	86.23%	60.45%	92.24%	82.50%	84.12%	64.21%
ZC	83.46%	57.81%	60.61%	88.48%	72.91%	65.05%
WAMP	90.26%	94.62%	37.18%	92.01%	83.17%	84.12%
VAR	86.48%	88.93%	66.13%	91.89%	41.78%	64.23%

Table 3.
Feature records for selected gestures at 250 mS window.

3.2 Classification

Regarding the neural network, created by using the Levenberg-Marquardt algorithm, a root mean squared error (RMSE) of 2.9437×10^{-9} was obtained, which was inferior to what was expected (10^{-9}) in only 16 training epochs (**Figure 14**).

The training correlation coefficient was 94.94% (**Figure 15**). The error in the training set (therefore the estimation of the real error) depends mostly on the exact sample, chosen for the training and the exact sample for the test (which are completely dependent on each other since they are mutually exclusive).

3.3 CAD design

The designed prototype was created as anthropomorphic hand and able to perform three types of hand grasping (tip, spherical, and cylindrical).

The direct and inverse kinematics of the prototype was developed based on the antrophormism of the robotic hand. **Figure 16** shows index finger prosthesis prototype model in order to calculate. The Denavit Hartenberg (DH) parameters. The dimensions of the phalanges are as follows: $L_1 = 2\,inch$, $L_2 = 1,37\,inch$, and $L_3 = 1\,inch$.

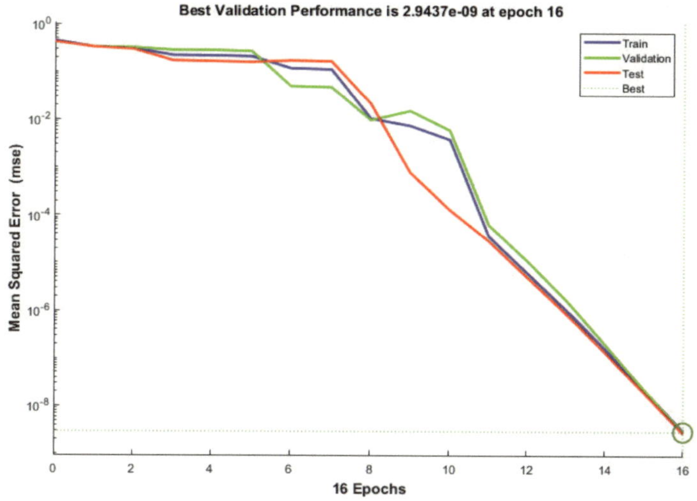

Figure 14.
Training algorithm used in ANN validation.

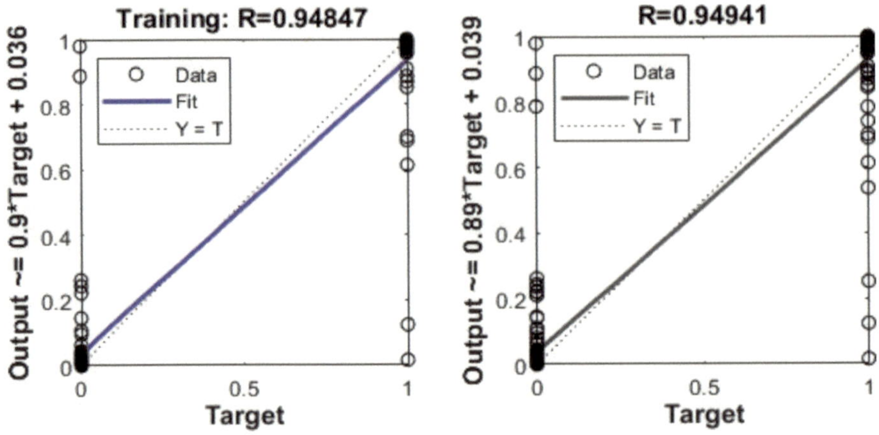

Figure 15.
Correlation between the experimental values and the ANN predicted values.

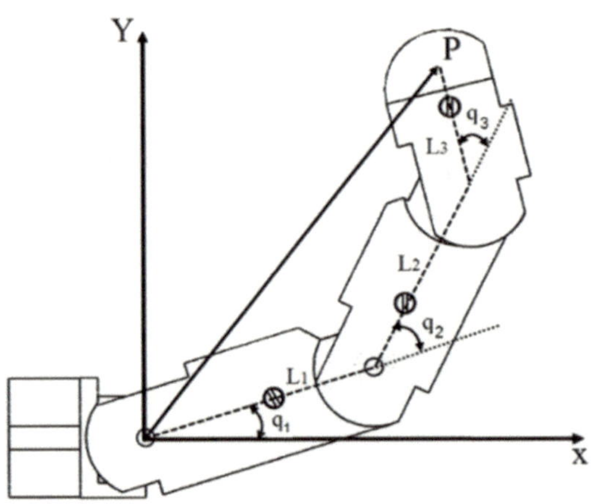

Figure 16.
Index finger prosthesis prototype model of a robotic hand.

The Denavit Hartenberg (DH) parameters of the finger are shown in **Table 4**:

DH parameters	Finger joints		
	1	2	3
q_i	q_1	q_2	q_3
d_i	0	0	0
a_i	L_1	L_2	L_3
α_i	0	0	0

Table 4.
Denavit Hartenberg (DH) parameters of the finger.

Direct kinematics allows knowing the position and orientation of the distal phalanx, which is:

$$P_x = L_3(C_1C_{23} - S_1S_{23}) + L_2C_{12} + L_1C_1 \tag{10}$$

$$P_y = L_3(S_1C_{23} - C_1S_{23}) + L_2S_{12} + L_1S_1 \tag{11}$$

Donde

$$S_1 = Sin(q_i), C_i = Cos(q_i), S_{ij} = Sin\left(q_i + q_j\right), C_{ij} = Cos\left(q_i + q_j\right) \quad (12)$$

The direct kinematics of the finger is

$$q_1 = \tan^{-1}\left(\frac{P_y}{P_x}\right) - \tan^{-1}\left(\frac{L_1 sin\,(q_2) + L_3 sin\,(q_2)}{L_1 + L_2 cos\,(q_2) + L_3 cos\,(q_2)}\right) \quad (13)$$

$$q_2 = \cos^{-1}\frac{\left(-2L_1L_2 + 2L_2L_3 \pm \sqrt{(2L_1L_2 + 2L_2L_3)^2 - 16L_1L_3\left(L_1^2 + L_2^2 + L_3^2 - P_x^2 - P_y^2 - 2L_1L_3\right)}\right)}{8L_1L_2} \quad (14)$$

and

$$q_3 = kq_2(14)\; k \approx \frac{7}{11} \quad (15)$$

The dynamic model of an n-articulation robot, which in Lagrange's equation can be written as:

$$M(q)\ddot{q} + C(q, \dot{q}) + G(q) = \tau \quad (16)$$

Where q is the vector of articulated variables, τ is the vector of generalized forces acting as the manipulating robot, $M(q)$ is the inertia matrix, $C(q, \dot{q})$ is the centripetal forces matrix, and $G(q)$ is the gravity vector [28]:

$$L(q, \dot{q}) = K(q, \dot{q}) - U(q) \quad (17)$$

$$\frac{d}{dt}\left(\frac{\partial L(q, \dot{q})}{\partial \dot{q}}\right) - \frac{\partial L(q, \dot{q})}{\partial q_i} = \tau_i\; i = 1, \ldots 3 \quad (18)$$

The kinetic energy of the finger can be expressed as

$$K_1 = \frac{1}{2} m_1 c_1^2 \dot{q}_1^2 + \frac{1}{2} I_1 \dot{q}_1^2 \quad (19)$$

$$\begin{aligned} K_2 = {} & \frac{1}{2} m_2 (C_2^2 \dot{q}_2^2 - 2C_2^2 \dot{q}_1\, \dot{q}_2 - 2C_2 l_1 Cos(q_2)\dot{q}_1\dot{q}_2 + C_2^2\dot{q}_1^2 + 2C_2 l_1 Cos(q_2)\dot{q}_1{}^2 + l_1\dot{q}_1{}^2) \\ & + \frac{1}{2} I_2 (\dot{q}_1 - \dot{q}_2)^2 \end{aligned} \quad (20)$$

$$\begin{aligned} K_3 = {} & \frac{1}{2} m_3 (2C_3 l_1 \dot{q}_1\, (\dot{q}_1 - \dot{q}_2 + \dot{q}_3 \cos\,(\dot{q}_2 - \dot{q}_3) \\ & + (2C_3 l_2\, Cos\,(q_3) + 2l_1 l_2\, Cos\,(q_2) + C_3^2 + l_1^2 + l_2^2)\dot{q}_1^2 \\ & + ((-4C_3 l_2\, Cos\,(q_3) - 2l_1 l_2\, Cos\,(q_2) - 2C_3^2 - 2l_2^2)\dot{q}_2^2 \\ & + 2C_3(C_3 + l_2\, Cos\,(q_3))\dot{q}_3)\dot{q}_1 + 2C_3 l_2\, Cos\,(q_3) + C_3^2 + l_2^2)\dot{q}_2^2 \\ & - 2C_3(l_2\, Cos\,(q_3) + C_3)\dot{q}_2\dot{q}_3 + C_3^2\dot{q}_3^2) + \frac{1}{2} I_3 (\dot{q}_1 - \dot{q}_2 + \dot{q}_3)^2 \end{aligned} \quad (21)$$

The potential energy in the analyzed finger can be expressed as

$$U_1 = -m_1 g C_1 Cos(q_1) \tag{22}$$

$$U_2 = -m_2 g l_1 Cos(q_1) - m_2 g C_2 Cos(q_1 - q_2) \tag{23}$$

$$U_3 = -m_3 g l_1 Cos(q_1) - m_3 g l_2 Cos(q_1 - q_2) + m_3 g C_3 Cos(q_1 - q_2 + q_3) \tag{24}$$

Finding solutions for Lagrange's equations, the dynamic model of the system is

$$\begin{aligned}
\tau_1 = {} & m_3 l_1 c_3 Cos(q_2 - q_3)(\ddot{q}_1 - \ddot{q}_2 + \ddot{q}_3) - m_3 l_1 C_3 Sin(q_2 - q_3)(\dot{q}_1 - \dot{q}_2 + \dot{q}_3)(\dot{q}_2 - \dot{q}_3) \\
& + m_3 l_1 c_3 Cos(q_2 - q_3)\ddot{q}_1 - m_3 l_1 C_3 Sin(q_2 - q_3)(\dot{q}_2 - \dot{q}_3)\dot{q}_1 \\
& + [-2m_3 l_2 C_3 Sin(q_3)\dot{q}_3 - 2l_1(m_2 c_2 - m_3 l_2) Sin(q_2)\dot{q}_2]\dot{q}_1 \\
& + [2m_3 l_2 Cos(q_3) + 2l_1(m_2 c_2 - m_3 l_2) Cos(q_2) + m_3(l_1^2 + l_2^2 + l_3^2) + m_1 C_1^2] + m_2 l_1^2 \\
& + m_2 c_2^2 + I_1 + I_2 + I_3]\ddot{q}_1 + [2m_3 l_2 C_3 Sin(q_3)\dot{q}_3 + l_1(m_2 c_2 - m_3 l_2) Sin(q_2)\dot{q}_2]\dot{q}_2 \\
& + [m_3 l_2 C_3 Cos(q_3) + m_3 C_3{}^2 + I_3]\ddot{q}_3 - m_3 l_2 C_3 Sin(q_3)\dot{q}_3{}^2 \\
& - [2m_3 l_2 C_3 Cos(q_3) + l_1(m_2 c_2 - m_3 l_2) Cos(q_2) + m_3(l_2^2 + C_3^2) + m_2 c_2{}^2 + I_2 + I_3]\ddot{q}_2 \\
& - (m_1 c_1 - m_1 l_1 - m_3 l_1) g \, Sin(q_1) + (m_2 C_2 - m_3 l_2) g \, Sin(q_1 - q_2) \\
& + m_3 c_3 g \, Sin(q_1 - q_2 + q_3)
\end{aligned} \tag{25}$$

$$\begin{aligned}
\tau_2 = {} & -m_3 l_1 c_3 Cos(q_2 - q_3)\ddot{q}_1 + m_3 l_1 c_3 Sin(q_2 - q_3)(\dot{q}_2 - \dot{q}_3)\dot{q}_1 \\
& + [2m_3 l_2 c_3 Sin\ (q_3)\dot{q}_3 + l_1(m_2 c_2 + m_3 l_2) Sin(q_2)\dot{q}_2]\dot{q}_1 \\
& - [2m_3 l_2 c_3 Cos\ (q_3) + l_1(m_2 c_2 + m_3 l_2) Cos(q_2) + m_3(l_2^2 + c_3^2) + m_2 c_2^2 + I_2 + I_3]\ddot{q}_1 \\
& - 2m_3 l_2 c_3 Sin\ (q_3)\dot{q}_2\dot{q}_3 + [2m_3 l_2 c_3 Cos(q_3) + m_3(l_2^2 + c_3^2) + m_2 c_2^2 + I_2 + I_3]\ddot{q}_2 \\
& - [m_3 l_2 c_3 Cos\ (q_3) + m_3 c_3^2 + I_3]\ddot{q}_3 + m_3 l_2 c_3 Sin(q_3)\,\dot{q}_3{}^2 \\
& + l_1(m_2 c_2 + m_3 l_2) Sin(q_2)[\dot{q}_1{}^2 - \dot{q}_1\dot{q}_2] - (m_2 c_2 + m_3 l_2) g \, Sin(q_1 - q_2) \\
& + m_3 l_1 c_3 Sin(q_2 - q_3)(\dot{q}_1 - \dot{q}_2 + \dot{q}_3)\dot{q}_1 - m_3 c_3 g \, Sin\ (q_1 - q_2 + q_3)
\end{aligned} \tag{26}$$

$$\begin{aligned}
\tau_3 = {} & m_3 l_1 c_3 Cos(q_2 - q_3)\ddot{q}_1 - m_3 l_1 c_3 Sin(q_2 - q_3)(\dot{q}_2 - \dot{q}_3)\dot{q}_1 + [m_3 c_3^2 + I_3]\ddot{q}_3 \\
& - m_3 l_2 c_3 Sin(q_3)(\dot{q}_1 - \dot{q}_2)\dot{q}_3 + [m_3 l_2 c_3 Cos\ (q_3) + m_3 c_3^2 + I_3](\ddot{q}_1 - \ddot{q}_2) \\
& - m_3 c_3\{-g Sin(q_1 - q_2 + q_3) + [l_1 Sin(q_2 - q_3)\dot{q}_1 - l_2 Sin(q_3)(\dot{q}_1 - \dot{q}_2)(\dot{q}_1 - \dot{q}_2 + \dot{q}_3)]\}
\end{aligned} \tag{27}$$

To follow the track of position trajectories, the PD control is used for gravity compensation (**Figure 17**) [22], where

$$\tau = K_p \hat{q} + K_v \dot{\hat{q}} + G(q) \tag{28}$$

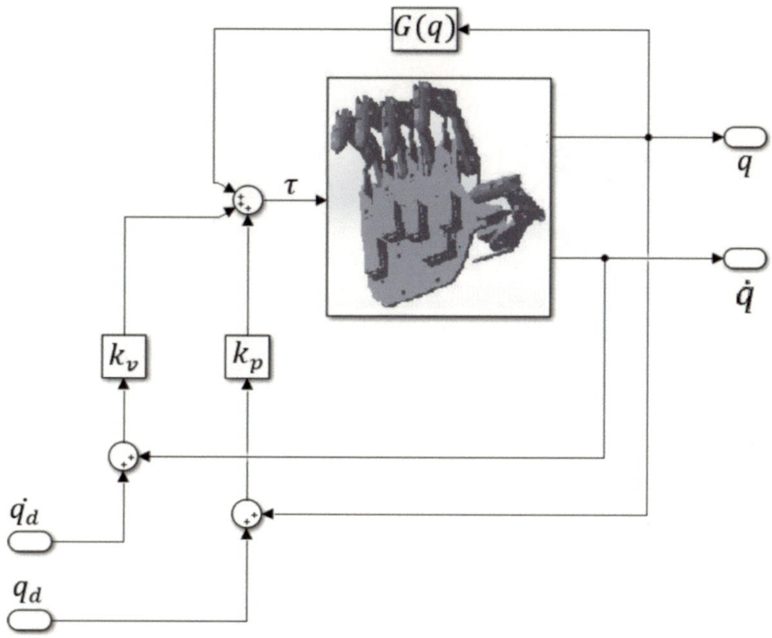

Figure 17.
Proportional derivative (PD) control with gravity compensation.

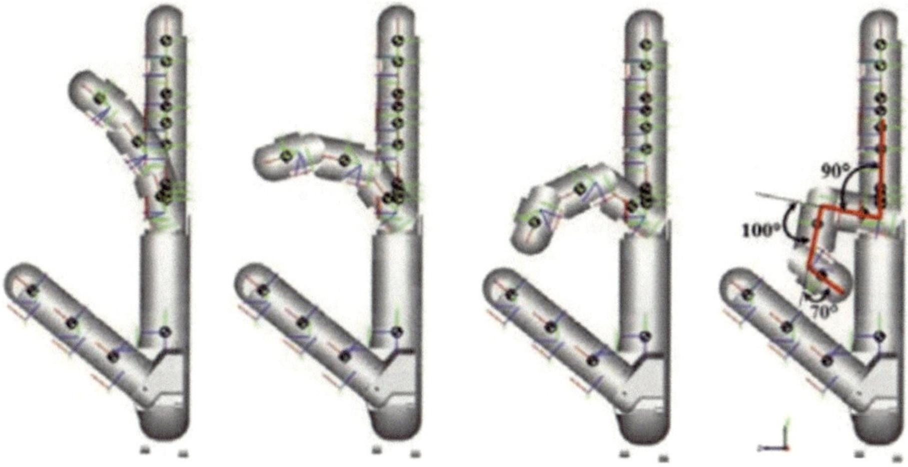

Figure 18.
PD control simulation in SimMechanics.

Figure 18 shows the SimMechanics tool is used to generate the trajectories of each of the fingers. Once the trajectories of each of the fingers have been generated, the workspace of each of them is generated.

3.4 Arduino connections to generate the interface with LabVIEW

Figure 19 shows the connection Arduino-computer and Arduino-servomotors as the fundamental relationships to get intercommunication and produce grasp

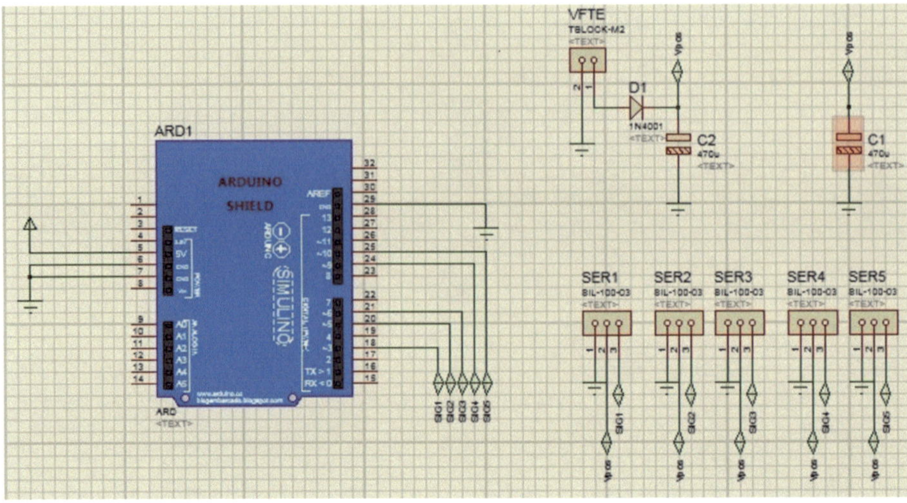

Figure 19.
Programming Arduino Uno, LabView, and DC motors.

movements like cylindrical, spherical, and tip. Figure also shows the Proteus package simulation.

Figure 20 shows the workspace of the index finger of the prototype robotic prosthesis generated from the SimMechanics. The implementation of the robotic hand prosthesis required an intensive learning of the different hand postures. A LabView application to perform the corresponding grasps will be carried out.

Figure 21 shows the flowchart of the developed application in LabView. Several tests with the anthropomorphic subactuated robotic hand were carried out in order to confirm if modeling task was correctly performed by fingers joints for specific hand gesture.

Figure 22 shows the trajectories that were generated with the developing software and implemented in LabView in order to reproduce the movement of the underactuated anthropomorphic robotic prosthesis.

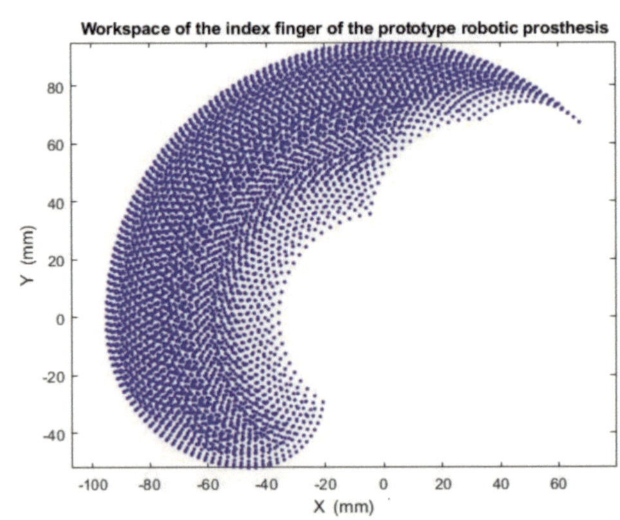

Figure 20.
Index finger workspace of the robotic prosthesis prototype.

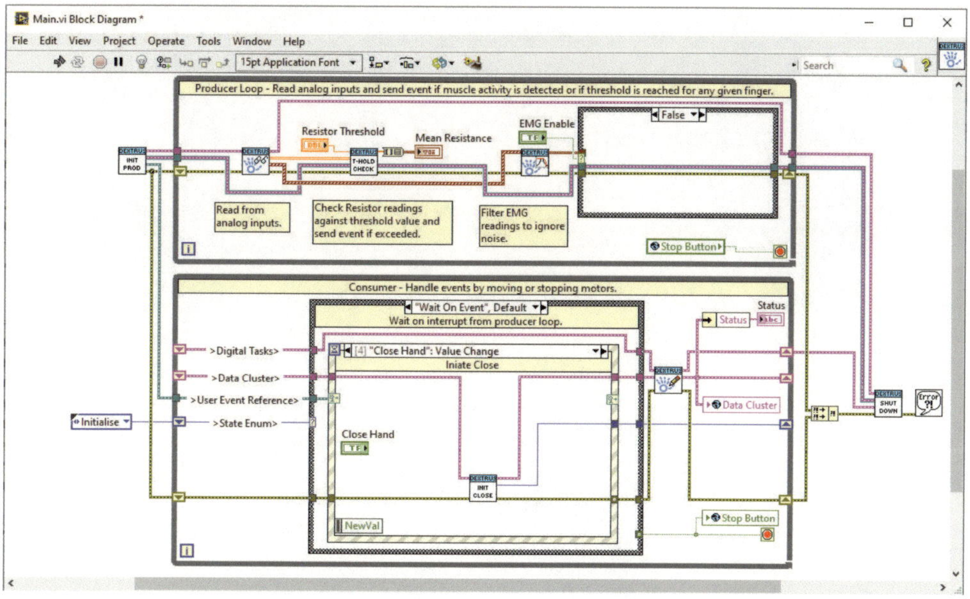

Figure 21.
Flowchart of the developed application in LabView.

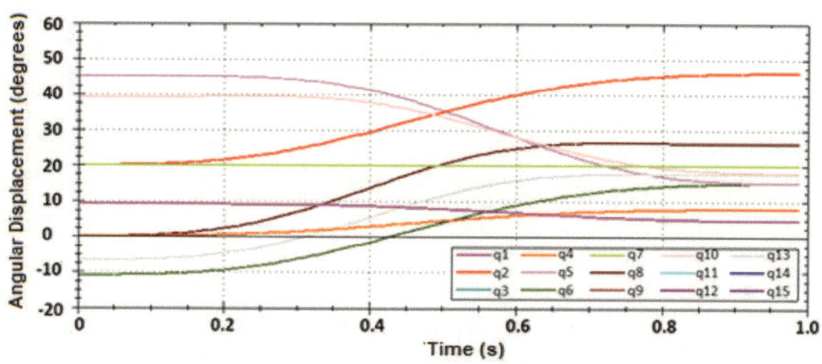

Figure 22.
Anthropomorphic underactuated finger trajectories.

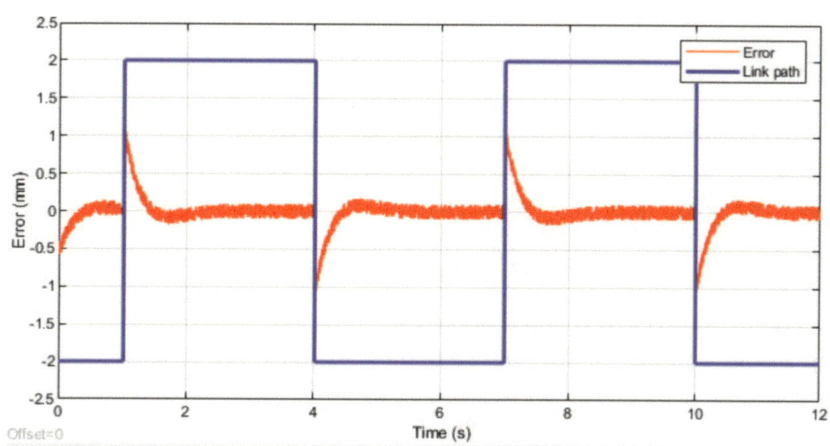

Figure 23.
Cartesian error in the PD control.

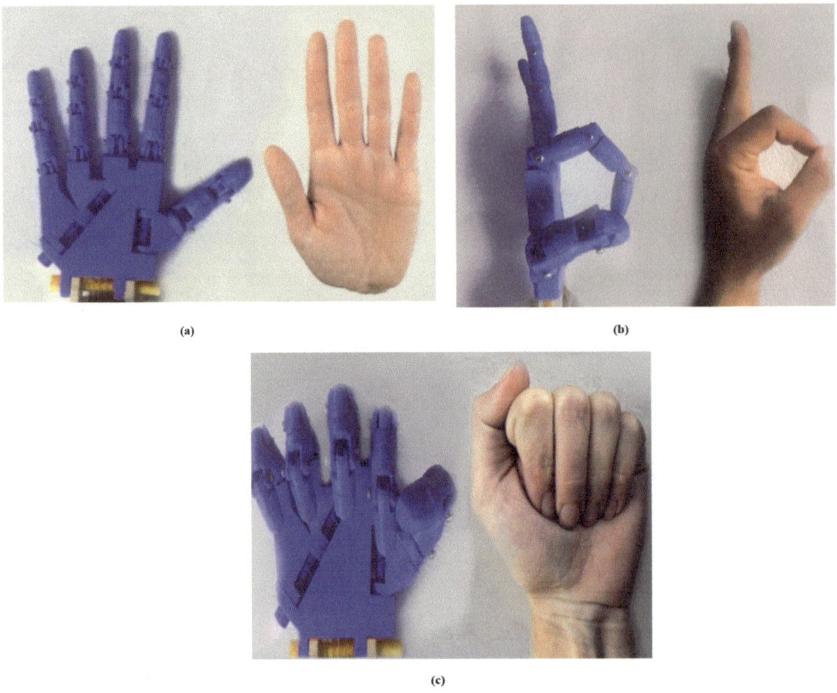

Figure 24.
Position of the fingers in different gestures. (a) Open hand, (b) precision grip, and (c) closed hand.

PD controller parameters tuning methods were implemented, which were tuned manually by trial and error, and then an automatic parameter adjustment was used minimizing the integral of the tracking error by minimum squares. The PD controller makes fingertip tracking possible, thus allowing flexion and extension motions in the finger, in a way that the finger gets to a point without an important overshoot on axis y of 1.85 mm in a shorter time than 0.05 s. As shown in **Figure 23**, the values obtained are son k = 1, ζ = 0.01, C = 0.12, γ = 0.0015, the gains found were Kp = 0.004 and Kd = 0.035, respectively.

Finally, **Figure 24** shows the position of the fingers according to the different gestures according to the control system designed.

4. Conclusions

The Myo armband is a wireless portable device developed by Thalmic Labs, capable of recording EMG through eight surface stainless steel electrodes, and has a sampling rate of 200 Hz. In addition, the Myo armband has an inertial unit of measure sensor (IMU) nine-axis, haptic feedback, and Bluetooth communication. These characteristics combined with a compact design, as it easily adjusts to the forearm, maintaining the distance between electrodes, lead to an acquisition system that is easier to use for prosthetic systems.

Mean absolute value (MAV), wavelength (WL), zero crossing (ZC), Wilson amplitude (WA), and variance were used to accomplish feature extraction by using a Myo armband device in different time series. The features extraction of the characteristics through the MAV allows the comparison between the values determined experimentally and predicted by the ANN, with a high level of effectiveness (94.94%).

Multilayer network topology was used to carry out the design of the artificial neural network (feedforward and back-propagation). The mean square error value of $1.2041x10^{-19}$ was obtained by using the Levenberg-Marquardt training algorithm; however, this value was lower than desired (10^{-3}) in only 16 training epochs.

A prototype of hand prostheses was developed based on the anthropometry, kinematics and dynamics of the hand joints, and the main dimensions of the joints as well as the fingers' trajectories to guarantee the different hand gestures. The direct and inverse kinematic model of the prototype robotic hand prosthesis based on the DH parameters was obtained. The simulations of the workspace and the PD control of the hand were performed by finding the Cartesian error set on the axis and 1.85 mm in a time less than 0.05 s. This allows the tracking of objectives attainable by the fingertips, developing movements of flexion and extension of the finger so that the finger reaches the point without an important overshoot.

A control system was developed based on the Arduino microcontroller architecture. The design system allows generating the joint trajectories of the hand prostheses prototype.

Author details

Ruthber Rodríguez Serrezuela[1]*, Roberto Sagaro Zamora[2] and Enrique Marañón Reyes[3]

1 Industrial Engineering, Corporación Universitaria del Huila, Neiva, Colombia

2 Mechanical and Design Engineering Department (M y D), Tribology Group, Universidad de Oriente, Cuba

3 Centre for Studies in Neurosciences, Images and Signals Processing (CENPIS), Universidad de Oriente, Cuba

*Address all correspondence to: ruthber.rodriguez@corhuila.edu.cu

References

[1] Bouchet A, Cuilleret J. Anatomía descriptiva, topográfica y funcional. Editorial Médica Panamericana; 1997

[2] Gallagher N, Maldonado SJ, Maffia Bizzozero S, Fernandez L. Impacto psicológico del trabajador amputado. 2013. Available from: http://dspace.uces.edu.ar:8180/dspace/bitstream/handle/123456789/2351/Impacto_Callagher_Maldonado_otros.pdf?sequence=3 [Accessed: 15 January 2020]

[3] Cortés MAR. 12. Evaluación y tratamiento psicológico de los amputados. In: Los amputados y su rehabilitación. México: Intersistemas, S.A.; 2016

[4] Mason MT, Salisbury JK Jr. Robot Hands and the Mechanics of Manipulation. Winston PH, Brady M, editors. United States; 1985

[5] Jacobsen S, Iversen E, Knutti D, Johnson R, Biggers K. Design of the Utah/MIT dextrous hand. In: Proceedings. 1986 IEEE International Conference on Robotics and Automation. Vol. 3. 1986. pp. 1520-1532

[6] Fukaya N, Asfour T, Dillmann R, Toyama S. Development of a five-finger dexterous hand without feedback control: The TUAT/Karlsruhe humanoid hand. In: 2013 IEEE/RSJ International Conference on Intelligent Robots and Systems (IROS). 2013. pp. 4533-4540

[7] Diftler MA, Mehling JS, Abdallah ME, Radford NA, Bridgwater LB, Sanders AM, et al. Robonaut 2-the first humanoid robot in space. In: 2011 IEEE International Conference on Robotics and Automation (ICRA). IEEE; 2011. pp. 2178-2183

[8] Chen Z, Lii NY, Wimböck T, Fan S, Liu H. Experimental evaluation of Cartesian and joint impedance control with adaptive friction compensation for the dexterous robot hand DLR-HIT II. International Journal of Humanoid Robotics. 2011;**8**(04):649-671

[9] Sun W, Kong J, Wang X, Liu H. Innovative design method of the metamorphic hand. International Journal of Advanced Robotic Systems. 2018;**15**(1):1729881417754154

[10] Available from: http://es.bebionic.com/ [Accessed: 15 January 2020]

[11] Pasquina P et al. Recent advances in bioelectric prostheses. Neurology: Clinical Practice. 2015;**5**(2):164-170

[12] Tov EY. Advanced Lectures on Machine Learning. Berlin, Heidelberg: Springer Berlin Heidelberg; 2003

[13] Akhmadeev K, Rampone E, Yu T, Aoustin Y, Le Carpentier É. A real-time gesture classification-using surface EMG to control a robotics hand. In: ENOC 2017. 2017

[14] Sathiyanarayanan M, Rajan S. MYO Armband for physiotherapy healthcare: A case study using gesture recognition application. In: 2016 8th International Conference on Communication Systems and Networks (COMSNETS). IEEE; 2016. pp. 1-6

[15] Dirgantara GP, Basari. Optimized circuit and control for prosthetic arm based on myoelectric pattern recognition via power spectral density analysis. In: AIP Conference Proceedings. Vol. 2092. AIP Publishing; 2019. p. 020013

[16] Calderon CA, Jaramillo L, Zuñiga J, Hernandez W, Rivas-Echeverría F. A Neural Network embedded system for real-time identification of EMG signals. In: 2018 IEEE International Conference on Automation/XXIII Congress of the

Chilean Association of Automatic Control (ICA-ACCA). IEEE; 2018. pp. 1-7

[17] Marque C, Bisch C, Dantas R, Elayoubi S, Brosse V, Perot C. Adaptive filtering for ECG rejection from surface EMG recordings. Journal of Electromyography and Kinesiology. 2005;**15**(3):310-315

[18] Vladimir BVF, Javier MCM, Evgeny AV, Lukyanov A, Emanuel MPL. Modelado y simulación del Robot Mitsubishi RV-2JA controlado mediante señales electromiográficas. Enfoque UTE. 2018;**9**(2):208-222

[19] Bekey GA, Goldberg KY. Neural Networks in Robotics. Vol. 202. Springer Science & Business Media; 2012

[20] Yamashita Y, Tani J. Emergence of functional hierarchy in a multiple timescale neural network model: A humanoid robot experiment. PLoS Computational Biology. 2008;**4**(11): e1000220

[21] Levine S, Pastor P, Krizhevsky A, Ibarz J, Quillen D. Learning hand-eye coordination for robotic grasping with deep learning and large-scale data collection. The International Journal of Robotics Research. 2018;**37**(4–5): 421-436

[22] Lima AAM, Araujo RM, dos Santos FAG, Yoshizumi VH, de Barros FK, Spatti DH, et al. Classification of hand movements from EMG signals using optimized MLP. In: 2018 International Joint Conference on Neural Networks (IJCNN). IEEE; 2018. pp. 1-7

[23] Vinstrup J, Calatayud J, Jakobsen MD, Sundstrup E, Jørgensen JR, Casaña J, et al. Hand strengthening exercises in chronic stroke patients: Dose-response evaluation using electromyography. Journal of Hand Therapy. 2018;**31**(1): 111-121

[24] Meeker C et al. EMG pattern classification to control a hand orthosis for functional grasp assistance after stroke. In: 2016 IEEE International Conference on Robotics and Automation (ICRA). 2016

[25] Bae J-H et al. Concurrent grasping and manipulation by arm-hand coordinated movements based on task-distribution. Advanced Robotics. 2005; **19**(4):401-434

[26] Yoon D, Lee G, Lee S, Choi Y. Underactuated finger mechanism for natural motion and self-adaptive grasping towards bionic partial hand. In: 6th IEEE RAS/EMBS International Conference on Biomedical Robotics and Biomechatronics (BioRob). IEEE; June 2016. pp. 548-553

[27] Roche AD. Clinical perspectives in upper limb prostheses: An update. Current Surgery Reports. 2019;7:5

[28] Nishad A, Upadhyay A, Pachori RB, Acharya UR. Automated classification of hand movements using tunable-Q wavelet transform based filter-bank with surface electromyogram signals. Future Generation Computer Systems. 2019;**93**:96-110

Chapter 5

Advanced Materials and Assembly Strategies for Wearable Biosensors: A Review

Eun Kwang Lee, Hocheon Yoo and Chi Hwan Lee

Abstract

Recent technological advances of soft functional materials and their assembly into wearable (i.e., on-skin) biosensors lead to the development of ground-breaking biomedical applications ranging from wearable health monitoring to drug delivery and to human-robot interactions. These wearable biosensors are capable of unobtrusively interfacing with the human skin and enabling long-term reliable monitoring of clinically useful biosignals associated with health and other conditions affecting well-being. Scalable assembly of diverse wearable biosensors has been realized through the elaborate combination of intrinsically stretchable materials including organic polymers or/and low-dimensional inorganic nanomaterials. In this Chapter, we review various types of wearable biosensors within the context of human health monitoring with a focus of their constituent materials, mechanics designs, and large-scale assembly strategies. In addition, we discuss the current challenges and potential future research directions at the end of this chapter.

Keywords: advanced functional materials, wearable biosensors, health monitoring systems, stretchable electronics, sensor technology

1. Introduction

Wearable sensor technology has evolved from traditionally fundamental measurement technology across science, engineering, and industry, and is now increasingly significant as a core method to advance human healthcare. To meet the requirements allowing for preventative health monitoring, diagnosis, and treatment, various types of wearable biosensors have been developed to capture the physical and electrophysiological biosignals (e.g., temperature, heart rate, respiration rate, electrodermal activity, and body motion) or biochemical responses (e.g., biomarkers in biofluids). Many of these wearable biosensors are required to remain in contact with the human skin for a prolonged period throughout the continuous monitoring of the biosignals. In this field, the largest continuing challenge is that rigid or semi-flexible forms of biosensors, particularly when integrated with wireless communication unit, are not compatible with the soft and irregular skin surface [1]. This mechanical mismatch results in discomfort to users as well as considerable noise signals during data collection. Recent advances in soft functional materials and assembly techniques have led to the development of mechanically stretchable and flexible biosensors that can be unobtrusively integrated into the human skin in

IntechOpen

a manner that complies with the natural motion of the wearer [2, 3]. The thin and flexible nature of these biosensors allows their conformal, seamless contact to the skin while simultaneously providing (i) excellent breathability and deformability for user comfort and (ii) durability to allow repeated attachment and detachment to the skin without irritating the wearer and damaging the devices. These aspects play a critical role in achieving high-fidelity recording of biosignals during long-term use in many clinical applications [4, 5].

According to the report by Grand View Research, Inc, the global market for wearable (i.e., on-skin) biosensors is anticipated to reach USD 2.86 billion by 2025 [6] at a phenomenal Compound annual growth rate (CAGR) of 38.8% during the forecast period (**Figure 1**) [6]. The wearable biosensors are a key component of electronic medical platform systems used by consumers as interest in real-time motion detection activity tracking grows. Furthermore, the wearable biosensors are emerging as a promising revolution that captures clinically important parameters form a distance and thereby reduces the patient's overall hospital cost. The manufacturers have incorporated contextual information and data to determine motion detection activities. Additionally, this analysis provides users with results that can be used to define their health and fitness goals [6]. This rapid interest over this market is likely to drive industry growth over the forecast period into advanced stages. The market of wearable biosensors in the field of health and fitness monitoring and diagnosis is gaining more attention due to their potential number of applications.

The wearable biosensors demand the following requirements. First, they require the ability to interface with the human skin with high compatibility, durability, and abrasion-resistant for the recording of biosignals with high-fidelity. Therefore, the conventionally-used semiconducting materials (e.g., silicon) remain impracticable. Second, they require an accurately operatable sensing system ('selectivity') that can differentiate between various environmental stimuli including mechanics, temperature, humidity, and various mechanical components such as atmospheric pressure, lateral deformation, shear, flexion, torsion, and vibration. Lastly, they require an affordable 'sensitivity' to detect the tiny biological signals through an appropriate amplification.

In this Book chapter, we overviewed various types of wearable biosensors tailored for the monitoring of mechanical, optical, and biochemical responses for human healthcare. We categorized the wearable biosensors according to their formfactors. In Section 3, we overviewed the functional materials used for these

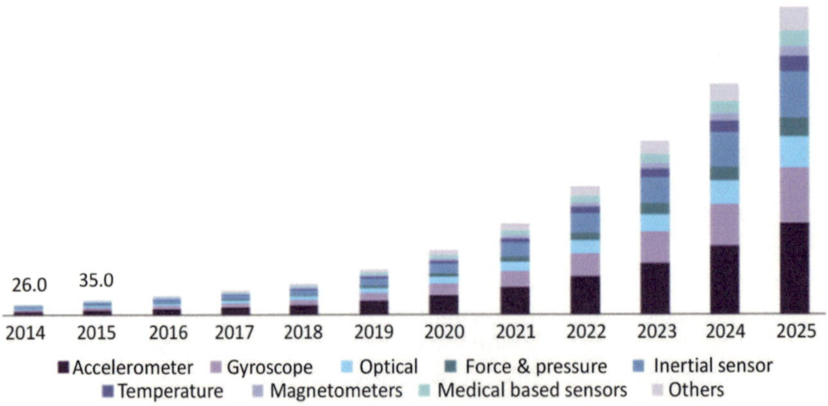

Figure 1.
A schematic graph that depicts continuous growth of wearable sensor market size. Adapted from Ref. [6].

biosensors, such as carbon-based nanomaterials and inorganic nanostructured materials, that provide tailored mechanical, electrical, or/and electrochemical properties. We also described the basic sensing mechanism (e.g. piezoresistive, piezocapacitive, iontronic, and piezoelectric sensing) of the wearable biosensors. In addition, we discussed organic field-effect transistor type of wearable biosensors, which can amplify small biological signals into large-signal information. In Section 4, we described various transduction systems according to their sensing mechanisms (e.g., electromechanical, optoelectrical and chemical sensing). In Section 5, we reviewed recently-reported assembly strategies to construct the wearable biosensors in a cost-effective manner. In Section 6, we discussed about future opportunity to further facilitate the commercialization of these wearable biosensors at a wider scale.

2. Types of wearable biosensors

Several human biosignals and stimuli should be concerned to display user's health conditions. For example, the assessment of biochemistry in biofluids (e.g., sweat, interstitial fluid, and blood) can provide fruitful information about personal health status and disease progression. In addition, both electrical and non-electrical biosignals such as electrooculography (EOG), mechanomyogram (MMG), electrocardiogram (ECG), electromyogram (EMG), galvanic skin response (GSR), magnetoencephalogram (MEG), and electroencephalogram (EEG) are useful indicators to offer the biosignal and info of a special tissue, organ, brain, or cellular system, such as the nervous system.

In addition to these internal vital signs, the on-skin detection of external harmful stimuli with a biosensor is also a critical issue. When it comes to the, the realm of wearable biosensing applications can be extended to motion detection, hazardous gas monitoring, disease diagnosis, and harmful UV-light detection (**Figure 2**). The sensing mechanisms of these sensors are diverse. In this Section, we will discuss several examples of chemical, optoelectronic and mechanical biosensors.

2.1 Wearable chemical biosensors

Sweat and sebum are representative human skin secretions that originate from the sweat glands in the dermal layer of the epidermis and therefore in-situ detection of these secretions on the skin is critically important for health monitoring. Sweat, a physiological aid for regulating body temperature, is secreted from the external glands. For example, sweat is a particularly useful sensing target due to the ease and presence of biomarkers associated with critical health conditions such as dehydration, physical exhaustion, mental stress and illness [13–15]. Sebum is secreted to lubricate human skin from Sebaceous glands. When sebum spreads up along the hair shaft, it is distributed over the surface of the skin, lubricating, and waterproofing the stratum corneum, the outer layer of the skin. It consists mostly of lipids. Those secretions can reflect the human health condition indirectly. Sebum provides antioxidant and antimicrobial lipids to the skin surface. Thus, proper secretion of sebum on the human skin surface increases the skin permeable barrier function. However, excess sebum frequently results in acne vulgaris. The acidic state of the skin pH is an essential factor in retaining the integrity of the skin-permeable barrier. It is reported that skin pH can be changed in skin diseases such as atopic dermatitis [16].

Wearable chemical biosensors that non-invasively analyze biofluids such as sweat, sebum, saliva, tears, and intermediate fluids provide the potential to

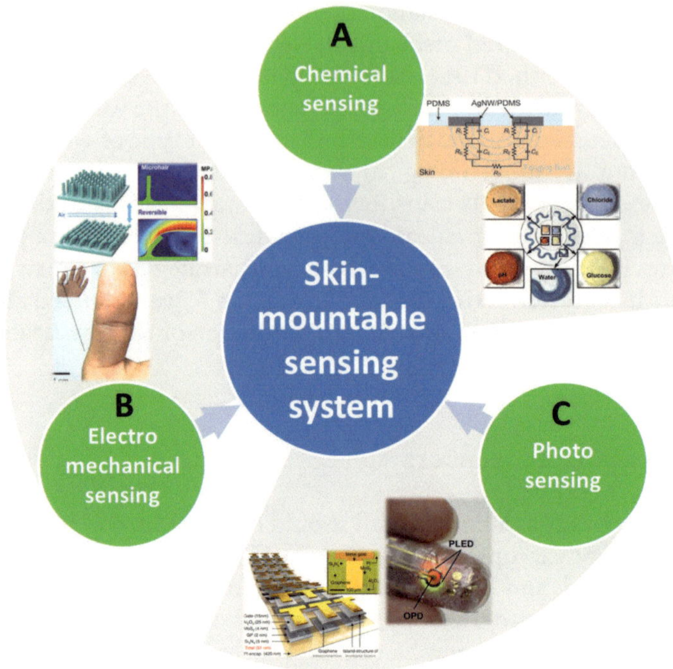

Figure 2.
A schematic diagram of wearable biosensors. (A) Wearable chemical biosensors. Adapted from Refs. [7, 8]. (B) Wearable photodetectors. Adapted from Refs. [9, 10]. (C) Wearable electromechanical biosensors. Adapted from Refs. [11, 12].

dramatically improve health condition evaluations by tracking changes in metabolic processes [17]. The sweat sample collection can be performed using an absorbent pad or a plastic microtube [18]. However, these methods are not compatible with remote monitoring and on-site use because they depend on cumbersome multi-step expensive benchtop hardware for sample preparation procedures and analysis. Recent advances in soft microfluidics, stretchable/flexible chemical sensing technologies form a basis of a new wearable sensor system that overcomes the limitations of this conventional approach [19]. The wearable sweat sensors are promising tools for continuous health and physiological monitoring. Among the various types of sweat sensors, optical detection utilizes photo-transmission techniques such as chromaticity, fluorescence, and light detection to provide an attractive strategy for measuring integrated chemical sensors due to cost efficiency and simplicity. Colorimetric sensors are also widely adopted in wearable sensor platforms, especially in case of the integrated microfluidic systems. Koh et al. demonstrated that a soft, flexible microfluidic platform based on silicon elastomer was recently developed, using colorimetric dyes to detect lactate, chloride, glucose, pH and loss of sweat [7]. The dye was located on top of the filter paper inserted into the micro reservoir. The lactate and glucose measurements were achieved by integrating enzymes into chromaticity-inducing reagents to enable the colorimetric readout sensing.

In terms of the detection of hazardous gases to human, Lee et al. demonstrated a flexible and transparent biosensor on polyethylene terephthalate (PET) that can detect 255 ppb NH_3 using spray-deposited single wall carbon nanotube (SWCNT) with Au nanoparticles in a reproducible manner [20]. The AuNP decoration of transparent SWCNT film through the use of an electron beam (e-beam) evaporation enhanced the performance of the gas sensor, which exhibited a high uniformity of the sensing behavior. The enhancement of this sensing performance was resulted from the carrier depletion zone control enabled by the combination structure of the AuNPs and the SWCNTs. The proposed sensor had a fast response time regarding NH_3 gas but did not fully recover at room temperature.

Lee et al. developed a patch-based, integrated system that combines non-invasive sweat glucose monitoring with microneedle-assisted therapy (**Figure 3**) [21]. The patch-based wearable/strip type single-use integrated systems include large-area porous metal based electrode, minimized sensor designs for stable sweat detection from small amounts of sweat, design patchable and disposable sensors to achieve practical application, multicycle operation of the sweat measuring control and absorption layer to collect efficiently sweat samples, a porous Au nanostructure film to maximize the surface-to-volume ratio to detect a tiny amount of glucose in sweat. This sweat sensor exhibited high performances in terms of sensitivity, multimodal sensing, and accuracy.

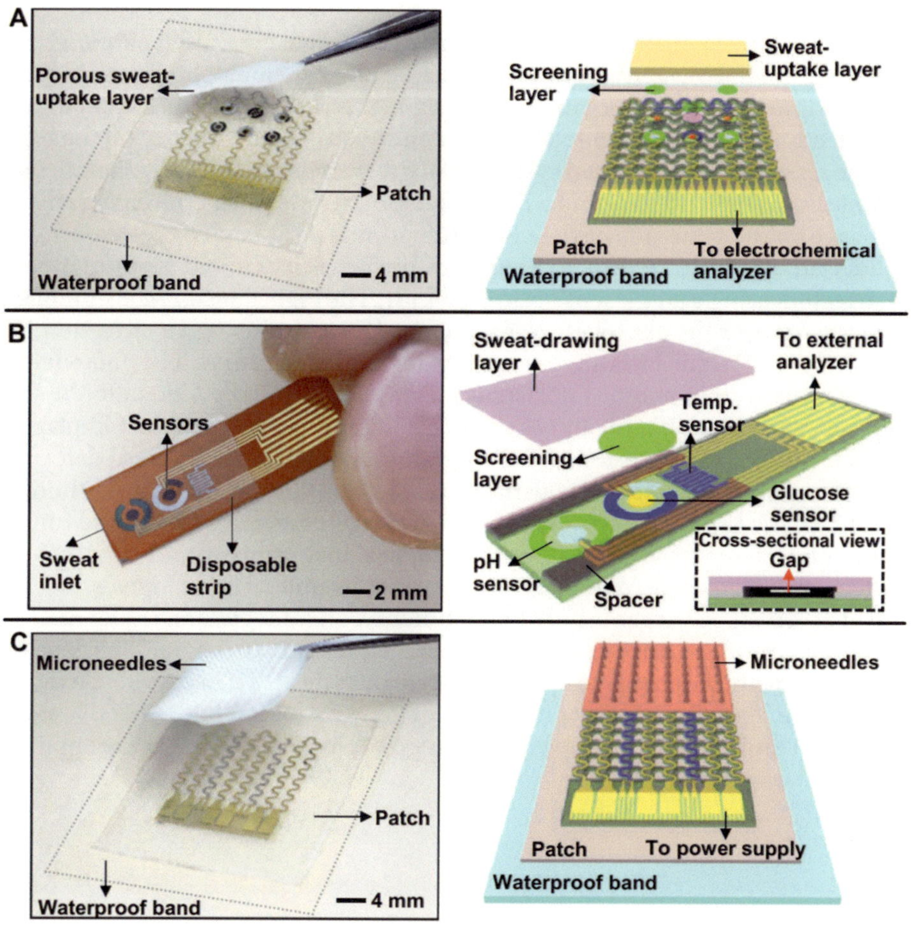

Figure 3.
(A) Optical camera image (top; dotted line, edges of the patch) and schematic (bottom) of the wearable sweat monitoring patch. A porous sweat-uptake layer is placed on a Nafion layer and sensors. (B) Optical camera image (top) and schematic (bottom) of the disposable sweat monitoring strip. (C) Optical camera image (top; dotted line, edges of the patch) and schematic (bottom) of the transdermal drug delivery device. Replacement-type microneedles are assembled on a three-channel thermal actuator. Adapted from Ref. [21].

2.2 Wearable optoelectronic sensors

Photodetector is a key device attached to the front end of the optical receiver that converts input optical signals into output electrical signals [22]. Especially in medical applications, optoelectronic devices are very useful as they are able to detect biometric signals and other clinical information non-invasively. Organic optoelectronic devices including organic light emitting diodes (OLEDs), organic photodetectors (OPDs), and organic phototransistors are in the spotlight in the area of medical devices as they provide a wide absorption spectrum and high photogeneration yield with easy-to-fabricate, lightweight, and flexible features [23].

Recently, OLEDs [24–30], polymer light-emitting diodes (PLEDs) [31–34], and OPDs [35–38] were fabricated on glass or plastic substrates, implementing a muscle contraction detector and transmission mode pulse oximeter. Moreover, OLEDs and organic photovoltaics were manufactured on 1-μm-thick ultra-thin films but were operated in N_2 box atmosphere [39, 40]. Realizing ultra-flexible optical sensor with an extended stability of surrounding conditions, allowing the sensors to integrate intimately and unnoticed on the skin, and to enable the application's cornucopia [10].

A representative non-invasive measurement system using pulsed oximetry characterizes peripheral oxygen saturation evaluated by oxyhemoglobin in the blood is shown in **Figure 4** [10]. An organic pulse oximeter with polymer LEDs and Si-based photodetectors were implemented based on pulse sensing and display on the human skin. The reflective pulse oxygen system used green and red LEDs to generate two wavelengths through fingers, and a light detector later measured the change in absorbance on the same side of the LED to determine peripheral oxygenation [10].

Choi et al. demonstrated an array of ultra-high-density curved MoS_2-graphene light detectors using a single lens optical unit [9]. The high-density MoS_2-graphene curved structure of the photodetector array was fabricated using an ultra-thin, soft material and strain-isolating/-releasing device architectures. The photodetector array and ultrathin neural-interfacing electrodes were embedded onto the soft flexible printed circuit board, accomplishing a human eye-inspired soft implantable optoelectronic device. The proposed device offered minimal mechanical deformation to the eye model, which were demonstrated by both experiments and finite element analysis (FEA) simulations. The wearable photodetector array and ultrathin neurointerference system reduced mechanical distortion of the retina and effectively stimulated the retinal nerve responded by optical input signals.

Ng et al. developed organic bulk heterojunction photodetectors having dark current as low as <1 nA cm^{-2} and efficient charge collection behavior. The development of a 4 μm-thick sensor layer using amorphous silicon TFTs provided a highly flexible image sensor operation with excellent performance as high as > 35% external quantum efficiency and noise equivalent power of 30 pW cm^{-2} at the applied reverse bias voltage of −4 V [41].

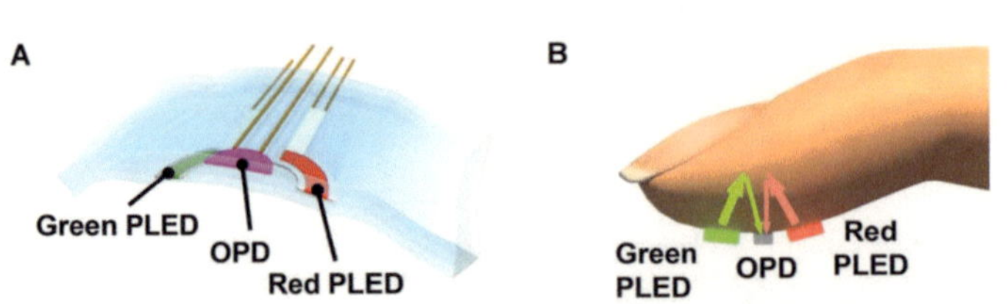

Figure 4.
Ultraflexible organic pulse oximeter. (A) Device structure of the pulse oximeter. (B) Operation principle of the reflective pulse oximeter. Adapted from Ref. [10].

2.3 Wearable electromechanical sensors

Various types of wearable electromechanical sensors have been developed by exploiting different sensing mechanisms such as piezoresistive, piezoelectric, capacitive and iontronic methods (**Figure 5**) [5, 42].

One of the simplest electronic devices is a piezoresistive, where a variation in resistance is recorded when the resistor is in contact with the human skin. In this piezoresistive mechanism, not only the value of the resistance but also several other parameters are assessed, including response time, recovery time and sensitivity. Since the resistors can be easily manufactured and characterized, they represent the most-widely-studied-device-structure for application detection, including flexible and wearable sensors [43].

Wearable capacitive sensors measure the change in the capacitance of a capacitor. The fabrication of these capacitive sensors is relatively simple (consecutive vertical stacking of metal/insulator/metal) and can detect various forms of mechanical force, such as strain, pressure, and touch.

Piezoelectricity defines as the accumulation of electrical changes in piezoelectric materials under mechanical stress. The piezoelectric-based sensors measure voltage change when electrical polarization induced by strain or pressure is generated.

Iontronic sensors are to form ionic-electronic interface at the nanoscale distance between the electrode and the electrolyte. When voltage is applied at each positive and negative electrodes, the corresponding counter ions accumulate at the interface of electrodes, resulting in an ultrahigh capacitance per unit-area. The capacitance of these iontronic sensors is at last 1000 times larger than that of metal oxide-based parallel plate capacitors. Thus, iontronic capacitance-type sensors are on the spotlight suitable for wearable electromechanical sensors due to its intrinsic high value of capacitance. The detailed working principle will discuss at Section 4 in detail.

Park et al. reported an array of ultra-thin consistent tactile detectors based on MoS_2 film of 2.2 cm × 2.2 cm. The integrated sensor with a graphene electrode provided excellent mechanically flexible endurance and optical transmittance in the visible light wavelength range. The proposed sensor device exhibited high sensitivity, good uniformity, and linearity with an excellent endurance of 10,000 cycles. The ultrathin tactile sensor was made on a plastic substrate, providing high stability of its operation performance even on various substrates including leather and a fingertip [11].

Investigations into the body-sensory system and tactile perception of human skin significantly enhanced the operation performance of rubber-based medical

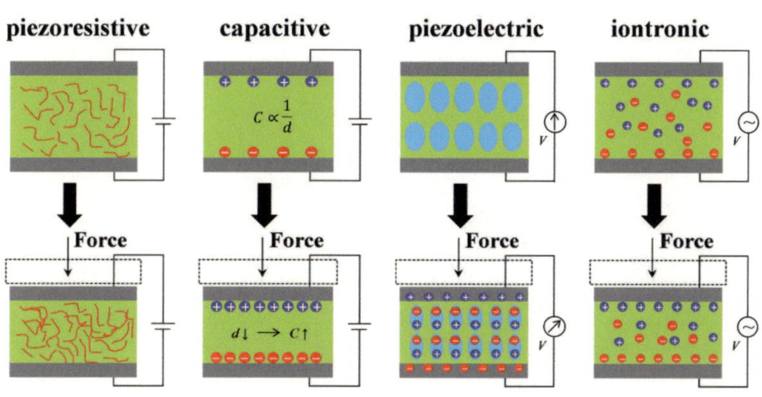

Figure 5.
An illustrative diagram demonstrating different types of mechanical sensing methods.

sensors and synthetic electronic skins [44–46]. Chun et al. demonstrated sensing device emulating hairy skin for multimodal detection. The thermal spray coating of graphene nanoplatelets (GNPs) enabled to fabricate the array of sensors and electrodes onto a flexible substrate. The percolation network array structure of GNP (5×5 cm^2, 16 pixels) was successfully able to detect the spatially applied pressures as well as locally varied temperature distribution, evaluating the human skin behavior. The microhairs in electronic devices were able to offer a mapping of electrical signals enabled by contactless air currents to identify the direction, angle of incidence, and intensity of the applied wind [12].

3. Materials used in wearable sensors

Due to the boost in the area of flexible and stretchable electronic materials, various wearable sensor devices have been demonstrated [47]. In order to integrate the wearable sensor with the human body, the mechanical properties of the sensor must be delicate and elastic, and it must be placed on the surface of human skin. Ordinarily, Silicon is the basic material of semiconductor hardware, but its modulus is about 10,000 times higher than that of human skin. Given the huge mechanical inconsistency, the most intuitive approach is to develop electronic materials (**Figure 6**) that are inherently soft to achieve mechanical compatibility and thus implement unrecognizable biosensors. Several review articles on material synthesis, structural engineering, and platform design were published [47–52].

3.1 Carbon-based nanomaterials

The carbon-based nanomaterials (CNM) discussed in this Chapter are materials with honeycomb lattice structures such as carbon nanotubes (CNTs), graphene

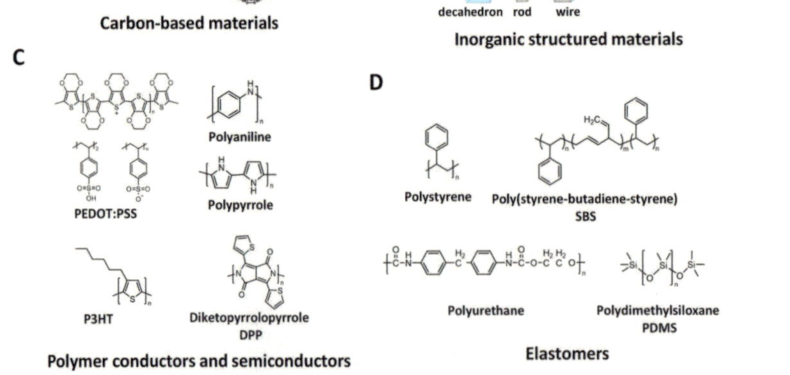

Figure 6.
Typical soft electronic materials for wearable sensors. (A) Carbon-based materials. Adapted from Ref. [53]. (B) Inorganic structured materials. Adapted from Ref. [54]. (C) Polymer conductors and semiconductors. (D) Elastomers.

(containing graphene oxide (GO) and reduced graphene oxide (rGO)), etc [55]. CNMs contain superior properties such as good electrical conductivity, excellent mechanical properties, high chemical and thermal stability, low toxicity. These excellent properties of CNMs have drawn great attention in wearable electronics [56, 57].

Cohen et al. demonstrated a high elasticity strain gauge using the capacitive detection of carbon nanotubes-based parallel electrodes separated by dielectric elastomer as shown in **Figure 7A** [58]. The device relies on the Poisson effect, so that the uniaxial strain creates a scaled strain so that the two transmissive electrodes come closer together. Even in the 3000-cycle test with 3% strain, the sensor's capacitance did not decrease.

Crumpled/wrinkled skin-like sensor using graphene for noninvasive and real-time pulsed sensing operation was demonstrated by Yang et al. (**Figure 7B**) [59]. The modification of PDMS (Polydimethyloxane) substrate stiffness achieves the optimal balance between acceptable linearity and high sensitivity, further realizing beat-to-beat radial pulse measurements for people of various ages and before and after motion.

A strain sensor device using a fish-scale-like graphene layer embedded on an elastic tape was accomplished by Liu et al. as shown in **Figure 7C** [60]. This configuration enabled graphene to form adjacent overlapping layers, realizing overlapping areas through reversible slip and consequently change contact resistance. Due to the fish-scale-like structure, this strain sensor was able to detect both stretching and bending deformation, as well as high performances including high sensitivity, low detection limit, wide range of deformation, excellent reliability and stability were achieved. This strain sensor can be manufactured by stretching/exhausting the composite film of rGO and elastic tape, so the process is simple, inexpensive, and has excellent energy saving and scalability.

By using dry spinning, Ryu et al. reported that they developed a strain sensor with an extremely elastic behavior based on highly oriented CNT fibers as shown in **Figure 7D** [61]. As The device was made of a flexible substrate, capable of measuring more than 900% strains with superior sensitivity and exhibited rapid response and good durability. Such sensors should be used extensively in applications involving large variants, including soft robotics. These devices can be adapted for normal strain gauge applications.

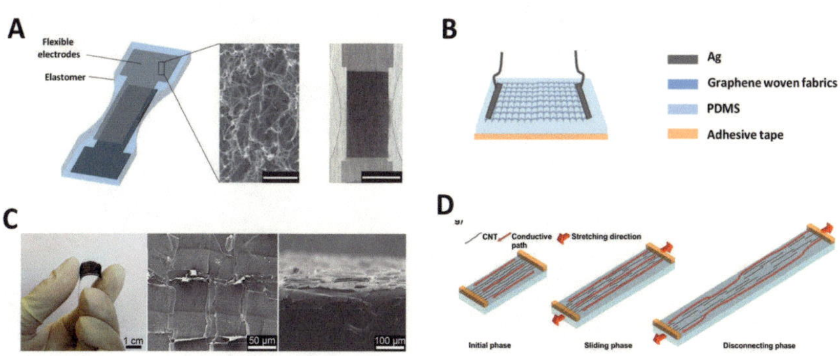

Figure 7.
Wearable biosensors based on carbon nanomaterials. (A) Design of a Poisson Capacitor. Adapted from Ref. [58] (From left to right) Schematic of our device geometry. SEM data demonstrating percolation of the CNTs within the electrode; scale bar is 500 nm. Close-up image of the sensing region of the device. (B) Schematic illustration of the pulse sensor. Adapted from Ref. [59]. (C) Fish-scale-like graphene-based (FSG) strain sensors. (From left to right) Photograph. Top view and cross-section view of SEM images. Adapted from Ref. [60]. (D) Schematic showing the morphology of a CNT fiber under strain; scale bar is 0.75 cm. Adapted from Ref. [61].

3.2 Inorganic nanostructured materials

Conventional silicon-based semiconductor devices are essential elements for real-time data processing and data transmission, but these silicon-based semiconductor devices are mostly composed on rigid chips. To solve this problem, the electronic component can be bonded on a rigid chip through micro- or macroscopic structural changes of materials, then, a wearable device can be manufactured through this approach [62].

Kaltenbrunner et al. developed a sensing system that enables to electronics of virtually unbreakable and imperceptible behaviors with ultrathin materials [63]. A sensing device of 2 mm thick layer was very light, reducing electronic waste, and this device was able to be applied to curves and dynamic surfaces (i.e., plastic wrap) (**Figure 8A**). Organic TFTs using ultra-high-density oxide gate dielectrics several nanometers thick at room temperature enable sophisticated large-area electronic foils with unprecedented mechanical and environmental stability. It can be crumpled like paper, with a radius of less than 5mm, which is repeatedly bent, providing an elongation rate of up to 230% in a pre-modified elastomer.

Silver nanoparticles from ultra-thin silver powder can be applied to the electronics sector due to their high conductivity [54]. Typically, the diameter of Ag nanoparticles is of hundreds of nanometers, but the shape of those particles is uneven [64–67].

On the other hand, silver nanowires (Ag NWs) are widely investigated over a long time due to their versatile electrical, chemical, and biological properties. Peng et al. demonstrated a triboelectric nanogenerator (TENG)-based e-skin which is highly conformal and stretchable, enough to attach on human skin. They have used nanofiber for breathability, biodegradability, sensitivity and Ag NWs for antibacterial activity [68]. The developed devices have been designed for the detection of physiological characteristics and movement states of the whole body (**Figure 8B**). A 3D nano-porous structure was formed by combining PLGA Tribune layer and PVA substrate and nanofiber.

3.3 Polymer conductors and semiconductors

Polymer conductor and semiconductor are crucial materials for the fabrication of wearable sensors due to their low-cost, solution-processability and easy-chemical modification. Intrinsically flexible electronic materials are building blocks of

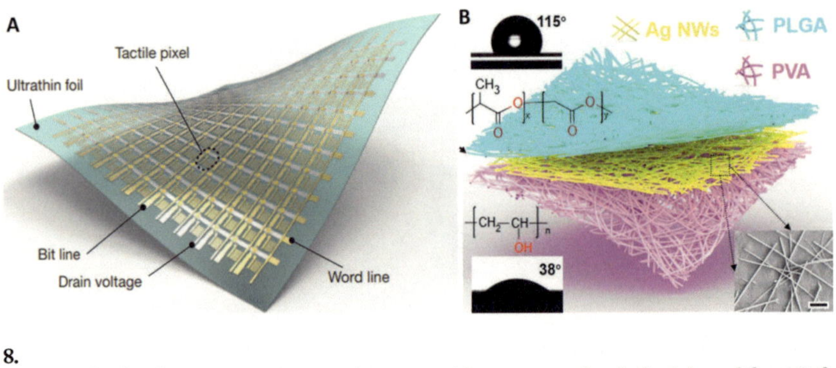

Figure 8.
(A) Illustration of a thin large-area active-matrix sensor with 12 × 12 tactile pixels. Adapted from Ref. [63]. (B) Schematic illustration of the three-dimensional network structure of the all-nanofiber TENG–based e-skin. The images of the water contact angle and molecular structure of PLGA and PVA are inserted on the top left and lower left, respectively. The surface SEM image of the Ag NW electrode is inserted on the lower right (scale bar, 2 μm). Adapted from Ref. [68].

wearable sensors which enable scalable and low-cost manufacturing, high-density device integration and large strain tolerance [69, 70].

Kim et al. reported that highly stretchable sensors and transistors that consist of intrinsically stretchable composite semiconductors and conductors [71] as shown in **Figure 9A**. They consist of three main materials: (1) Stretchable semiconductor: P3HT nanofibrils (P3HT-NF)-filled PDMS, (2) Stretchable conductor: PDMS filled with AuNP-AgNW, (3) Stretchable gate dielectric: ions gel. (DoS) electronics are demonstrated (**Figure 9B**), which is deformable, conformal, customizable robust against the human motion. After drawing the electronic ink on desired surfaces, dried ink is strongly attached onto the surface that allows ultra-conformality [72]. Drawn-on-Skin (DoS) electronics were combined with simple fabrication avoiding from dedicated equipment. In addition, these devices can be stacked onto another electronic composite layer on diverse surfaces. Ink, pen, and stencil act as a tool kit for making a variety of DoS electronics that can be mechanically modified and customized to curved textured skins.

3.4 Elastomer

What is another important material in wearable sensor are elastomers which are polymers with viscoelasticity (i.e., both viscosity and elasticity). Elastomers have weak intermolecular forces, generally low Young's modulus and high failure strain compared with other materials. Main strategy to construct a conductive elastomer is to combine elastomers and metallic nanomaterials for stretchability and conductivity. By optimizing the material design, elastomer-to-metallic nanomaterial composition ratio and fabrication processes of the metallic nanocomposites, stretchable conductors with exceptionally conductive and stretchable properties can be realized [73].

Maintaining electrical conductivity of the stretchable conductor during certain strain or tension is a critical parameter in the application of the wearable device. Usually, the electrical pathway in the composite materials should be formed in the composite. Various techniques, such as structural optimization of the nanomaterial, welding between the metallic nanomaterials (**Figure 10A**) [74], and additives [75], have been adopted In order to enhance the conductivity, (**Figure 10B**).

As the thickness decreases, the bending stiffness decreases at a rate of 3 times faster when the thickness of the elastomer is reduced to obtain a highly flexible wearable device. Elasticity can be obtained through various strategies for example fractal interconnect design, free deformation wavy configuration, bridge structure and serpentine structure [50, 76–84].

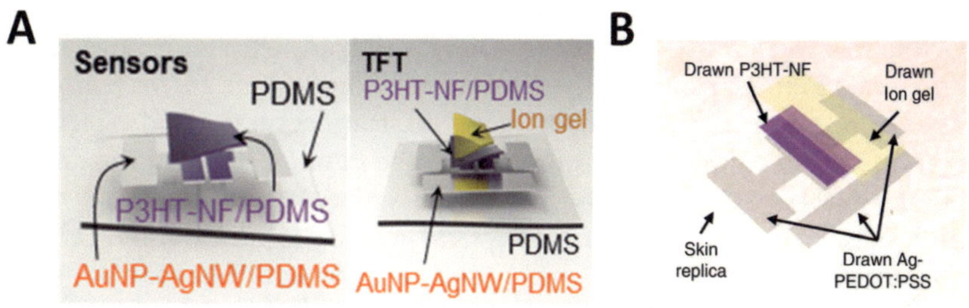

Figure 9.
(A) Schematic illustrations of a sensor (left) and a TFT (right), consisting of AuNP-AgNW conductors, P3HTNF/PDMS semiconductor composite, and ion gel dielectric vertically stacked on a PDMS substrate. Adapted from Ref. [71]. (B) Schematic of the DoS transistor based on the Ag-PEDOT:PSS ink as the conductor, P3HT-NF ink as the semiconductor, and ionic gel ink as the dielectric. Adapted from Ref. [72].

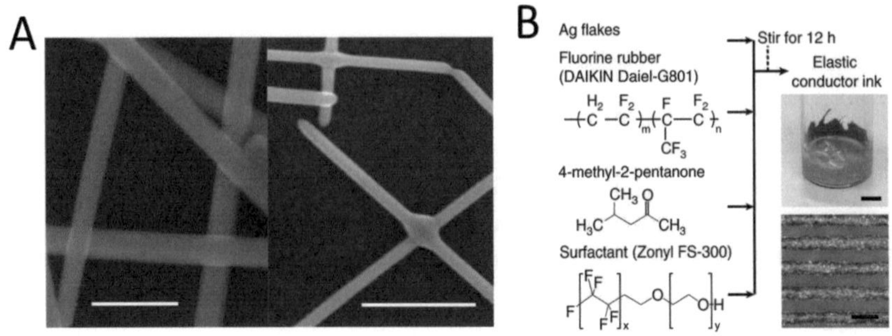

Figure 10.
(A) (Left) Plan-view SEM image of silver nanowire junctions before illumination. Scale bar is 200 nm. (Right) Plan-view SEM image of silver nanowire junctions after optical welding with a tungsten halogen lamp. Scale bar is 500 nm. Adapted from Ref. [74]. (B) Fabrication process of elastic conductor ink. Upper picture, elastic conductor ink. Scale bar, 10 μm. Lower picture, printed elastic conductor with high resolution. Scale bar, 100 mm. Adapted from Ref. [75].

The representative elastomers for the stretchability of wearable sensors are poly(styrene-butadiene-styrene) (SBS), polyurethane, polydimethylsiloxane (PDMS) and hydrogel polymer materials. Those elastomers are usually used as substrates or a matrix while embedding nanoparticles, nanowires, nanosheets in wearable electronics. Liquid conductors such as gallium metal alloys are less reactive and non-toxic, thus, they are utilized in microfluidic channels of wearable sensors [52, 85]. Hydrogel and polymer have high biocompatibility but relatively low conductivity, limiting performance, and many hydrogels suffer from stiffness over time due to drying. Conventional biocompatible materials usually combine hydrogel and polymer with nanomaterials and were constructed as composite materials to enhance performance and stability. When using nanomaterials such as CNT, care should be taken by encapsulating inside the elastic system to prevent potential health problems [86, 87]. Advances of biocompatible materials was required to improve breathability and stability for pragmatic use [62].

Especially, hydrogel is a 3D structure of hydrophilic polymers, which has been widely applied as a biomaterial due to their biocompatibility with human skin surface. Conductive hydrogel can be synthesized by combining hydrogel polymer with nanostructured metal or conductive polymer (**Figure 11A**) [88]. The synthesis of hydrogel involves physical and chemical crosslinking at a molecular level. Two type of cross-linked hydrogel, physically or chemically cross-linked hydrogels can be considered. Physically cross-linked one usually has self-healing properties but poor mechanical properties (**Figure 11B**) [89]. Chemically cross-linked one has high mechanical properties that withstands physical deformation but no mechanical self-healing properties [90]. Several recent approaches of structure fabrication include a dual network and sliding cross-link, which adjusts the Young's moduli from kilopascals to megapascals [91–93]. However, hydrogels suffer from dehydration and debonding. Encapsulation using elastomers on the hydrogels or the surface modification using supramolecules can be applied to avoid the dehydration and debonding [94].

Reliable signal acquisition from biophysical activity is paramount in the assessment of wearable sensors. Continuous physical movement of human body and dynamic skin surface condition facilitate detachment of wearable sensors during the signal acquisition. Thus, facile chemical and physical approaches have been adapted to achieve for the robust attachment of wearable sensor on arbitrary human skin surface under investigation. Yuk et al. investigated a simple yet effective strategy of inserting a cross-linked hydrophilic polymer (hydrogel skin) into various polymer

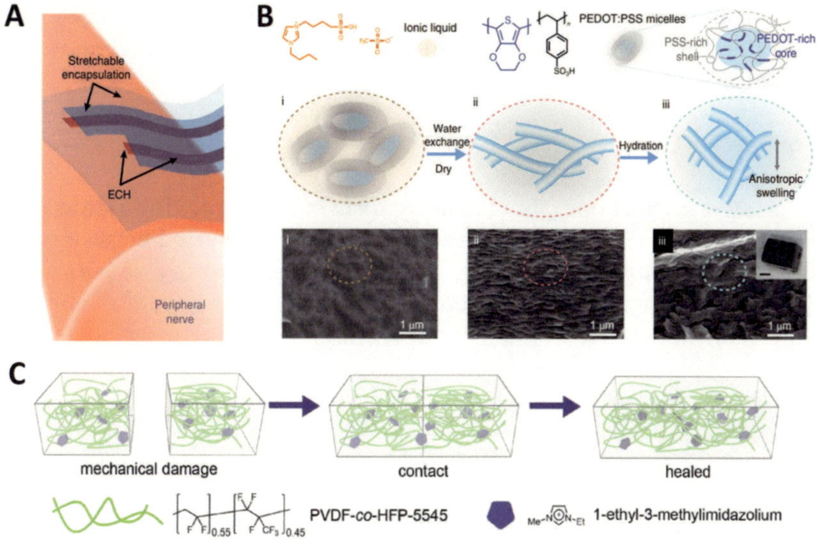

Figure 11.
(A) Schematic of the bioelectronic interface between a peripheral nerve and soft conductor electrodes and insulation materials. (B) Schematic of the stepwise PEDOT:PSS ECH synthesis process and SEM images showing morphological changes in each step during the synthesis of an ECH. An ionic liquid, 4-(3-butyl-1-imidazolio)-1-butanesulfonic acid triflate, was blended with the PEDOT:PSS solution and subsequently dried to form an ion gel (i); ionic liquid is exchanged with water and then dried at room temperature (ii); the dried sample exhibits aligned and interconnected microstructures that swell in water to form the ECH (iii). The interconnected PEDOT polymer network in the ECH results in a continuous electronic conductive pathway. Scale bar, 1 mm for the inset of (iii), which is an optical image of a hydrated ECH. Adapted from Ref. [88]. (C) Design concept for a transparent, self-healing, highly stretchable ionic conductor using ion–dipole interaction as the dynamic motif and demonstration of healing process and chemical structure of polymer and imidazolium cation. Adapted from Ref. [89].

surfaces, including silicon rubber, polyurethane, PVC, nitrile rubber and natural rubber, to facilitate the robust attachment of hydrogel and device interfaces. Due to the unique combination of soluble initiators absorbed on the polymer surface and hydrogel pregel initiators dissolved in hydrogel solutions, hydrogel skin is placed on the surface and adapted to the complex and fine geometry of the polymer substrate [95]. Hydrogel skins provided tissue-like softness with excellent mechanical rigidity, low friction, anti-easing performance and ion conductivity.

Yuk et al. also reported fabrication of bio-compatible dry double-sided tape (DST). The bio-compatible DST consists of biopolymer and crosslinked poly(acrylic acid) [96]. The authors attached an elastic strain sensor to a beating porcine heart to evaluate thermal motion that can serve as a versatile platform for wearables and implantable devices. In addition, they demonstrated possible applications using ex vivo models and the combination of DST and biosensors. This DST offered advantages over conventional tissue adhesives and sealants, such as fast adhesive formation, strong adhesion performance, flexibility, storage, and ease of use.

4. A variety of transduction systems for Wearable biosensors

To obtain physiological information or signals from the human body using skin-mounted bio-sensors, they are mainly composed of stretchable or flexible materials. Generally, flexible substrates, electrodes, and sensing materials are three essential parts of skin-mounted biosensors. More importantly, appropriate device systems, architectures, and sensing mechanisms should be combined with relevant electronic materials. In this Section, we mainly review widely used sensing mechanisms and architectures. [43, 97].

4.1 Piezoresistive type

Piezoresistive sensors operate as a mechanism of a pressure input into a resistance change output (**Figure 5A**). The active material is inserted between two electrodes in this resistive-type sensor. The active materials provide both sufficient charge transport ability for electrical current flow as well as good elasticity to offer various mechanical deformation during operation.

4.2 Piezocapacitive type

Piezocapacitive sensors can be obtained by a mechanism of a change in in the capacitance of a parallel plate capacitor as a function of the applied pressure stress (**Figure 5B**). Piezocapacitive sensors include three main components: electrode, substrate, and active material sandwiched by two electrodes. As a variation of the external pressure input, the capacitance varies, providing a detection of the target pressure sensing.

4.3 Piezoelectric type

Piezoelectricity defines as the phenomenon that occurs when positive and negative charges are localized when mechanical stress is applied, or vice versa (**Figure 5C**). The piezoelectric sensors are desirable for measuring the dynamic variation of the pressure or force. The output voltage produced by the sensor is impulsive and does not apply to static sensing.

4.4 Iontronic type

Supercapacitive iontronic pressure sensors convert the pressure input into the output of constant-capacity change. This type of pressure sensor enhances the compression effect by utilizing the formation of an electron double layer (EDL) at the dielectric layer and contact electrode. In other words, ionic gel with numerous positive and negative ions are spatially trapped between the two electrodes. The positive and negative ions are attracted to the negative and positive respectively, forming two EDLs as an increase of the applied voltage. The operating mechanism of this type of sensor depends on changes in the area between the electrode and the active material, as shown in **Figure 5D**. Increasing the contact area under certain pressure, positive or negative ions are induced, resulting in increased capacitance values [98].

4.5 Organic field-effect transistor type

Organic TFT-based sensors offer biosignals-sensing operation such as cell activity. In general, two major categories of organic TFTs are used for bio-sensing applications. Electrochemical doping and de-doping are the main reactions in an organic electrochemical transistor (OECT) to modulate ionic species to the active channel materials. Meanwhile, the capacitive field effect is the main reaction of electrolyte gate organic field effect transistor (EGOFET) at the interface of organic semiconductor and electrolyte [99].

Gualandi et al. reported a fully textile, wearable biosensor based on an OECT (**Figure 12**) using PEDOT: PSS conducting polymer. The fabricated OECT sensors can detect three biomolecules (ascorbic acid, adrenaline, and dopamine) by the reduction-oxidation reaction. Their performance is similar to normal OECTs. These results demonstrate that OECT can be established on a 3D-networked fiber substrate [100].

4.6 Photosensing type

Near-infrared (IR)-response organic light detector (OPD) has been investigated due to its potential applications of health monitoring, remote control, artificial vision, optical communication, and night vision. Especially, the short exposure of near-IR on human skin is not toxic and near-IR can propagate under tissue at ranges of 4 mm. Thus, near-IR is proper for skin-mountable health monitoring devices [101]. Furthermore, narrowband detection of near IR light between ≈700 and 1300 nm is highly desirable for biomedical sensing. Park et al. demonstrated high-performance skin-mountable near-IR OPDs which are mechanically conformable for the application of health care electronics [101]. The OPD (thinner than 3 μm) exhibits stable operation under conditions of mechanical deformation (10^3 times bending). Thanks to its balanced properties of high responsivity and stable mechanical conformability, the IR sensor device showed superior sensitivity in the near-IR region when it is under operation in a skin-conformal photoplethysmogram sensor compared to that of an existing rigid substrate device of the glass.

4.7 Chemical sensing type

The biochemical signal of the human body significantly varies depending on the health condition of the subject. Biomarker concentrations range from complex patterns and other time scales, i.e., time-to-time fluctuations in metabolites, hormonal and inflammatory changes, from neuron synapses to millisecond spikes in ions and neurotransmitters.

Over the years, continuous wearable technology for non-invasive monitoring has been developed. Imani et al. developed wearable devices that could measure chemical and electrophysiological signals simultaneously in the single patch. The hybrid wearable, called Chem-Phys patch, consists of three-electrode ammeter lactate biosensors and two ECG electrodes printed on the screen, enabling simultaneous real-time measurements of lactate and ECG as shown in **Figure 13** [102].

Nightingale et al. demonstrated a fully integrated wearable microfluid sensor, which not only provides accurate, precise, and powerful fluid sampling and control but also provides on-site chemical tests that use water droplets as microreactors [103].

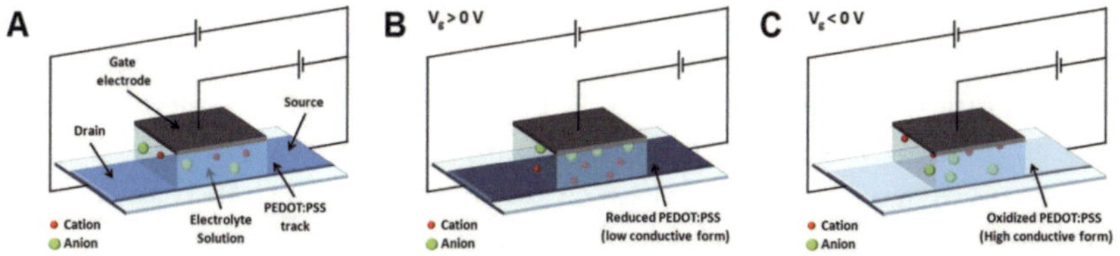

Figure 12.
OECT working principle. Scheme of an OECT (A) operating in conditions of low (B) and high (C) conductivity of the channel. Adapted from Ref. [100].

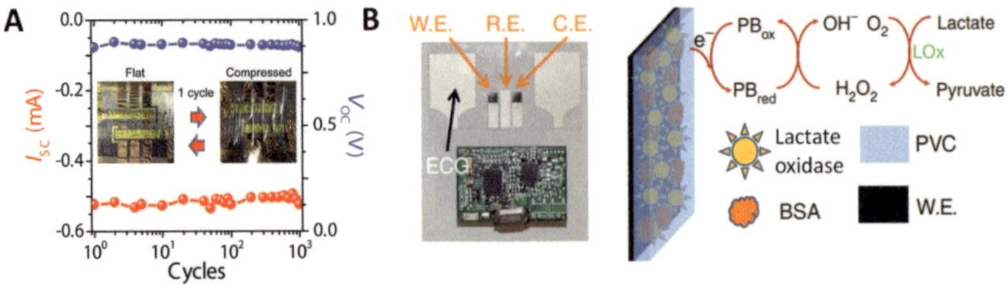

Figure 13.
(A) Cyclic stretching test of near-IR-OPD. The stretching cycle test was conducted at 100% tensile strain for 10^3 cycles. Adapted from Ref. [101]. (B) (Left) Image of a Chem–Phys patch along with the wireless electronics. (Right) Schematic showing the lactate oxidase-based lactate biosensor along with the enzymatic and detection reactions. Adapted from Ref. [102].

5. Device fabrication and assembly strategies

As device-manufacturing technology is actively being developed, skin-mounted biosensors have attracted scientific and industrial attention to everyday applications such as e-skin, health testing, underwater sensing, and interaction between people and machines [104]. In this subsection, we review the novel fabrication strategies for wearable sensors.

Skin-mounted electronic devices should be established on flexible substrates with reasonable fabrication costs. In particular, the ability to realize flexible or wearable thin film-based sensors provides much freedom for target substrates. One of the most promising and powerful candidates to produce low-cost skin-mounted bio-sensors is ink-jet printing, and due to its ultra-low-cost, non-vibration, and environmentally friendly fairness, it is an appropriate strategy to implement commercial thin-film devices and systems [105]. Ink-jet printing originated from the graphic art industry for mass production of standard products including fabrics and papers. In addition, advanced printing machines and inks solutions can produce on large-area products with low-cost and high-printing-speeds on the order of 10 m s^{-1}.

Holbery et al. demonstrated a demand (DOD) inkjet printing technique to fabricate touch sensors on polyethylene terephthalate (PET) substrates. The commercially available Poly(3,4-ethylenedioxythiophene): poly(styrenesulfonate) (PEDOT: PSS) solution and thermally curable methylsiloxane serves as transparent electrodes and dielectric, respectively. The resistance and transparency of PEDOT: PSS electrode gradually decreases from 20.8 to 6.9 kΩ and from 85 to 75%, respectively [106].

Inkjet printing supplies pressure pulses to the fluid-filled chamber, depleting ink drops on demand and triggering pulses through heat evaporation, sound perturbation, or piezoelectric operation. However, inkjet printing using thermal steam, acoustic perturbation, or piezoelectric operation lacks inkjet droplet control function of the inkjet nozzle in a controlled manner, making it challenging to print high resolution [107]. In particular, in electrohydrodynamic (EHD) jet printing, electric fields are applied between deposition nozzles and substrate to induce moving ions of ink to accumulate on the liquid surface. Because of the Coulombic repulsion of ions at the edge of the ink, the hemispherical meniscus turns into a conical shape (Taylor cone). Thus, a smaller diameter of inkjet resolution than that of the nozzle is obtained during EHD jet printing Compared to normal inkjet printing and aerosol printing which has limited resolution (~ tens of micrometer), few hundred resolutions (nearly 700 nm) can be realized using EHD jet printing [108].

Lee et al. reported three different transfer-printing (TP) methods for nanowire (NW) based devices [109]. Fundamentally, NWs on donor substrate is likely to be

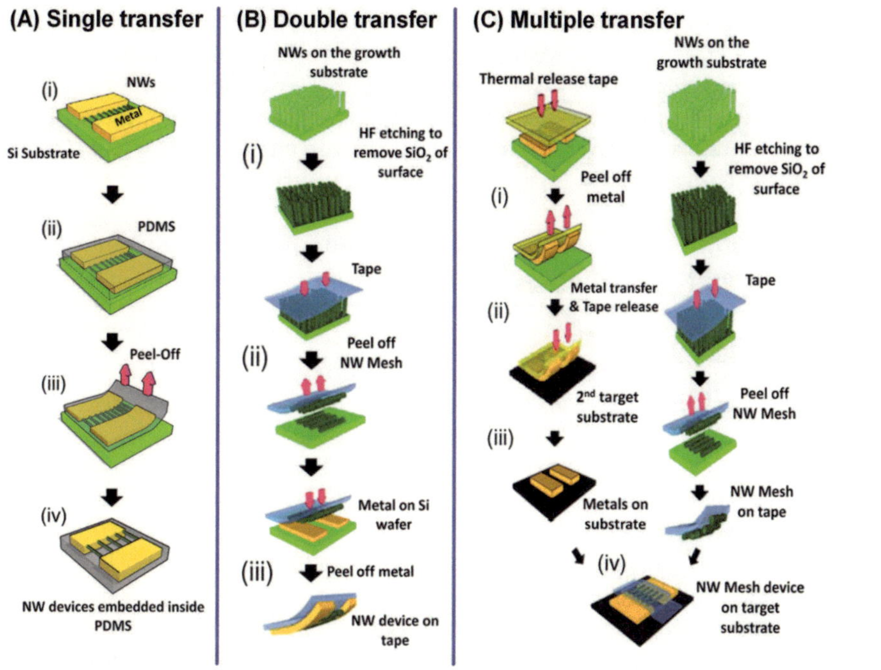

Figure 14.
Various transfer printing technique. (A) STP method on PDMS (Prefabricated NW devices → Deposition of liquid PDMS and curing → Peel off PDMS/NW devices → NW devices embedded inside PDMS). (B) DTP method (NWs on the growth substrate → HF etching to remove the native SiO_2 of NWs → Pressing down a tape to the NWs → Peel off the tape with NW mesh → Pressing down the tape/NW mesh to the prefabricated electrodes → 2nd Peel-off → NW device on the tape). (C) MTP method (1st column: pressing down a thermal release tape to the prefabricated electrodes → Peel off the thermal release tape with electrodes → Pressing down the thermal release tape/ electrodes to a target substrate → The thermal release tape is thermally released at 90°C; 2nd column: NWs on the growth substrate → HF etching to remove the native SiO_2 of NWs → Pressing down a tape to the NWs → Peel off the tape with NW mesh → Assembling of the tape/NW and the transferred electrodes). Adapted from Ref. [109].

transferred onto acceptor substrates which have stronger adhesion force than that of donor substrate (**Figure 14**). (1) Single transfer printing (STP) enables fabricated NW devices on a Si wafer to be transferred onto a PDMS substrate through a single peel-off step. (2) Double transfer printing (DTP) required a two-times transfer process from NWs and electrodes to fabricate devices. (3) Multiple transfer printing (MTP) includes the transfer of multiple electrodes using thermal release tapes on both flexible and rigid substrates.

Inganäs et al. demonstrated the additive technique for producing all translucent and flexible polymer photodetectors with a wide area. PEDOT: PSS electrodes were printed on a flexible PET film substrate through roll-to-roll (RTR). The printed PEDOT: PSS electrodes were served as both cathode and anode by a coating of Polyethylenimine (PEI) on PEDOT: PSS. After the spin-coating of an active layer on top of PEDOT: PSS and PEDOT: PSS/PEI, the two multi films were laminated through a hot-pressing roller (120°C). The fabricated all-polymeric photodetector also demonstrated mechanical durability [110].

6. Future opportunities

As part of the era of digital health, widespread use and deployment of wearable sensors should overcome specific technical challenges. One such challenge is the biological receptor in wearable chemical biosensors. Since the signal transducer material and technologies of wearable chemical biosensors have already been considerably advanced, a major obstacle that hinders the development of the wearable chemical biosensors field may be not a signal transducer material, but a biological material. A diversity of target materials is narrow in current biological receptors and needs to be improved in terms of material stability, selectivity, bonding power, and production cost.

Ideal wearable sensors are physically small and can store important personal health data; therefore, biosensors and personal health data may be lost. The development of more secure and encryption technologies is desired to keep personal privacy and security.

The personal calibration of the wearable sensor is also one of the main challenges. Everybody has different personal health conditions (e.g. diet, family medical history and genetics). Therefore, symptoms of early diagnosis may vary from person-to-person. It is necessary to develop hardware and software that can comprehensively interpret human health through the development of artificial intelligence, as well as calibration of personal health status. Although artificial intelligence's big data could be used to interpret an individual's health, the patient's disease should not be immediately evaluated through other people's precedents using wearable sensors. In addition, since individual's body shape and skin surface condition are all different, research that combines 3D printing technology to create a wearable sensor according to the individual's condition might be an interesting direction for further research.

7. Outlook and conclusions

Wearable sensors and portable point-of-care medical devices are getting intensive attention from academic and industry societies. However, intensive understanding and studies of biosensing mechanisms, transduction mechanisms from biosignal to an electrical signal, and proper device platforms for specified medical purposes are prior to the commercialization of wearable sensors. Although those technical developments have been made for the last decades, social understanding from society and medical approval and its prerequisite is at infancy. Accelerating personalization in one's lifestyle (currently due to Coronavirus Disease-19, COVID-19, and increasing interests in personal health care), point-of-care, and self-medical assessment will get attention more and more.

Recently, enormous development in soft electronic materials and advanced fabrication strategies have rendered to materialize wearable sensors. Wearable sensors can be applied in not only biosensing but also a lot of fields such as medical, industrial process, environmental monitoring, and military. The medical field is currently one of the most in-demand fields. By utilizing free movement of the sensors and their immediate recognition characteristics, it is possible to use drugs and perform rapid treatment for critically ill patients those who have issues in blood sugar, pregnancy hormones, cancer cells, cholesterol, lactic acid, and urea and etc. In addition, wearable sensors could be utilized in environmental monitoring field for the detection of environmental toxic substances in large areas rapidly and efficiently. The pollution in air, water and soil can be minimized for comfortable living environment. For example, the detection of environmental substances such as environmental hormones (dioxin), biological oxygen demand (BOD) of wastewater, heavy metals, and pesticides, can lead to an advanced life quality on human society. In the military, wearable sensors would allow for the detection of various biological sources. These can be used as a weapon that might drive mass destruction such as sarin and anthrax, which requires fast analysis time. In addition to that, miniaturized wearable sensor would also allow for a maximized range of motion for direct use.

In summary, it is still unobvious to best match the architectures of wearable sensors to which diagnostic tasks. Moreover, a wearable sensor that is functional in the lab may not be of use in the field or clinic for several reasons. Multidisciplinary research involving life science, engineering, and physics needs to be performed simultaneously to construct more reliable and affordable wearable biosensors.

Acknowledgements

C.H.L. acknowledge funding supports from the National Institute of Health (NIH) National Institute of Biomedical Imaging and Bioengineering (NIBIB: 1R21EB026099-01A1).

Conflict of interest

The authors declare no conflict of interest.

Author details

Eun Kwang Lee[1†], Hocheon Yoo[2†] and Chi Hwan Lee[3*]

1 Weldon School of Biomedical Engineering, Purdue University, West Lafayette, IN 47907, USA

2 Electronic Engineering, Gachon University, 1342 Seongnam-daero, Seongnam 13120, South Korea

3 Weldon School of Biomedical Engineering, School of Mechanical Engineering, School of Materials Engineering, Purdue University, West Lafayette, IN 47907, USA

*Address all correspondence to: lee2270@purdue.edu

† These authors contributed equally.

References

[1] Yuk H, Lu B, Zhao X. Hydrogel bioelectronics. Chemical Society Reviews. 2019;**48**:1642-1667. DOI: 10.1039/C8CS00595H

[2] Lee Y, Kim J, Joo H, Raj MS, Ghaffari R, Kim D-H. Wearable Sensing Systems with Mechanically Soft Assemblies of Nanoscale Materials. Advanced Materials Technologies. 2017;**2**:1700053. DOI: 10.1002/admt.201700053

[3] Saifullah DA, Sahidayana MM, Farina M, Fatimah I. Potential applications of human artificial skin and electronic skin (e-skin): a review. Bioinspired, Biomimetic and Nanobiomaterials. 2018;**7**:53-64. DOI: 10.1680/jbibn.17.00002

[4] Kim D-H, Lu N, Ma R, Kim Y-S, Kim R-H, Wang S, et al. Epidermal Electronics. Science. 2011;**333**:838. DOI: 10.1126/science.1206157

[5] Lee EK, Kim MK, Lee CH. Skin-Mountable Biosensors and Therapeutics: A Review. Annual review of biomedical engineering. 2019;**21**:299-323. DOI: 10.1146/annurev-bioeng-060418-052315

[6] Global Wearable Sensors Market Size, Industry Report, 2018-2025 [Internet]. 2018. Available from: https://www.grandviewresearch.com/industry-analysis/global-wearable-sensor-market [Accessed: 2020-09-10]

[7] Koh A, Kang D, Xue Y, Lee S, Pielak RM, Kim J, et al. A soft, wearable microfluidic device for the capture, storage, and colorimetric sensing of sweat. Science Translational Medicine. 2016;**8**:366ra165. DOI: 10.1126/scitranslmed.aaf2593

[8] Yao S, Myers A, Malhotra A, Lin F, Bozkurt A, Muth JF, et al. A Wearable Hydration Sensor with Conformal Nanowire Electrodes. Advanced Healthcare Materials. 2017;**6**:1-8. DOI: 10.1002/adhm.201601159

[9] Choi C, Choi MK, Liu S, Kim MS, Park OK, Im C, et al. Human eye-inspired soft optoelectronic device using high-density MoS2-graphene curved image sensor array. Nature Communications. 2017;**8**:1664. DOI: 10.1038/s41467-017-01824-6

[10] Yokota T, Zalar P, Kaltenbrunner M, Jinno H, Matsuhisa N, Kitanosako H, et al. Ultraflexible organic photonic skin. Science Advances. 2016;**2**. DOI: 10.1126/sciadv.1501856

[11] Park M, Park YJ, Chen X, Park Y-K, Kim M-S, Ahn J-H. MoS2-Based Tactile Sensor for Electronic Skin Applications. Advanced Materials. 2016;**28**:2556-2562. DOI: 10.1002/adma.201505124

[12] Chun S, Son W, Choi C, Min H, Kim J, Lee HJ, et al. Bioinspired Hairy Skin Electronics for Detecting the Direction and Incident Angle of Airflow. ACS Applied Materials & Interfaces. 2019;**11**:13608-13615. DOI: 10.1021/acsami.9b01427

[13] Mena-Bravo A, de Castro MDL. Sweat: A sample with limited present applications and promising future in metabolomics. Journal of Pharmaceutical and Biomedical Analysis. 2014;**90**:139-147. DOI: 10.1016/j.jpba.2013.10.048

[14] Calderon-Santiago M, Priego-Capote F, Turck N, Robin X, Jurado-Gamez B, Sanchez JC, et al. Human sweat metabolomics for lung cancer screening. Analytical and Bioanalytical Chemistry. 2015;**407**:5381-5392. DOI: 10.1007/s00216-015-8700-8

[15] Adewole OO, Erhabor GE, Adewole TO, Ojo AO, Oshokoya H,

Wolfe LM, et al. Proteomic profiling of eccrine sweat reveals its potential as a diagnostic biofluid for active tuberculosis. Proteomics Clinical Applications. 2016;**10**:547-553. DOI: 10.1002/prca.201500071

[16] Lim S, Shin J, Cho Y, Kim KP. Dietary Patterns Associated with Sebum Content, Skin Hydration and pH, and Their Sex-Dependent Differences in Healthy Korean Adults. Nutrients. 2019;**11**:12. DOI: 10.3390/nu11030619

[17] Heikenfeld J. Non-invasive Analyte Access and Sensing through Eccrine Sweat: Challenges and Outlook circa 2016. Electroanalysis. 2016;**28**:1242-1249. DOI: 10.1002/elan.201600018

[18] Hammond KB, Turcios NL, Gibson LE. Clinical evaluation of the macroduct sweat collection system and conductivity analyzer in the diagnosis of cystic fibrosis. The Journal of Pediatrics. 1994;**124**:255-260. DOI: 10.1016/S0022-3476(94)70314-0

[19] Bandodkar A. J., W. J. Jeang, R. Ghaffari, J. A. Rogers, in *Annual Review of Analytical Chemistry*, Vol. 12, 2019, 1-22.

[20] Lee KH, Scardaci V, Kim HY, Hallam T, Nolan H, Bolf BE, et al. Highly sensitive, transparent, and flexible gas sensors based on gold nanoparticle decorated carbon nanotubes. Sensors and Actuators B-Chemical. 2013;**188**:571-575. DOI: 10.1016/j.snb.2013.07.048

[21] Lee H, Song C, Hong YS, Kim MS, Cho HR, Kang T, et al. Wearable/disposable sweat-based glucose monitoring device with multistage transdermal drug delivery module. Science Advances. 2017;**3**:e1601314. DOI: 10.1126/sciadv.1601314

[22] Hui R., Chapter 4 - Photodetectors. In: R. Hui. Introduction to Fiber-Optic Communications, DOI: 10.1016/B978-0-12-805345-4.00004-4

[23] Simone G, Dyson MJ, Meskers SCJ, Janssen RAJ, Gelinck GH. Organic Photodetectors and their Application in Large Area and Flexible Image Sensors: The Role of Dark Current. Advanced Functional Materials. 2020;**30**:1904205. DOI: 10.1002/adfm.201904205

[24] Fujisaki Y, Nakajima Y, Takei T, Fukagawa H, Yamamoto T, Fujikake H. Flexible Active-Matrix Organic Light-Emitting Diode Display Using Air-Stable Organic Semiconductor of Dinaphtho 2, 3-b: 2 ', 3 '-f thieno 3, 2-b -thiophene. Ieee Transactions on Electron Devices. 2012;**59**:3442-3449. DOI: 10.1109/ted.2012.2220968

[25] Nakajima Y, Nakata M, Takei T, Fukagawa H, Motomura G, Tsuji H, et al. Development of 8-in. oxide-TFT-driven flexible AMOLED display using high-performance red phosphorescent OLED. Journal of the Society for Information Display. 2014;**22**:137-143. DOI: 10.1002/jsid.227

[26] Reineke S, Lindner F, Schwartz G, Seidler N, Walzer K, Lussem B, et al. White organic light-emitting diodes with fluorescent tube efficiency. Nature. 2009;**459**:234-U116. DOI: 10.1038/nature08003

[27] Uoyama H, Goushi K, Shizu K, Nomura H, Adachi C. Highly efficient organic light-emitting diodes from delayed fluorescence. Nature. 2012;**492**:234. DOI: 10.1038/nature11687

[28] Aizawa N, Pu YJ, Watanabe M, Chiba T, Ideta K, Toyota N, et al. Solution-processed multilayer small-molecule light-emitting devices with high-efficiency white-light emission. Nature Communications. 2014;**5**. DOI: 10.1038/ncomms6756

[29] Zhang QS, Li B, Huang SP, Nomura H, Tanaka H, Adachi C. Efficient blue organic light-emitting diodes employing thermally activated delayed fluorescence. Nature Photonics. 2014;**8**:326-332. DOI: 10.1038/nphoton.2014.12

[30] Udagawa K, Sasabe H, Cai C, Kido J. Low-Driving-Voltage Blue Phosphorescent Organic Light-Emitting Devices with External Quantum Efficiency of 30%. Advanced Materials. 2014;**26**:5062-5066. DOI: 10.1002/adma.201401621

[31] Burroughes JH, Bradley DDC, Brown AR, Marks RN, Mackay K, Friend RH, et al. Light-Emitting-Diodes Based on Conjugated Polymers. Nature. 1990;**347**:539-541. DOI: 10.1038/347539a0

[32] Gustafsson G, Cao Y, Treacy GM, Klavetter F, Colaneri N, Heeger AJ. Flexible Light-Emitting-Diodes Made from Soluble Conducting Polymers. Nature. 1992;**357**:477-479. DOI: 10.1038/357477a0

[33] Png RQ, Chia PJ, Tang JC, Liu B, Sivaramakrishnan S, Zhou M, et al. High-performance polymer semiconducting heterostructure devices by nitrene-mediated photocrosslinking of alkyl side chains. Nature Materials. 2010;**9**:152-158. DOI: 10.1038/nmat2594

[34] Liang JJ, Li L, Niu XF, Yu ZB, Pei QB. Elastomeric polymer light-emitting devices and displays. Nature Photonics. 2013;**7**:817-824. DOI: 10.1038/nphoton.2013.242

[35] Rauch T, Boberl M, Tedde SF, Furst J, Kovalenko MV, Hesser GN, et al. Near-infrared imaging with quantum-dot-sensitized organic photodiodes. Nature Photonics. 2009;**3**:332-336. DOI: 10.1038/nphoton.2009.72

[36] Gong X, Tong MH, Xia YJ, Cai WZ, Moon JS, Cao Y, et al. High-Detectivity Polymer Photodetectors with Spectral Response from 300 nm to 1450 nm. Science. 2009;**325**:1665-1667. DOI: 10.1126/science.1176706

[37] Baeg KJ, Binda M, Natali D, Caironi M, Noh YY. Organic Light Detectors: Photodiodes and Phototransistors. Advanced Materials. 2013;**25**:4267-4295. DOI: 10.1002/adma.201204979

[38] Park S, Kim SJ, Nam JH, Pitner G, Lee TH, Ayzner AL, et al. Significant Enhancement of Infrared Photodetector Sensitivity Using a Semiconducting Single-Walled Carbon Nanotube/C-60 Phototransistor. Advanced Materials. 2015;**27**:759-765. DOI: 10.1002/adma.201404544

[39] White MS, Kaltenbrunner M, Glowacki ED, Gutnichenko K, Kettlgruber G, Graz I, et al. Ultrathin, highly flexible and stretchable PLEDs. Nature Photonics. 2013;**7**:811-816. DOI: 10.1038/nphoton.2013.188

[40] Kaltenbrunner M, White MS, Glowacki ED, Sekitani T, Someya T, Sariciftci NS, et al. Ultrathin and lightweight organic solar cells with high flexibility. Nature Communications. 2012;**3**. DOI: 10.1038/ncomms1772

[41] Ng TN, Wong WS, Chabinyc ML, Sambandan S, Street RA. Flexible image sensor array with bulk heterojunction organic photodiode. Applied Physics Letters. 2008;**92**. DOI: 10.1063/1.2937018

[42] Liu D, Hong G. Wearable Electromechanical Sensors and Its Applications. In: Nasiri N, editor. Wearable Devices - the Big Wave of Innovation. IntechOpen. DOI: 10.5772/intechopen.85098

[43] Wearable Organic Nano-sensors. In: Flexible and Wearable

Electronics for Smart Clothing, DOI: 10.1002/9783527818556.ch1

[44] Boutry CM, Negre M, Jorda M, Vardoulis O, Chortos A, Khatib O, et al. A hierarchically patterned, bioinspired e-skin able to detect the direction of applied pressure for robotics. Science Robotics. 2018;**3**:9. DOI: 10.1126/scirobotics.aau6914

[45] Chortos A, Liu J, Bao ZA. Pursuing prosthetic electronic skin. Nature Materials. 2016;**15**:937-950. DOI: 10.1038/nmat4671

[46] Wang S. H., J. Xu, W. C. Wang, G. J. N. Wang, R. Rastak, F. Molina-Lopez, et al. Skin electronics from scalable fabrication of an intrinsically stretchable transistor array. Nature. 2018;**555**:83-+. DOI: 10.1038/nature25494

[47] Rim YS, Bae SH, Chen H, De Marco N, Yang Y. Recent Progress in Materials and Devices toward Printable and Flexible Sensors. Advanced Materials. 2016;**28**:4415-4440. DOI: 10.1002/adma.201505118

[48] Wang CF, Wang CH, Huang ZL, Xu S. Materials and Structures toward Soft Electronics. Advanced Materials. 2018;**30**:49. DOI: 10.1002/adma.201801368

[49] Choi S, Lee H, Ghaffari R, Hyeon T, Kim DH. Recent Advances in Flexible and Stretchable Bio-Electronic Devices Integrated with Nanomaterials. Advanced Materials. 2016;**28**:4203-4218. DOI: 10.1002/adma.201504150

[50] Rogers JA, Someya T, Huang YG. Materials and Mechanics for Stretchable Electronics. Science. 2010;**327**:1603-1607. DOI: 10.1126/science.1182383

[51] Choi S, Han SI, Kim D, Hyeon T, Kim DH. High-performance stretchable conductive nanocomposites: materials, processes, and device applications. Chemical Society Reviews. 2019;**48**:1566-1595. DOI: 10.1039/c8cs00706c

[52] Matsuhisa N, Chen XD, Bao ZA, Someya T. Materials and structural designs of stretchable conductors. Chemical Society Reviews. 2019;**48**:2946-2966. DOI: 10.1039/c8cs00814k

[53] Thune E., C. Strunk, Quantum Transport in Carbon Nanotubes. In: G. Cuniberti, K. Richter, G. Fagas. Introducing Molecular Electronics, DOI: 10.1007/3-540-31514-4_14

[54] Zhang P, Wyman I, Hu J, Lin S, Zhong Z, Tu Y, et al. Silver nanowires: Synthesis technologies, growth mechanism and multifunctional applications. Materials Science and Engineering: B. 2017;**223**:1-23. DOI: 10.1016/j.mseb.2017.05.002

[55] Wang C, Xia K, Wang H, Liang X, Yin Z, Zhang Y. Advanced Carbon for Flexible and Wearable Electronics. Advanced Materials. 2019;**31**:1801072. DOI: 10.1002/adma.201801072

[56] Chen K, Gao W, Emaminejad S, Kiriya D, Ota H, Nyein HYY, et al. Printed Carbon Nanotube Electronics and Sensor Systems. Advanced Materials. 2016;**28**:4397-4414. DOI: 10.1002/adma.201504958

[57] Jang H, Park YJ, Chen X, Das T, Kim MS, Ahn JH. Graphene-Based Flexible and Stretchable Electronics. Advanced Materials. 2016;**28**:4184-4202. DOI: 10.1002/adma.201504245

[58] Cohen DJ, Mitra D, Peterson K, Maharbiz MM. A Highly Elastic, Capacitive Strain Gauge Based on Percolating Nanotube Networks. Nano Letters. 2012;**12**:1821-1825. DOI: 10.1021/nl204052z

[59] Yang TT, Jiang X, Zhong YJ, Zhao XL, Lin SY, Li J, et al. A Wearable

and Highly Sensitive Graphene Strain Sensor for Precise Home-Based Pulse Wave Monitoring. Acs Sensors. 2017;**2**:967-974. DOI: 10.1021/acssensors.7b00230

[60] Liu Q, Chen J, Li YR, Shi GQ. High-Performance Strain Sensors with Fish-Scale-Like Graphene-Sensing Layers for Full-Range Detection of Human Motions. ACS Nano. 2016;**10**:7901-7906. DOI: 10.1021/acsnano.6b03813

[61] Ryu S, Lee P, Chou JB, Xu RZ, Zhao R, Hart AJ, et al. Extremely Elastic Wearable Carbon Nanotube Fiber Strain Sensor for Monitoring of Human Motion. ACS Nano. 2015;**9**:5929-5936. DOI: 10.1021/acsnano.5b00599

[62] Xu C, Yang Y, Gao W. Skin-Interfaced Sensors in Digital Medicine: from Materials to Applications. Matter. 2020;**2**:1414-1445. DOI: 10.1016/j.matt.2020.03.020

[63] Kaltenbrunner M, Sekitani T, Reeder J, Yokota T, Kuribara K, Tokuhara T, et al. An ultra-lightweight design for imperceptible plastic electronics. Nature. 2013;**499**:458-463. DOI: 10.1038/nature12314

[64] Wiley B, Sun YG, Mayers B, Xia YN. Shape-controlled synthesis of metal nanostructures: The case of silver. Chemistry-a European Journal. 2005;**11**:454-463. DOI: 10.1002/chem.200400927

[65] Xia YN, Xiong YJ, Lim B, Skrabalak SE. Shape-Controlled Synthesis of Metal Nanocrystals: Simple Chemistry Meets Complex Physics? Angewandte Chemie-International Edition. 2009;**48**:60-103. DOI: 10.1002/anie.200802248

[66] Xia YN, Xia XH, Peng HC. Shape-Controlled Synthesis of Colloidal Metal Nanocrystals: Thermodynamic versus Kinetic Products. Journal of the American Chemical Society. 2015;**137**:7947-7966. DOI: 10.1021/jacs.5b04641

[67] Sau TK, Rogach AL, Jackel F, Klar TA, Feldmann J. Properties and Applications of Colloidal Nonspherical Noble Metal Nanoparticles. Advanced Materials. 2010;**22**:1805-1825. DOI: 10.1002/adma.200902557

[68] Peng X, Dong K, Ye CY, Jiang Y, Zhai SY, Cheng RW, et al. A breathable, biodegradable, antibacterial, and self-powered electronic skin based on all-nanofiber triboelectric nanogenerators. Science Advances. 2020;**6**:10. DOI: 10.1126/sciadv.aba9624

[69] Trung TQ, Lee N-E. Recent Progress on Stretchable Electronic Devices with Intrinsically Stretchable Components. Advanced Materials. 2017;**29**:1603167. DOI: 10.1002/adma.201603167

[70] Liang JJ, Li L, Chen D, Hajagos T, Ren Z, Chou SY, et al. Intrinsically stretchable and transparent thin-film transistors based on printable silver nanowires, carbon nanotubes and an elastomeric dielectric. Nature Communications. 2015;**6**:10. DOI: 10.1038/ncomms8647

[71] Kim HJ, Sim K, Thukral A, Yu CJ. Rubbery electronics and sensors from intrinsically stretchable elastomeric composites of semiconductors and conductors. Science Advances. 2017;**3**:8. DOI: 10.1126/sciadv.1701114

[72] Ershad F, Thukral A, Yue JP, Comeaux P, Lu YT, Shim H, et al. Ultra-conformal drawn-on-skin electronics for multifunctional motion artifact-free sensing and point-of-care treatment. Nature Communications. 2020;**11**:13. DOI: 10.1038/s41467-020-17619-1

[73] Joo H, Jung D, Sunwoo S-H, Koo JH, Kim D-H. Material Design and Fabrication Strategies for Stretchable Metallic Nanocomposites. Small.

2020;**16**:1906270. DOI: 10.1002/smll.201906270

[74] Garnett EC, Cai WS, Cha JJ, Mahmood F, Connor ST, Christoforo MG, et al. Self-limited plasmonic welding of silver nanowire junctions. Nature Materials. 2012;**11**:241-249. DOI: 10.1038/nmat3238

[75] Matsuhisa N, Kaltenbrunner M, Yokota T, Jinno H, Kuribara K, Sekitani T, et al. Printable elastic conductors with a high conductivity for electronic textile applications. Nature Communications. 2015;**6**:11. DOI: 10.1038/ncomms8461

[76] Zhang YH, Fu HR, Su YW, Xu S, Cheng HY, Fan JA, et al. Mechanics of ultra-stretchable self-similar serpentine interconnects. Acta Materialia. 2013;**61**:7816-7827. DOI: 10.1016/j.actamat.2013.09.020

[77] Zhang YH, Huang YG, Rogers JA. Mechanics of stretchable batteries and supercapacitors. Current Opinion in Solid State & Materials Science. 2015;**19**:190-199. DOI: 10.1016/j.cossms.2015.01.002

[78] Lu CF, Li M, Xiao JL, Jung I, Wu J, Huang YG, et al. Mechanics of Tunable Hemispherical Electronic Eye Camera Systems That Combine Rigid Device Elements With Soft Elastomers. Journal of Applied Mechanics-Transactions of the Asme. 2013:**80**. DOI: 10.1115/1.4023962

[79] Su YW, Liu ZJ, Wang SD, Ghaffari R, Kim DH, Hwang KC, et al. Mechanics of stretchable electronics on balloon catheter under extreme deformation. International Journal of Solids and Structures. 2014;**51**:1555-1561. DOI: 10.1016/j.ijsolstr.2014.01.008

[80] Shi XT, Xu RX, Li YH, Zhang YH, Ren ZG, Gu JF, et al. Mechanics Design for Stretchable, High Areal Coverage GaAs Solar Module on an Ultrathin Substrate. Journal of Applied Mechanics-Transactions of the. Asme. 2014;**81**. DOI: 10.1115/1.4028977

[81] Gao L, Zhang YH, Zhang H, Doshay S, Xie X, Luo HY, et al. Optics and Nonlinear Buckling Mechanics in Large-Area, Highly Stretchable Arrays of Plasmonic Nano structures. ACS Nano. 2015;**9**:5968-5975. DOI: 10.1021/acsnano.5b00716

[82] Ma Q, Cheng HY, Jang KI, Luan HW, Hwang KC, Rogers JA, et al. A nonlinear mechanics model of bio-inspired hierarchical lattice materials consisting of horseshoe microstructures. Journal of the Mechanics and Physics of Solids. 2016;**90**:179-202. DOI: 10.1016/j.jmps.2016.02.012

[83] Yuan JH, Shi Y, Pharr M, Feng X, Rogers JA, Huang YG. A Mechanics Model for Sensors Imperfectly Bonded to the Skin for Determination of the Young's Moduli of Epidermis and Dermis. Journal of Applied Mechanics-Transactions of the. Asme. 2016;**83**. DOI: 10.1115/1.4033650

[84] Su YW, Ping XC, Yu KJ, Lee JW, Fan JA, Wang B, et al. In-Plane Deformation Mechanics for Highly Stretchable Electronics. Advanced Materials. 2017:**29**. DOI: 10.1002/adma.201604989

[85] Byun SH, Sim JY, Zhou ZA, Lee J, Qazi R, Walicki MC, et al. Mechanically transformative electronics, sensors, and implantable devices. Science Advances. 2019;**5**. DOI: 10.1126/sciadv.aay0418

[86] Zhao YL, Xing GM, Nanotoxicology ZFC. Are carbon nanotubes safe? Nature Nanotechnology. 2008;**3**:191-192. DOI: 10.1038/nnano.2008.77

[87] Maynard AD. Are we ready for spray-on carbon nanotubes? Nature Nanotechnology. 2016;**11**:490-491. DOI: 10.1038/nnano.2016.99

[88] Liu YX, Liu J, Chen SC, Lei T, Kim Y, Niu SM, et al. Soft and elastic hydrogel-based microelectronics for localized low-voltage neuromodulation. Nature Biomedical Engineering. 2019;**3**:58-68. DOI: 10.1038/s41551-018-0335-6

[89] Cao Y, Morrissey TG, Acome E, Allec SI, Wong BM, Keplinger C, et al. A Transparent, Self-Healing, Highly Stretchable Ionic Conductor. Advanced Materials. 2017;**29**:9. DOI: 10.1002/adma.201605099

[90] Annabi N, Tamayol A, Uquillas JA, Akbari M, Bertassoni LE, Cha C, et al. 25th Anniversary Article: Rational Design and Applications of Hydrogels in Regenerative Medicine. Advanced Materials. 2014;**26**:85-124. DOI: 10.1002/adma.201303233

[91] Sun JY, Zhao XH, Illeperuma WRK, Chaudhuri O, Oh KH, Mooney DJ, et al. Highly stretchable and tough hydrogels. Nature. 2012;**489**:133-136. DOI: 10.1038/nature11409

[92] Sun TL, Kurokawa T, Kuroda S, Bin Ihsan A, Akasaki T, Sato K, et al. Physical hydrogels composed of polyampholytes demonstrate high toughness and viscoelasticity. Nature Materials. 2013;**12**:932-937. DOI: 10.1038/nmat3713

[93] Bin Imran A, Esaki K, Gotoh H, Seki T, Ito K, Sakai Y, et al. Extremely stretchable thermosensitive hydrogels by introducing slide-ring polyrotaxane cross-linkers and ionic groups into the polymer network. Nature Communications. 2014;**5**. DOI: 10.1038/ncomms6124

[94] Yuk H., T. Zhang, S. T. Lin, G. A. Parada, X. H. Zhao. Tough bonding of hydrogels to diverse non-porous surfaces. Nature Materials. 2016;**15**:190-+. DOI: 10.1038/nmat4463

[95] Yu Y, Yuk H, Parada GA, Wu Y, Liu XY, Nabzdyk CS, et al. Multifunctional "Hydrogel Skins" on Diverse Polymers with Arbitrary Shapes. Advanced Materials. 2019;**31**(9). DOI: 10.1002/adma.201807101

[96] Yuk H., C. E. Varela, C. S. Nabzdyk, X. Y. Mao, R. F. Padera, E. T. Roche, et al. Dry double-sided tape for adhesion of wet tissues and devices. Nature. 2019;**575**:169-+. DOI: 10.1038/s41586-019-1710-5

[97] Huang Y, Fan X, Chen S-C, Zhao N. Emerging Technologies of Flexible Pressure Sensors: Materials, Modeling, Devices, and Manufacturing. Advanced Functional Materials. 2019;**29**:1808509. DOI: 10.1002/adfm.201808509

[98] Lin MF, Xiong JQ, Wang JX, Parida K, Lee PS. Core-shell nanofiber mats for tactile pressure sensor and nanogenerator applications. Nano Energy. 2018;**44**:248-255. DOI: 10.1016/j.nanoen.2017.12.004

[99] Wang NX, Yang AN, Fu Y, Li YZ, Yan F. Functionalized Organic Thin Film Transistors for Biosensing. Accounts of Chemical Research. 2019;**52**:277-287. DOI: 10.1021/acs.accounts.8b00448

[100] Gualandi I, Marzocchi M, Achilli A, Cavedale D, Bonfiglio A, Fraboni B. Textile Organic Electrochemical Transistors as a Platform for Wearable Biosensors. Scientific Reports. 2016;**6**:10. DOI: 10.1038/srep33637

[101] Park S, Fukuda K, Wang M, Lee C, Yokota T, Jin H, et al. Ultraflexible Near-Infrared Organic Photodetectors for Conformal Photoplethysmogram Sensors. Advanced Materials. 2018;**30**:8. DOI: 10.1002/adma.201802359

[102] Imani S, Bandodkar AJ, Mohan AMV, Kumar R, Yu SF, Wang J, et al. A wearable chemical-electrophysiological hybrid biosensing system for real-time health and fitness monitoring. Nature Communications. 2016;**7**(7). DOI: 10.1038/ncomms11650

[103] Nightingale AM, Leong CL, Burnish RA, Hassan SU, Zhang Y, Clough GF, et al. Monitoring biomolecule concentrations in tissue using a wearable droplet microfluidic-based sensor. Nature Communications. 2019;**10**:12. DOI: 10.1038/s41467-019-10401-y

[104] Ding Y-R, Xue C-H, Fan Q-Q, Zhao L-L, Tian Q-Q, Guo X-J, et al. Fabrication of superhydrophobic conductive film at air/water interface for flexible and wearable sensors. Chemical Engineering Journal. 2021;**404**:126489. DOI: 10.1016/j.cej.2020.126489

[105] Chung S, Cho K, Lee T. Recent Progress in Inkjet-Printed Thin-Film Transistors. Advanced Science. 2019;**6**:27. DOI: 10.1002/advs.201801445

[106] Ma S, Ribeiro F, Powell K, Lutian J, Møller C, Large T, et al. Fabrication of Novel Transparent Touch Sensing Device via Drop-on-Demand Inkjet Printing Technique. ACS Applied Materials & Interfaces. 2015;**7**:21628-21633. DOI: 10.1021/acsami.5b04717

[107] Minemawari H, Yamada T, Matsui H, Tsutsumi J, Haas S, Chiba R, et al. Inkjet printing of single-crystal films. Nature. 2011;**475**:364-367. DOI: 10.1038/nature10313

[108] Wu CS, Tetik H, Cheng J, Ding WB, Guo HY, Tao XT, et al. Electrohydrodynamic Jet Printing Driven by a Triboelectric Nanogenerator. Advanced Functional Materials. 2019;**29**:8. DOI: 10.1002/adfm.201901102

[109] Lee CH, Kim DR, Zheng X. Fabricating nanowire devices on diverse substrates by simple transfer-printing methods. Proceedings of the National Academy of Sciences. 2010. DOI: 10.1073/pnas.0914031107

[110] Xu X, Zhou X, Zhou K, Xia Y, Ma W, Inganäs O. Large-Area, Semitransparent, and Flexible All-Polymer Photodetectors. Advanced Functional Materials. 2018;**28**:1805570. DOI: 10.1002/adfm.201805570

Section 3

Mathematical Assessment on Biosensors

Chapter 6

Ultra-Precise MEMS Based Bio-Sensors

Vinayak Pachkawade

Abstract

This chapter evaluated the state-of-the art MEMS sensors used for bio sensing applications. A new class of resonant micro sensor is studied. A sensor structure based on the array of weakly coupled resonators is presented. It is shown that due to the weak coupling employed between the resonators in an array manifest ultra-high sensitivity of the output to the added analytes/biomolecules. Due to the highly-precise output of such bio-sensors, minimum detectable mass in the range of sub-actogram is also possible using such MEMS sensors. Analytical modeling of such micro biosensors is presented in this chapter to understand the key performance parameters. Furthermore, role of these new classes of MEMS resonant biosensors operating at ambient temperature and/or pressure is also discussed.

Keywords: MEMS biosensor, bioelectronics, micro sensors for biological applications, biochemical analyte detection and identification using MEMS

1. Introduction

In recent years, there has been a growing interest in the development and implementation of innovative solutions in the form of a miniaturized bio-sensors. In this regard, in the MEMS community emphasis has been given to design and fabricate highly sensitive, and precise biomass sensors. These bio-sensors are used for detection, identification and measurement of either single and/or multi-analyte/s at lower cost, size, weight, and power consumption. Moreover, resonant devices are widely popular as a sensor for various chemical/biological applications [1]. In the context of biomass sensing, typical examples of resonant sensing include mass identification or detection [2–7]. A key attribute of these sensors is that the output signal is the variation/shift in the resonant frequency (Δf) of a vibrating structure that is subjected to small perturbations in the structural parameters i.e. effective mass/stiffness. Additional features of this method of detection are simple mechanical design, semi-digital nature of the signal (thus using simple frequency measurement system such as frequency counter and not requiring additional analog-to-digital (A/D) conversion circuit), ultra-high resolution [8–10], (up to 10^{-15} grams scale [11–13] and up to 10^{-18} grams scale [14–17]). There are however also a challenge associated with the resonant sensor employing only one resonator; firstly, maximum theoretical frequency shift based parametric sensitivity, $\Delta f/f$ is limited to 1/2 [18]. Sensors of these types are prone to environmental shifts such as pressure and/or temperature. Furthermore, these types of sensors, when used as a mass sensor are able to detect only one type of material (target analyte) at a time thus

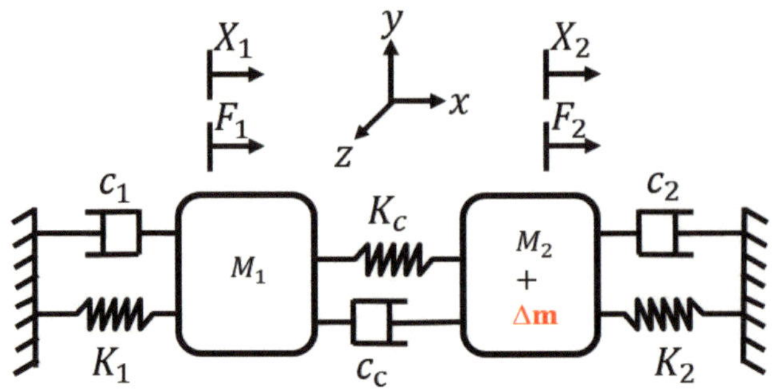

Figure 1.
A schematic representation of a 2-DoF coupled resonant mass-spring-damper system to be used as a high-sensitivity biomass detector/identifier sensor. In a symmetric design, it is assumed that $M_1 = M_2 = M$, $K_1 = K_2 = K$. *A mass perturbation,* Δm *is added onto the mass* M_2*, causing system imbalance, leading to the energy localization/confinement and mode shape change. Mode-shape change is utilized as the output of the sensor.*

avoiding the possibility to rapidly detect and differentiate multiple biochemical analytes in parallel [19].

In the past few years, in the MEMS community, a paradigm shift is observed in the design and implementation of micromechanical resonating sensors. A new perspective is presented in using *1-d* chain of a coupled resonating proof masses, more familiarly refereed as multi degree-of-freedom (m-DoF) array, coupled resonator (CR) array, weakly coupled resonators (WCR) or mode-localized sensors [20–28]. **Figure 1** shows a representative schematic for such system. In this class of a sensors, coupling between the vibrating proof masses is constituted either electrostatically or mechanically. These sensors attribute an ultra-high parametric sensitivity (up to three to four orders high in magnitude) [29]. Such elevated levels of sensitivities are manifested via a novel transduction principle, i.e. sensing magnitude of vibrational energy exchange between the moving proof masses that are subject to a small disruption introduced into the system. This disruption serves to alter an effective mass, Δm of one of the proof mass element in a chain (see **Figure 1**). Primarily, due to relatively higher parametric sensitivities, m-DoF coupled resonators are emerging as an alternative and promising resonant sensing solution.

Other acknowledged advantages of weakly-coupled resonating sensors are linearity (attributed to high sensitivity, relative immunity against responding to common mode noise for example, ambient pressure and/or temperature [30–32] and the parallel detection capability in the context of the mass sensing applications [33–36]. These characteristics make mode-localized coupled resonators effective. For the obvious advantages as given, m-DoF coupled resonant sensors are being pursued over conventional method of resonant sensing, i.e. sensing the frequency shift, Δf of a single resonating device.

2. Theory

A viable method to understand the operation of the mode-localized CR is its analysis through the transfer function model. The transfer function analysis enables to understand the system-level behavior of a biosensor unit. **Figure 1** shows a lumped parameter model of a 2 DoF mass-spring-damper system in the context of CR biosensor. It shows proof masses, M_i, mechanical spring constant, K_i and the damping coefficients, c_i, (i = 1, 2). The c_c models the damping force between the two resonating proof masses. Two proof masses are coupled through another spring, K_c as shown. A displacement of the proof mass, x_i (i = 1, 2) in response to the applied force, F_i (i = 1, 2) is also indicated. Based on the free body diagram, a set of governing differential equations of motion for 2-DoF mass-spring-damper can be used to derive the theoretical transfer function. Subsequently, an expressions for mode-frequencies, ω_i and modal amplitudes/amplitude ratio (AR) as a function of applied disorder in the mass, δ_m can be obtained.

Following assumptions hold true for a symmetric device- $M_1 = M_2 = M$, $K_1 = K_2 = K$ and $c_1 = c_2 = c$. Forcing vectors F_i acting on the proof masses are the harmonic excitation (drive) forces that cause displacements, x_i, assumed to occur at one frequency. Quantities δ_m and κ are normalized perturbation to the mass and normalized coupling factor, given as $\delta_m = \Delta m/M$ and $\kappa = K_c/K$, respectively. When system experiences imbalance into the initial symmetry *i.e.*, $\Delta m \neq 0$, governing set of equations of motion for the two-coupled proof masses is given as follows:

$$M\ddot{x}_1 + (c + c_c)\dot{x}_1 + (K + K_c)x_1 - c\dot{x}_2 - K_c x_2 = F_1(t) \tag{1}$$

$$(M + \Delta m)\ddot{x}_2 + (c + c_c)\dot{x}_2 + (K + K_c)x_2 - c\dot{x}_1 - K_c x_1 = F_2(t) \tag{2}$$

By operating the system in vacuum, the impact of the following can be reduced, i) damping force of individual proof mass and ii) damping force that occurs between two proof masses, hence $c_1 = c_2 = c_c = 0$ can be assumed for the simplified analysis. Therefore, (1) and (2) can be modified as below:

$$M\ddot{x}_1 + (K + K_c)x_1 - K_c x_2 = F_1(t) \tag{3}$$

$$(M + \Delta m)\ddot{x}_2 + (K + K_c)x_2 - K_c x_1 = F_2(t) \tag{4}$$

By applying a Laplace Transform to Eqs. (3) and (4), following expressions are obtained:

$$G_{11}(s)X_1(s) - G_{12}(s)X_2(s) = F_1(s) \tag{5}$$

$$G_{22}(s)X_2(s) - G_{21}(s)X_1(s) = F_2(s), \tag{6}$$

where

$$G_{11}(s) = s^2 M + (K + K_c) \tag{7}$$

$$G_{12}(s) = G_{21}(s) = K_c \tag{8}$$

$$G_{22}(s) = s^2(M + \Delta m) + (K + K_c) \tag{9}$$

In Eq. (6), set $F_2(s) = 0$, and derive an expression for $X_1(s)$ and $X_2(s)$ to use these values back in Eq. (5). An output transfer function is then obtained as follows:

$$G_1(s) = \frac{X_1(s)}{F_1(s)} = \frac{G_{22}(s)}{G_{11}(s)G_{22}(s) - G_{12}(s)G_{21}(s)} \tag{10}$$

$$G_2(s) = \frac{X_2(s)}{F_1(s)} = \frac{G_{21}(s)}{G_{11}(s)G_{22}(s) - G_{12}(s)G_{21}(s)} \tag{11}$$

Similar procedure can be applied to obtain an expression for $G_3(s) = \frac{X_1(s)}{F_2(s)}$ and $G_4(s) = \frac{X_2(s)}{F_2(s)}$. Using the values of $G_{11}(s)$, $G_{12}(s)$ $G_{21}(s)$ and $G_{22}(s)$ derived earlier in Eq. (7) through (9), following equations are obtained

$$G_1(s) = \frac{X_1(s)}{F_1(s)} = \frac{s^2(M + \Delta m) + K_\alpha}{s^4 M(M + \Delta m) + s^2 K_\alpha[M + (M + \Delta m)] + K_\alpha^2 - K_c^2} \quad (12)$$

$$G_2(s) = \frac{X_2(s)}{F_1(s)} = \frac{K_c}{s^4 M(M + \Delta m) + s^2 K_\alpha[M + (M + \Delta m)] + K_\alpha^2 - K_c^2} \quad (13)$$

Here $K_\alpha = (K + K_c)$. Using $s = j\omega$, Eqs. (12) and (13) can be modified to attain

$$G_1(j\omega) = \frac{X_1(j\omega)}{F_1(j\omega)} = \frac{-\omega^2(M + \Delta m) + K_\alpha}{\omega^4 M(M + \Delta m) - \omega^2 K_\alpha(2M + \Delta m) + K_\alpha^2 - K_c^2} \quad (14)$$

$$G_2(j\omega) = \frac{X_2(j\omega)}{F_1(j\omega)} = \frac{K_c}{\omega^4 M(M + \Delta m) - \omega^2 K_\alpha(2M + \Delta m) + K_\alpha^2 - K_c^2} \quad (15)$$

A denominator of Eqs. (14) and (15) is given by

$$\omega^4 M(M + \Delta m) - \omega^2 K_\alpha(2M + \Delta m) + K_\alpha^2 - K_c^2 = 0 \quad (16)$$

Eq. (16) is the characteristic equation of 2 DoF coupled system. Roots of Eq. (16) can be given as

$$\omega_{ip}^2 \approx \frac{K_\alpha(2M + \Delta m) - \sqrt{\Delta m^2 K_\alpha^2 M^2 + 4K_c^2(M^2 + \Delta m)}}{2M^2} \quad (17)$$

$$\omega_{op}^2 \approx \frac{K_\alpha(2M + \Delta m) + \sqrt{\Delta m^2 K_\alpha^2 M^2 + 4K_c^2(M^2 + \Delta m)}}{2M^2} \quad (18)$$

Here, ω_{ip}^2 and ω_{op}^2 are in-phase and out-of-phase natural mode frequencies of the device. With $\Delta m = 0$, Eqs. (17) and (18) take the form $\omega_{ip}^2 = \frac{K}{M}$ and $\omega_{op}^2 = \frac{K+2K_c}{M}$. Dividing (14) by (15), amplitude ratio (AR) is obtained as

$$\frac{H_1(j\omega)}{H_2(j\omega)} = \frac{-\omega^2(M + \Delta m) + K_\alpha}{K_c} \quad (19)$$

By substituting the values of ω in Eq. (19), the expression for mode AR as a function of mass perturbation, Δm is obtained as follows:

$$\frac{H_1(j\omega_{ip})}{H_2(j\omega_{ip})} = \frac{-\left(\frac{K(2M+\Delta m) - \sqrt{\Delta m^2 K_\alpha^2 M^2 + 4K_c^2(M^2+\Delta m)}}{2M^2}\right)(M + \Delta m) + K_\alpha}{K_c} \quad (20)$$

$$\frac{H_1(j\omega_{ip})}{H_2(j\omega_{ip})} = \frac{-\left(\frac{K(2M+\Delta m) + \sqrt{\Delta m^2 K_\alpha^2 M^2 + 4K_c^2(M^2+\Delta m)}}{2M^2}\right)(M + \Delta m) + K_\alpha}{K_c} \quad (21)$$

With $\Delta m = 0$, Eq. (20) and (21) take the form as

$$\frac{H_1(j\omega_{ip})}{H_2(j\omega_{ip})} = 1; \frac{H_1(j\omega_{op})}{H_2(j\omega_{op})} = -1 \quad (22)$$

Eq. (22) represents initial balanced condition of a two CR.

2.1 Analytical models

Figure 2 represents the analytical plots of the 2-DoF CR sensor system. In **Figure 2(a)**, mode-frequencies as a function of induced mass disorder is shown. Lower resonant frequency of the out-of-phase mode indicates that a design uses an electrical coupling between the two resonators. With $\delta_m = 0$, two resonant frequencies are closely spaced apart (frequency separation determined by the value of the coupling spring constant, *Kc* used in the system). However, when $\delta_m \neq 0$, resonant mode-frequencies veer away from each other as the magnitude of the δ_m is increased. In **Figure 2(b)**, similar trend can be observed, where, amplitude ratio (AR) as a function of induced mass disorder is shown. Slopes of the curves in each graphs determine the sensitivity of mode-frequencies and AR to the normalized mass perturbation into the system. The theoretical sensitivity norms (in the context of the mass perturbations, Δm) for the amplitude ratio (AR), eigenstate and the resonant frequency used in CR sensors are expressed as below:

$$\left(\frac{x1}{x2}\right)_{ji} = \left|\frac{r_n - r_0}{r_0}\right| \approx \left|\frac{\Delta m}{2K_c}\right| \tag{23}$$

$$(x)_{ji} = \frac{|a_n - a_0|}{|a_0|} \approx \left|\frac{\Delta m}{4K_c}\right| \tag{24}$$

$$\left(f_{ji}\right) = \frac{|f_n - f_0|}{|f_0|} \approx \left|\frac{\Delta m}{2m_{eff}}\right| \tag{25}$$

for j^{th} resonator (j = 1, 2) at i^{th} mode of the frequency response (i = 1, 2), respectively. For the electrostatic coupling between the two resonators, an effective value of the coupling spring is given by $K_c = -(\Delta v^2)\frac{\varepsilon_0 A}{g^3}$, where Δv refers the potential difference between the two masses, g is capacitive gap, ε is permittivity and A is the cross sectional area of the parallel-plate capacitor.

Figure 3 shows a plot of AR variation as a function of mass perturbation. Two different values of coupling spring, K_c are used. For lower effective value of the coupling spring, K_c = 100 *N/m*, (coupling factor, κ = 0.00075), higher changes in the AR can be extracted (relatively higher slope). This aspect shows the tunable characteristic of a sensitivity in a CR biosensor unit. In **Figure 4**, different forms of the

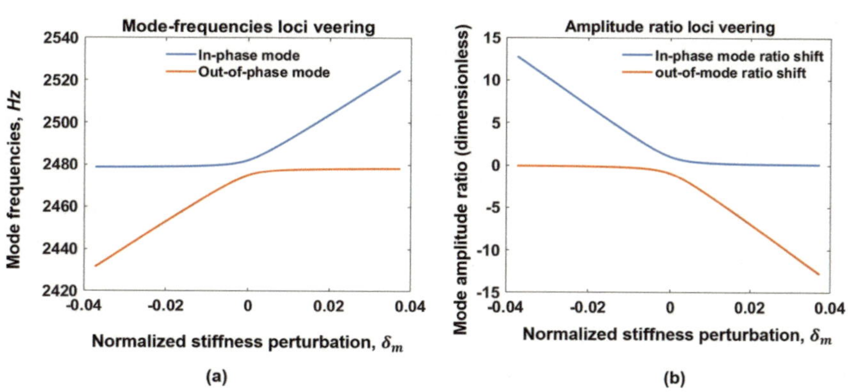

Figure 2.
Mode-frequencies and AR veering phenomenon observed in CR mode-localized mass sensors. δ_m *is the applied normalized mass perturbation. Slope of the AR curves determined the sensitivity. Lower value of the coupling spring,* K_c *enhances sensitivity to the mass perturbation for the AR output.*

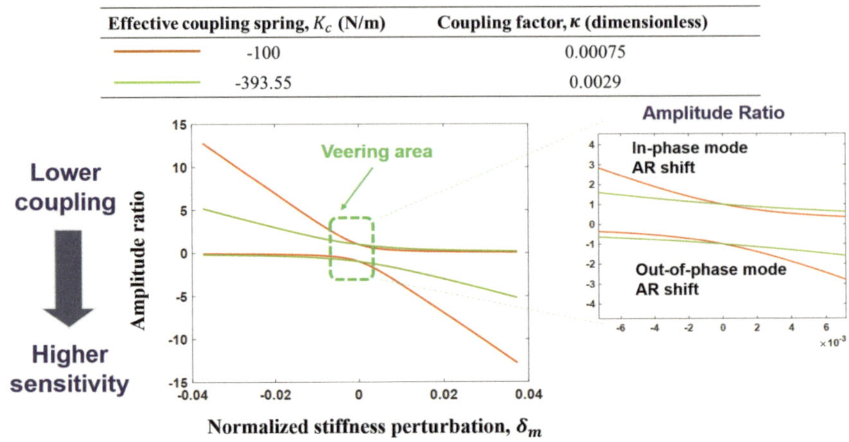

Figure 3.
Amplitude ratio (AR) curve veering in 2-DoF mode-localized coupled resonators mass sensors. The lower coupling factor κ leads to higher changes in the AR when the normalized perturbation δ_m is applied.

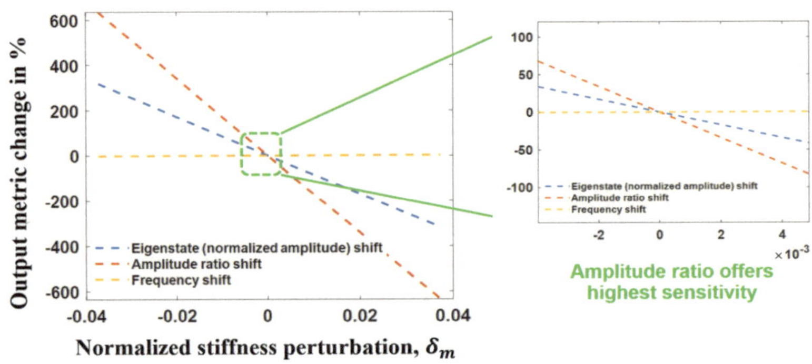

Figure 4.
Different types of the outputs with coupled resonators (CR) sensors. The amplitude ratio (AR) shift shows the highest percentage changes as a function of the mass perturbation, δ_m.

outputs (as expressed in (23) through (25)) are compared against the values of applied mass perturbations in a 2-DoF CR sensor system. As seen, the AR output offers the highest achievable sensitivity. Therefore, AR sensing is the preferred method of the sensing in CR biosensor system. It can be written that $S_{R_i} > S_{a_i} \gg S_{f_i}$. Here, S_{R_i}, $S_{a_{ji}}$ and S_{f_i} denote the *theoretical maximum sensitivity* for AR, amplitude and frequency for j^{th} resonator (j = 1, 2) at the ith mode of the frequency response (i = 1, 2), respectively. Another way to understand the operation of a 2-DoF CR biosensor is through its output frequency response. **Figure 5** shows an output response of resonator 1 and 2 in a 2-DoF coupled resonant (CR) mass biosensor system. As two resonators are used in the CR system, two peaks appear in the output response. Initially, assuming a symmetric system (i.e. $M_1 = M_2 = M$, $K_1 = K_2 = K$), j^{th} resonator (j = 1, 2) vibrate with equal amplitudes at the ith mode (i = 1, 2) of the output response. After the mass disorder, δ_m is introduced, it is observed that vibration amplitudes of the jth resonator (j = 1, 2) at the ith mode (i = 1, 2) of the output response change. An amplitude shift is denoted by Δ_a. The frequency shift, Δf at both the modes is also seen. After the mass perturbation, for the resonator 1, vibration amplitude is seen decreased at the first mode, whereas amplitude is seen increased at the second mode.

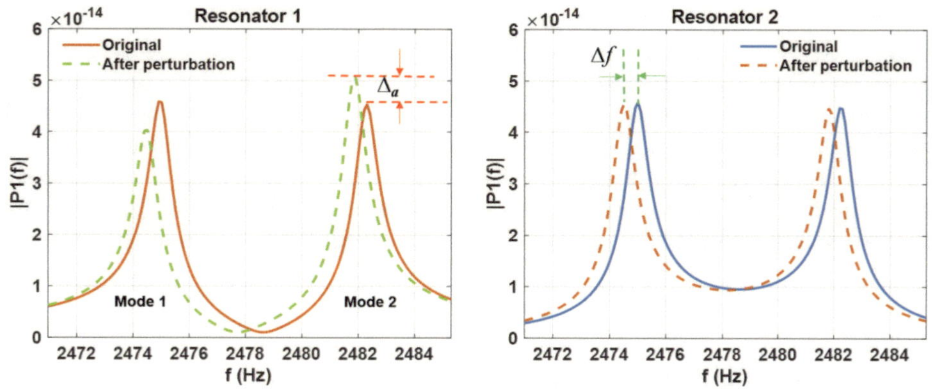

Figure 5.
The output response of a 2-DoF coupled resonator mode-localized design used for biomass sensing applications. Due to the mass addition or removal process, initial eigenmodes and eigen-frequencies of the jth resonator (j = 1, 2) change due to the mode-localization. Changes in the amplitudes, Δ_a are found to be 2 to 3 orders high in magnitude than that of the corresponding changes into the frequencies, Δf at the ith mode (i = 1, 2) of the output response.

2.2 Frequency response and a finite element model (FEM)

Figure 6(a) shows a frequency response (bode diagram) of a 2-DoF CR system. **Figure 6(b)** shows a COMSOL mode shape simulation for a designed geometry of a two mechanically coupled resonators. A structural mechanics module of COMSOL Multiphysics [37] can be used to design CR sensor and simulate for the mode shape

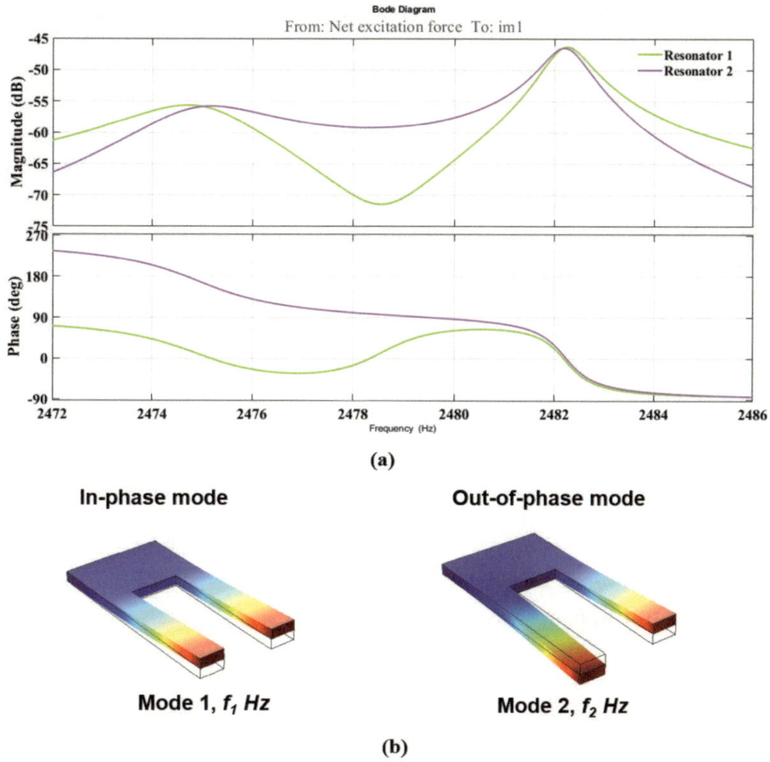

Figure 6.
Output frequency response (bode diagram) of the CR sensor showing the two modes of a 2-DoF sensor. A finite element model is also depicted to determine the mode shape and resonant frequencies of the design. Note the swapping of the two modes as per the coupling used in the sensor.

and eigen-frequencies of the design. As seen from the FEM results, for mode 1, vibrating elements (cantilevers) move in the same direction (in-phase mode) and the same amplitudes [1, 1]. For mode 2, both the cantilevers move in opposite direction (out-of-phase mode) and the same amplitudes [1,-1]. The two simulated mode frequencies are f_1 and f_2 for mode 1 (in-phase) and mode 2 (out-of-phase), respectively. As the FEM illustrates, the coupling used in the design is mechanical. If the coupling used in the design is electrical, out-of-phase mode precedes the in-phase mode as seen in the bode diagram (note the phase difference of the two resonators).

3. Case studies in m-DoF resonant mass sensing

In this section, different types of MEMS ultra-precise sensors based on the m-DoF CR architecture are discussed. In MEMS resonant biosensors, a surface of the micromechanical resonator is coated with a sensitive thin film. A resonant frequency shift is monitored as a result of adsorption/absorption of the target analyte/s [19]. In the same framework, CR structures are used as a mass sensors owing to the enhanced mass sensitivity and parallel monitoring of multiple analyte/s.

3.1 Study I

For the first time, it was proposed that a vibration mode localization can be used to demonstrate an elevated mass sensitivity [36]. A fabricated prototype is shown in **Figure 7(a)**. In this work, two nearly identical mechanically coupled gold-foil microcantilevers were used. For the experimentation, borosilicate microspheres (mean diameter of 4.9 μm with a mass of $\approx$154 pg were added on cantilever 2. Piezoelectric shaker was used for the driving scheme for the sensor. A laser doppler vibrometer was used to capture the tip velocities at different locations of individual cantilevers. An output plot as seen in **Figure 7(b)** was obtained to show eigenstate variation as a function of normalized mass perturbation, δ_m. With Δm = 0, vibration amplitudes of cantilevers 1 and 2 at two mode frequencies (i.e. two distinct modes as in-phase and out-of-phase) are seen. Uneven amplitudes for both the cantilevers at both the modes are result of fabrication mismatch. With $\Delta m \neq 0$, vibration amplitudes of both the cantilevers change at both the modes. With mass added to cantilever 2, amplitudes of both the resonators at both the modes are seen to be increased. Amplitude of resonator 1 is relatively higher than amplitude of resonator 2 at the first mode (at lower frequency in the response). Amplitude of resonator 2 is relatively higher than amplitude of resonator 1 at the second mode (at the higher frequency in the response). A relatively larger shift (either in amplitude or resonant frequency) indicates vibration energy is localized to that particular cantilever at the mode of operation. With a mass differential (Δm) in the system, resonant frequencies of both the cantilevers at both the modes also change. However, relative changes in the amplitudes are orders of magnitude higher than the changes in frequencies. This work experimentally demonstrated about two orders higher in magnitude relative changes into the eigenstates (5–7%) than relative changes in the frequencies (0.01%). Enhanced sensitivity of eigenstates to the added mass was attributed to the decreased scaled coupling strength, κ between the two cantilevers. Each eigenstate is the normalized vector formed by the amplitudes of the two vibrating elements (cantilevers) at a corresponding resonance frequency. In the same work, mass removal from the cantilever surface resulted in return of eigenstates to their original values.

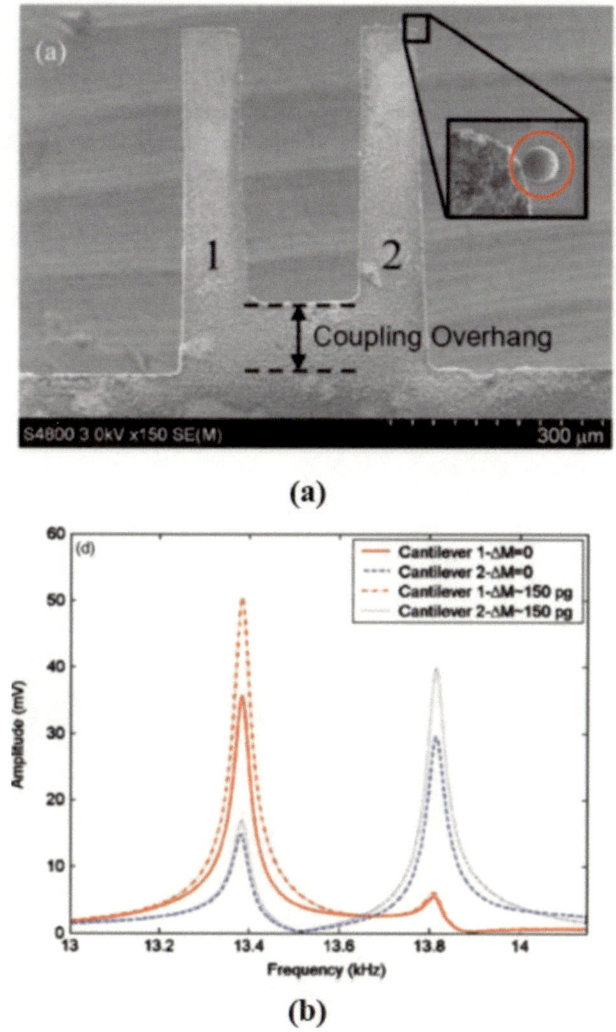

Figure 7.
Ultrasensitive mass sensor using a mode localization in coupled microcantilevers (a) fabricated prototype and (b) amplitude-frequency response of a fabricated prototype before and after the mass imbalance introduced into the system [33]. Reprinted from [33] with the permission of AIP Publishing.

3.2 Study II

Moreover, using an array of polysilicon microcantilevers (up to 15) it is possible to record up to 3 orders higher changes in eigenstate based output of the sensor [35]. In an array of cantilevers, each pattern of eigenmode shifts is unique. Therefore, by examining an experimentally measured pattern of eigenmode shifts it is possible to determine to which cantilever a target analyte particle has adhered. A mass sensitivity of up to two orders higher was found as opposed to the previous work [36] reported by the same group. A mass sensitivity of up to three orders higher was found as opposed to relative frequency shifts. It is therefore feasible to design coupled resonant (CR) microstructures and use eigenmode as an output metric for enhanced parametric sensitivity over resonant sensors that use frequency shift output. However, it is also evident that merely adding the number of resonators in a 1-dimensional (1-*d*) chain does not necessarily increase the parametric sensitivity in proportion.

3.3 Study III

In a study, an array of four micro beams, S_1-S_4 are attached to a common shuttle mass, SM for the detection and identification of multiple analytes [19, 38]. Geometrical asymmetry in the micro beams (length mismatch) assured sufficient separation of individual resonant peaks (as seen in **Figure 8(a)**) at the corresponding eigenmode frequencies in the output response. An output response of the fabricated prototype along with mode shapes are shown in **Figure 8(a)**. A capillary tube containing the specific polymer solutions was interfaced to one or all of the micro beams to functionalize them for vapor detection. Specifically, toluene and methanol, and toluene/methanol mixtures were used with the polymers to prepare analyte concentration for the functionalization of the surface of the microbeam/s in an

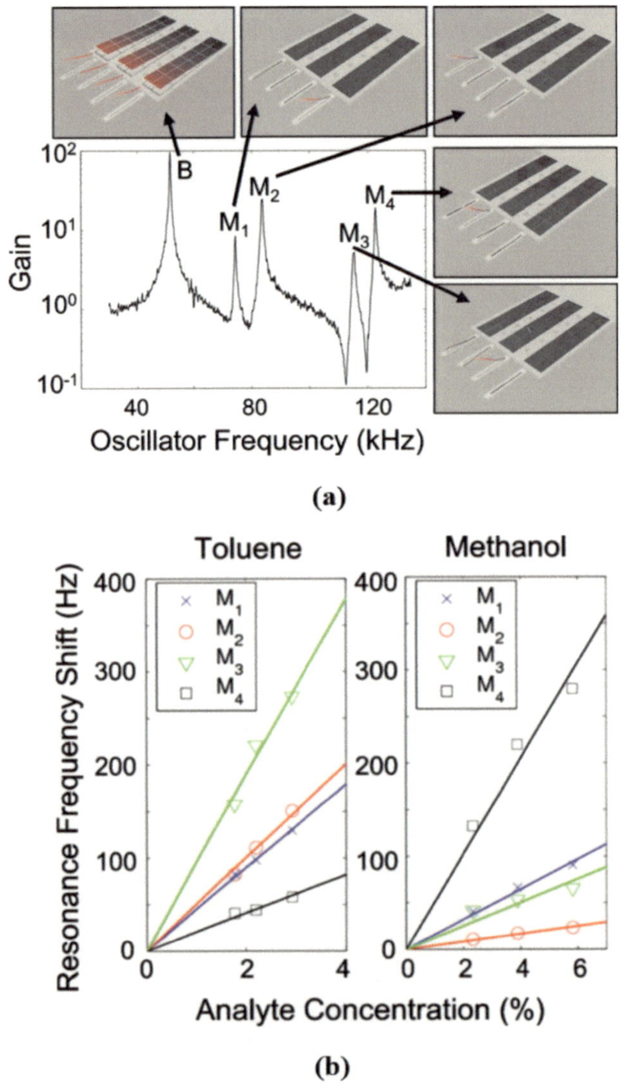

Figure 8.
Frequency response of the single input single output scheme in an array of coupled micro beams. (a) Composite response indicated by B and the individual mode-frequencies (M1-M4) of the mode-localized micro beams upon mass absorption due to the added analyte concentration. Also shown are the resonant mode shapes of the system. (b) Resonant frequency shifts of the four individual modes as a function of added mass concentration of the analyte. Slopes of the curve determine the sensitivity to the analyte, also making it possible to identify particular vapor concentration. Reprinted from [38] with the permission of AIP Publishing.

DOI: http://dx.doi.org/10.5772/intechopen.93931

array. The functionalized prototype was excited to motion by the piezoelectric actuator operating at a pressure level of 200 *Torr*. As shown in **Figure 8(b)**, a single output signal (resonant frequency shifts of all micro beams as a function of analyte concentration in %) was measured optically from the SM to obtain the composite response due to the mode-localization. Detection process is as follows: i) measure the resonance frequencies, M1-M4 (without added mass) in the pure nitrogen gas, ii) introduce an analyte and wait for the absorption to reach steady state, iii) measure the resonance frequencies once more, and determining the resulting frequency shifts. In this experiment, the frequency shift of each localized microbeam mode (M1-M4) was determined for various analyte concentrations (**Figure 8(b)**). As observed from **Figure 8(b)**, M3 shows the highest sensitivity to the toluene, whereas, M4 exhibits highest sensitivity to the added mass concentration of the methanol. Knowing the shifts of the two most sensitive microbeam modes M3 and M4 and their sensitivities from **Figure 8(b)**, the concentrations of methanol and toluene in the vapor were estimated to be 2.8% and 2.0%, respectively, and found in good agreement with the actual concentrations of 2.3% methanol and 2.3% toluene.

3.4 Study IV

In the recent study, 'Fano resonances' were observed in purely mechanical systems constituted by an array of nano and microcantilever resonators [39]. An array of micro/nano-scale cantilevers were used for mass sensing. A fabricated prototype and the output response is shown in **Figure 9**. Nanoscale cantilevers (thickness of 100 *nm*) fabricated of silicon nitrate were excited with piezoelectric disk shaker. A laser optical based detection was performed with sub-picometer resolution. Cantilevers here are directly connected to the bulk silicon without any suspended overhang at the base. As a consequence, each cantilever resonance is said to be identified by the main resonance curve (Lorentzian curve). No other resonant peak (entangled states due to coupling) are observed in the output response. Instead, due to an interference between the tails of the Lorentzian curve and the resonance peaks of the other cantilevers in an array, it was said that fano-peaks appeared at the corresponding resonant frequencies of the other cantilevers in an array (**Figure 9(b)**). Increased sensitivity (i.e. being able to measure smallest change in mass, Δm of up to 5 *pg*, Δm m/Q) of fano-resonances was attributed to their exhibited relatively higher quality factor, Q (10× than the main resonance

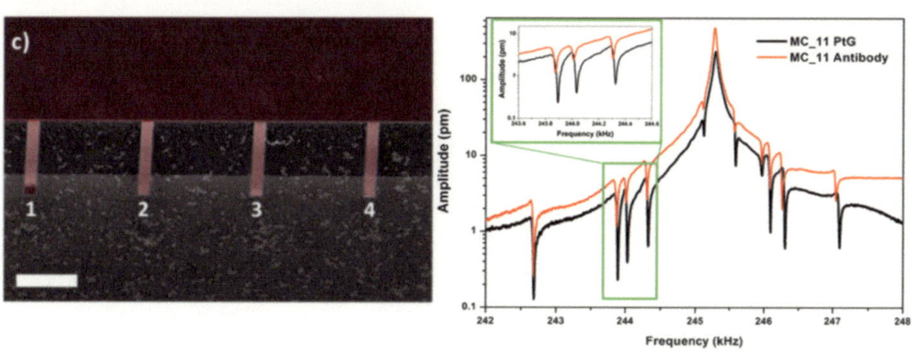

(a) **(b)**

Figure 9.
Fabricated prototype (a) and (b) vibration spectra of one cantilever in an array. Up to 9 cantilevers, not shown here were used in this work to propose a single and fast measurement scheme for cantilever arrays using Fano-resonance analysis [39]. Reprinted from [39] with the permission of Springer Nature under creative commons licenses.

peak). A negative shift in the resonant frequencies of all the 'Fano-resonances' was observed as the results of parallel mass loading on all the cantilevers in an array. Therefore, a single, fast measurement scheme (parallelization) was proposed to characterize the frequency response of one cantilever in an array. Several configurations of micro/nano scale cantilever arrays were fabricated and experimental results were given along with the theory model.

4. Common-mode-rejection in resonant mass sensors

Mode-localized sensors that utilize an array of ideally identical, weakly coupled, vibrating microstructural elements are shown to be relatively immune to the false output. Environmental factors (such as ambient pressure [30, 32], temperature [31, 40]) and/or nonspecific bindings (in case of mass sensing) influence all the vibrating elements uniformly. These factors as mentioned ideally does not affect the eigenmodes of the system, while shifts in the resonance frequencies still occur. One of the early work addressing the common-mode rejection of mode-localized sensor is given in [30]. As shown in **Figure 1**, in a 2-DoF WCR sensor, induced mismatch (Δm) affects one of the resonator. This is called a mass differential mode of operation. However, environmental variable such as temperature or pressure affects both the resonators simultaneously, which is termed as common-mode behavior of the micromechanical mode-localized sensors. It is found that, the mode-localized sensor is efficient in rejecting a common-mode noise (temperature and pressure) to the first order.

Table 1 provides a comparative performance summary (in terms of the attainable mass sensitivity and minimum detectable mass) of the ultra-precise and highly sensitive resonant mass sensors.

Reference	Output used	Relative sensitivity [a]	Minimum detectable mass, Δm	DoF	Material used
[36]	eigenstates	5% to 7% (higher than frequency shift output)	154 *pg*	2	borosilicate microspheres
[26]	eigenstates	3 orders higher	13.5 *pg*	2	platinum patches
[19, 38]	Frequency shift	NA	NA	4	polymer solutions
[41]	Frequency shift	NA	1.42×10^{-14} *kg*	3	NA
[42]	eigenstates	7000	10 *pg*	3	polystyrene micro-spheres
[39]	Frequency shift	NA	5 *pg*	4	NA
[43]	AR	34,361	2.1 *ng*	2	NA
[24]	AR	2.5%/*pg* (estimated via numerical model)	6 *pg*	2	NA
[44]	AR (Atmospheric pressure test)	25.31 (two orders higher than frequency shift output)	180 *ng*	3	Nanoparticles used
[34]	Eigenstates/ frequency shifts	NA	NA	4	Thermally killed bacteria

[a]Relative sensitivity is the ratio of sensitivity of eigenstate/s or AR output to the sensitivity of frequency shift output.

Table 1.
Mode-localized mass sensors summary.

5. Conclusion

In this chapter, the state-of-the-art in MEMS resonant sensor is studied. Numerical models were presented to understand the operation of the ultra-precise, high sensitivity devices used for the bio applications. Key performance parameters such as mass sensitivity was derived for the different available outputs in the CR resonant mass sensors. From the recent case studies and a comparative analysis as provided in **Table 1**, it can be concluded that CR resonant biosensor is emerging as a new sensing standard in the MEMS community.

Abbreviations and nomenclature

MEMS	Micro-electromechnical systems
m-DoF	multi-degree of freedom
CR	Coupled resonators
WCR	Weakly coupled resonators
A/D	Analog-to-digital converter
AR	Amplitude ratio
M_i	Proof mass *gram*
K_i	Mechanical spring constant *N/m*
c_i	Damping *Ns/m*
F	Forcing term *N*
x	Displacement of the proof mass *m*
K_c	Coupling spring constant (electrical) *N/m*
κ	Coupling factor *Unitless*
Δm	Mass perturbation *gram*
δ	Normalized perturbation *Unitless*
δ_m	Normalized mass perturbation *Unitless*
ω_{ip}	In-phase mode frequency *rad/sec*
ω_{op}	Out-of-phase mode frequency *rad/sec*
$\left(\frac{x1}{x2}\right)_{ji}$	Amplitude ratio of the jth resonator at the ith mode of the frequency response *Unitless*
$(x)_{ji}$	Amplitude of the jth resonator at the ith mode of the frequency response *V*
$\left(f_{ji}\right)$	Resonant frequency of the jth resonator at the ith mode of the frequency response *Hz*
Δf	Frequency shift *Hz*
Δ_a	Amplitude shift *V*
$\Delta f/f$	Frequency shift (normalized) *Unitless*
S_{R_i}	Sensitivity of AR shift to the normalized mass perturbation $V/V/\delta_m$
$S_{a_{ji}}$	Sensitivity of amplitude shift to the normalized mass perturbation V/δ_m
S_{f_i}	Sensitivity of frequency shift to the normalized mass perturbation Hz/δ_m

Author details

Vinayak Pachkawade
University of Liege, Belgium

*Address all correspondence to: vpachkawade@uliege.be

References

[1] Wasisto HS, Merzsch S, Waag A, Uhde E, Salthammer T, Peiner E. Airborne engineered nanoparticle mass sensor based on a silicon resonant cantilever. Sensors Actuators, B Chem. 2013;

[2] Zhang H, Kim ES. Micromachined acoustic resonant mass sensor. J Microelectromechanical Syst. 2005;

[3] Burg TP, Mirza AR, Milovic N, Tsau CH, Popescu GA, Foster JS, et al. Vacuum-packaged suspended microchannel resonant mass sensor for biomolecular detection. J Microelectromechanical Syst. 2006;

[4] Zhang W, Baskaran R, Turner KL. Effect of cubic nonlinearity on auto-parametrically amplified resonant MEMS mass sensor. Sensors Actuators, A Phys. 2002;

[5] Park K, Kim N, Morisette DT, Aluru NR, Bashir R. Resonant MEMS mass sensors for measurement of microdroplet evaporation. J Microelectromechanical Syst. 2012;

[6] Lee JEY, Bahreyni B, Zhu Y, Seshia AA. Ultrasensitive mass balance based on a bulk acoustic mode single-crystal silicon resonator. Appl Phys Lett. 2007;

[7] Li L. Simulation of Mass Sensor Based on Luminescence of Micro/Nano Electromechanical Resonator. IEEE Electron Device Lett. 2017;

[8] Jin D, Liu J, Li X, Liu M, Zuo G, Wang Y, et al. Tens femtogram resoluble piezoresistive cantilever sensors with optimized high-mode resonance excitation. In: Proceedings of 1st IEEE International Conference on Nano Micro Engineered and Molecular Systems, 1st IEEE-NEMS. 2006.

[9] Zou X, Thiruvenkatanathan P, Seshia AA. A high-resolution micro-electro-mechanical resonant tilt sensor. Sensors Actuators, A Phys. 2014;

[10] Zou X, Thiruvenkatanathan P, Seshia AA. Micro-electro-mechanical resonant tilt sensor with 250 nano-radian resolution. In: 2013 Joint European Frequency and Time Forum and International Frequency Control Symposium, EFTF/IFC 2013. 2013.

[11] Gupta A, Akin D, Bashir R. Single virus particle mass detection using microresonators with nanoscale thickness. Appl Phys Lett. 2004;

[12] Sone H, Okano H, Hosaka S. Picogram mass sensor using piezoresistive cantilever for biosensor. In: Japanese Journal of Applied Physics, Part 1: Regular Papers and Short Notes and Review Papers. 2004.

[13] Ilic B, Czaplewski D, Zalalutdinov M, Craighead HG, Neuzil P, Campagnolo C, et al. Single cell detection with micromechanical oscillators. J Vac Sci Technol B Microelectron Nanom Struct. 2001;

[14] Baek IB, Byun S, Lee BK, Ryu JH, Kim Y, Yoon YS, et al. Attogram mass sensing based on silicon microbeam resonators. Sci Rep. 2017;

[15] Davis ZJ, Boisen A. Aluminum nanocantilevers for high sensitivity mass sensors. Appl Phys Lett. 2005;

[16] Ekinci KL, Huang XMH, Roukes ML. Ultrasensitive nanoelectromechanical mass detection. Appl Phys Lett. 2004;

[17] Ono T, Esashi M. Magnetic force and optical force sensing with ultrathin silicon resonator. Rev Sci Instrum. 2003;

[18] Giessibl FJ. A direct method to calculate tip-sample forces from frequency shifts in frequency-modulation

atomic force microscopy. Appl Phys Lett. 2001;

[19] DeMartini BE, Rhoads JF, Shaw SW, Turner KL. A single input-single output mass sensor based on a coupled array of microresonators. Sensors Actuators, A Phys. 2007;

[20] Li L, Zhang YP, Ma CC, Liu CC, Peng B. Anti-symmetric mode vibration of electrostatically actuated clamped-clamped microbeams for mass sensing. Micromachines. 2020;

[21] Liang J, Hao Y, Kang H, Ruan B, Chang H. A Mode-Localized Voltmeter with Resolution of 46.8 Nanovolts. In: 2019 20th International Conference on Solid-State Sensors, Actuators and Microsystems and Eurosensors XXXIII, TRANSDUCERS 2019 and EUROSENSORS XXXIII. 2019.

[22] Manav M, Srikantha Phani A, Cretu E. Mode Localization and Sensitivity in Weakly Coupled Resonators. IEEE Sens J. 2019;

[23] Pandit M, Zhao C, Sobreviela G, Du S, Zou X, Seshia A. Utilizing energy localization in weakly coupled nonlinear resonators for sensing applications. J Microelectromechanical Syst. 2019;

[24] Rabenimanana T, Walter V, Kacem N, Le Moal P, Bourbon G, Lardiès J. Mass sensor using mode localization in two weakly coupled MEMS cantilevers with different lengths: Design and experimental model validation. Sensors Actuators, A Phys. 2019;

[25] Tao G, Choubey B. A simple technique to readout and characterize coupled MEMS resonators. J Microelectromechanical Syst. 2016;

[26] Thiruvenkatanathan P, Yan J, Woodhouse J, Aziz A, Seshia AA. Ultrasensitive mode-localized mass sensor with electrically tunable parametric sensitivity. Applied Physics Letters. 2010.

[27] Venstra WJ, Van Leeuwen R, Van Der Zant HSJ. Strongly coupled modes in a weakly driven micromechanical resonator. Appl Phys Lett. 2012 Dec 10; 101(24).

[28] Zhang H, Chang H, Yuan W. Characterization of forced localization of disordered weakly coupled micromechanical resonators. Microsystems Nanoeng. 2017;

[29] Zhao C, Wood GS, Xie J, Chang H, Pu SH, Kraft M. A Three Degree-of-Freedom Weakly Coupled Resonator Sensor with Enhanced Stiffness Sensitivity. J Microelectromechanical Syst. 2016;

[30] Thiruvenkatanathan P, Yan J, Seshia AA. Common mode rejection in electrically coupled MEMS resonators utilizing mode localization for sensor applications. In: 2009 IEEE International Frequency Control Symposium Joint with the 22nd European Frequency and Time Forum. 2009.

[31] Zhong J, Yang J, Chang H. The temperature drift suppression of mode-localized resonant sensors. In: Proceedings of the IEEE International Conference on Micro Electro Mechanical Systems (MEMS). 2018.

[32] Zhang H, Zhong J, Yuan W, Yang J, Chang H. Ambient pressure drift rejection of mode-localized resonant sensors. In: Proceedings of the IEEE International Conference on Micro Electro Mechanical Systems (MEMS). 2017.

[33] Chellasivalingam M, Pandit M, Kalberer M, Seshia AA. Ultra-fine Particulate Detection using Mode-localized MEMS Resonators. In: IFCS/EFTF 2019 - Joint Conference of the IEEE International Frequency Control Symposium and European Frequency and Time Forum, Proceedings. 2019.

[34] Marquez S, Alvarez M, Plaza JA, Villanueva LG, Dominguez C, Lechuga

LM. Asymmetrically coupled resonators for mass sensing. Appl Phys Lett. 2017;

[35] Spletzer M, Raman A, Sumali H, Sullivan JP. Highly sensitive mass detection and identification using vibration localization in coupled microcantilever arrays. Appl Phys Lett. 2008;

[36] Spletzer M, Raman A, Wu AQ, Xu X, Reifenberger R. Ultrasensitive mass sensing using mode localization in coupled microcantilevers. Appl Phys Lett. 2006;

[37] COMSOL. COMSOL Multiphysics® Modeling Software. Comsol. 2016;

[38] DeMartini BE, Rhoads JF, Zielke MA, Owen KG, Shaw SW, Turner KL. A single input-single output coupled microresonator array for the detection and identification of multiple analytes. Appl Phys Lett. 2008;

[39] Stassi S, Chiadò A, Calafiore G, Palmara G, Cabrini S, Ricciardi C. Experimental evidence of Fano resonances in nanomechanical resonators. Sci Rep. 2017;

[40] Pandit M, Zhao C, Sobreviela G, Seshia AA. Immunity to Temperature Fluctuations in Weakly Coupled MEMS Resonators. In: Proceedings of IEEE Sensors. 2018.

[41] Hajhashemi MS, Bahreyni B. Characterization of disturbances in systems of coupled micro-resonator arrays. IEEE Sens J. 2012;

[42] Wang DF, Li X, Yang X, Ikehara T, Maeda R. Enhancing amplitude changes by mode localization in trio cantilevers with mass perturbation. J Micromechanics Microengineering. 2015;

[43] Wood GS, Zhao C, Pu SH, Boden SA, Sari I, Kraft M. Mass sensor utilising the mode-localisation effect in an electrostatically-coupled MEMS resonator pair fabricated using an SOI process. Microelectron Eng. 2016;

[44] Wang Y, Zhao C, Wang C, Cerica D, Baijot M, Xiao Q, et al. A mass sensor based on 3-DOF mode localized coupled resonator under atmospheric pressure. Sensors Actuators, A Phys [Internet]. 2018;279(June):254–62. Available from: https://doi.org/10.1016/j.sna.2018.06.028

Chapter 7

Microfluidic Adsorption-Based Biosensors: Mathematical Models of Time Response and Noise, Considering Mass Transfer and Surface Heterogeneity

Ivana Jokić

Abstract

Adsorption-based microfluidic sensors are promising tools for biosensing. Advanced mathematical models of time response and noise of such devices are needed in order to improve the interpretation of measurement results, and to achieve the optimal sensor performance. Here the mathematical models are presented that take into account the coupling of processes that generate the sensor signal: adsorption–desorption (AD) of the target analyte particles on the heterogeneous sensing surface, and mass transfer (MT) in a microfluidic chamber. The response kinetics and AD noise (which determines the ultimate sensing performance) of protein biosensors are analyzed, assuming practically relevant analyte concentrations, sensing surface areas and MT parameters. The condition is determined under which MT significantly influences the sensor characteristics relevant for reliable analyte detection and quantification. It is shown that the development of improved mathematical models of sensor temporal response and noise can be used as one of strategies for achieving better sensing performance.

Keywords: microfluidic biosensor, surface heterogeneity, mass transfer, adsorption–desorption noise, mathematical model

1. Introduction

Microfluidic adsorption-based biosensors are promising devices for real-time, in-situ and low-cost analysis of samples taken from the environment, food or living organisms, enabling detection of the presence and measurement of the amount of target biological specimens: biomolecules (such as proteins or DNA fragments), microorganisms, or other biological structures [1–3]. Such sensors are highly sensitive, capable of operation with small sample quantities, and also small, lightweight and energy efficient, thus being especially suitable for autonomous, portable and distributed sensing applications [4–6]. Due to such characteristics, development of microfluidic sensors is very significant for environmental protection, medicine, agriculture, food inspection, public healthcare and security, and other fields, where they can substitute large and expensive laboratory equipment, typically located far from the place where the samples are taken for the analysis. They also enable the development of new fields of biosensor applications, such as the personalized medical point-of-care diagnostics, telemedicine, wearable sensors etc. [7–9].

In order to utilize the great potential of adsorption-based microfluidic biosensors for practical applications, research is performed aiming to enable optimization of their performance. The increase of sensitivity and response rate of the sensors, better selectivity, lowering of the minimal detectable concentration, higher reliability of measurement results ant their more accurate interpretation, as well as the research and development of new measurement methods, which enable obtaining of more information about one or multiple adsorbed substances at the same time, are of great practical significance. In that sense, of particular interest is to know the dependence of the temporal response and the sensor noise on the parameters of the sensing element, the measurement system, and the experimental conditions, which requires the development and application of mathematical models that take into account physical processes and phenomena relevant for generating the response and its fluctuations. The adsorption and desorption (AD) processes are inevitably taken into account in modeling of the response and noise, since they are fundamental for sensor operation, and are also the source of adsorption–desorption noise, which sets the fundamental limits of detection and quantification of the analyte. In structures of micrometer and nanometer dimensions, AD noise can dominantly determine the values of minimal detectable and quantifiable signal, as well as other limiting sensor performances, especially in the case of low analyte concentration [10–20]. In various cases, apart from the AD process of the target analyte, different additional processes influence the sensor response kinetics and noise, so it is necessary to take them into account in mathematical models.

The objective of this work is to present mathematical models of the temporal response and adsorption–desorption noise of microfluidic adsorption-based biosensors, that take into account the processes responsible for the generation of the sensor signal: adsorption–desorption of the target analyte particles on the heterogeneous sensing surface, and mass transfer (MT) in a microfluidic chamber. Section 2 presents the mathematical models of the sensor temporal response, while Section 3 describes the AD noise models, developed for the cases considered in Section 2. In Section 4, the results will be presented of the temporal response analysis, and of the analysis of AD noise of protein biosensors, both performed by using of the models presented in Sections 2 and 3, assuming practically relevant analyte concentrations, sensing surface areas and MT parameters. The conclusions will be summarized in Section 5.

2. Mathematical models of sensor temporal response

In adsorption-based biosensors (e.g. SPR (*Surface Plasmon Resonance*), resistive graphene-based, CNT (*Carbon NanoTube*) or NWFET (*NanoWire Field Effect Transistor*), SAW (Surface Acoustic Wave), FBAR (*thin Film Bulk Acoustic wave Resonator*), microcantilever sensors) detection of the target analyte and measurement of its concentration are based on the change of a measurable parameter of the sensing element, caused by analyte adsorption on the active surface [21–28]. Namely, the adsorption leads to the change of some of the sensing element's physical parameters (e.g. the mechanical strain or mechanical structure's mass, the effective density of the surface layer or its conductivity, the refraction index, the distribution of electric charges on the surface), which changes at least one measurable parameter of the sensor (e.g. the deflection or the resonant frequency of the mechanical structure; the amplitude, frequency or phase of surface or bulk acoustic waves in mechanical sensors; the resistance or current in electrical sensors; the intensity, reflection, transmission, or absorption of light in optical sensors).

Here, the term "temporal response of adsorption-based sensors" will be used to denote the temporal change of a certain physical parameter of the sensing element, which is induced by analyte adsorption. At any given time, that change is determined by the number of analyte particles bound to the sensing surface, and that number depends on the target analyte concentration in the sample. This enables the measurement of the concentration of the target substance to be performed by measuring the change of the physical parameter. Therefore, the mathematical model of the sensor temporal response is based on the model of the time evolution of the number of adsorbed particles as a function of analyte concentration, assuming that there is a known (preferably linear) relation between the two quantities.

In the analyses of microfluidic biosensors time response, which have been published in the literature, it is often assumed that the change of the number of adsorbed particles occurs only due to the AD process of the target substance, and the interpretation of experimental results is performed according to that [29, 30]. This simplified interpretation of the events occurring on the sensing surface is justified under the conditions that ensure a negligible influence of other processes, and assume a homogeneous adsorption surface. Analyses that include some of the additional effects that also influence the current number of adsorbed target particles are less abundant in the existing literature. For example, the mass transfer process of target adsorbate particles in a reaction chamber, toward or away from adsorption sites on the sensing surface, coupled with the AD process, is considered in [31–33]. Competitive AD processes of target and competitor substances are analyzed in [34, 35]. An example of the analysis encompassing multiple phenomena is the research of adsorption processes of two or three analytes on the surface of the same sensor, coupled with mass transfer processes of corresponding particles [36–38]. Sensing surface heterogeneity and mass transfer processes in biosensors are considered within the analysis of sensor models response in [30, 36, 39], where the need is emphasized for taking into account both of these factors simultaneously while creating experiments and interpreting the measurement results.

In this section, first the starting system of equations will be presented that model the change of the number of adsorbed particles on a sensing surface with an arbitrary number of different adsorption sites, and take into account mass transfer processes of analyte particles in the sensor chamber. Subsequently, simplified physical models will be defined and presented by suitable equations for certain cases of practical significance, in a similar way as in [39]. Also, conditions will be defined under which the application of the approximate models is justified. The case of adsorbing surface with two types of adsorption sites will be particularly considered.

2.1 Starting equations

It is assumed that the sensing element of a sensor is in a microfluidic reaction chamber of a rectangular cross-section, with the sample to be analyzed flowing through it. In **Figure 1** (left) a schematic representation is given of the chamber and the sensing element, with the designations of dimensions and coordinate axes. During the laminar fluid flow, a parabolic velocity profile is formed in the chamber (the profile belongs to the z = const. plane, and it is constant in the z-axis direction in the adsorbing surface zone).

On the sensor's active surface the recognition and binding of the target analyte occurs. Adsorption–desorption and mass transfer are the key processes for binding of particles to the sensing surface. The former is the process of binding of the

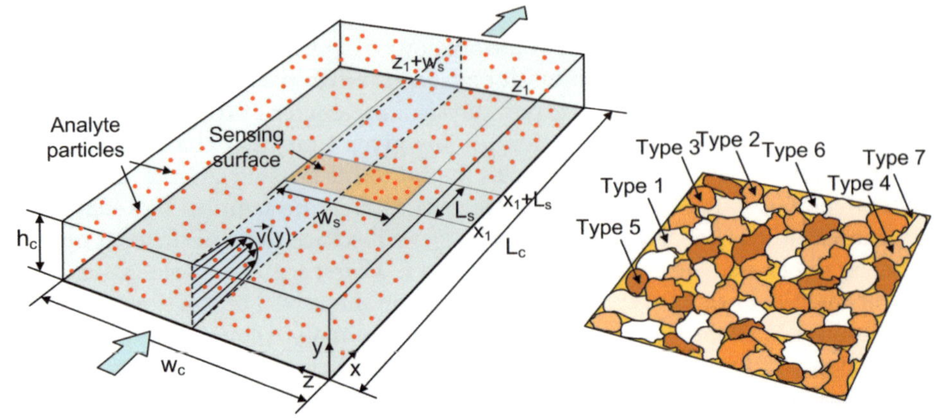

Figure 1.
Left: Schematic representation of a sensor flow-through reaction chamber of rectangular cross-section: geometry of the system with designations of dimensions and coordinate axes. The shaded longitudinal section in the z = const. plane, whose boundaries are denoted by a dashed line, shows the convection velocity profile (the case of laminar fluid flow). Right: Part of the heterogeneous sensing surface that contains multiple (e.g. 7, as shown) types of adsorption sites of different affinities toward the target analyte.

analyte particles to surface adsorption sites due to a certain affinity, and unbinding from them. The latter encompasses the processes (convection and diffusion) by which the analyte particles are transported through the microfluidic chamber to or from the binding sites. The coupling of these processes determines the spatial and temporal dependence of the analyte concentration in the chamber.

In the analysis, it is assumed that the adsorption occurs in a single layer only, that only one analyte particle can be adsorbed on an adsorption site, and that the probability of adsorption on any given site (or desorption from it), does not depend on the occupancy of adjacent sites. In the case of a homogeneous sensing surface (in the sense of the affinity toward the target analyte particles), the AD process is characterized by a single pair of adsorption and desorption rate constants, k_a and k_d.

The active surface of affinity-based sensors is often not comprised of uniform adsorption sites to which the particles of the target analyte bind [30, 40]. The reason for this can be a non-uniform surface morphology or chemical composition, or the existence of multiple possible binding sites for analyte particles due to the material structure on the molecular scale. In more detail, the presence of various defects, irregularities, cavities, pores, impurities, contaminants, different functional groups on the surface, etc. are some of numerous features that constitute the surface heterogeneity. Materials in the form of flakes with specific binding sites on edges and basal planes, such as liquid-phase exfoliated graphene [41], are also an example of a heterogeneous sensing surface. When a surface is functionalized with specific capturing probes for the target analyte, adsorption sites heterogeneity can be manifested through nonspecific binding of analyte particles to the surface. An adsorption surface can also be heterogeneous due to uneven binding of functionalizing entities (e.g. non-uniform orientation of capturing proteins when attached to the surface), which influences the affinity toward the analyte, and the efficiency of its binding. Whatever the reason, a heterogeneous sensing surface can be characterized by different affinities of different surface sites for the analyte particles binding. The analyte's AD process is then characterized by a certain distribution of adsorption and desorption rate constants across the surface, and it is described by a model that takes into account the surface non-uniformity.

If we assume that there is n types of adsorption sites on the surface, the surface heterogeneity can be described by a discrete set of n values of adsorption energies for the given analyte, thus yielding n pairs of adsorption and desorption rate constants (k_{ai}, k_{di}), $i = 1,2 \dots n$. Adsorption of a single analyte on n types of adsorption sites, randomly distributed across the adsorbing surface of a microfluidic sensor, is mathematically described by $n + 1$ equations, and by boundary and initial conditions. One of the equations is the convection-diffusion equation (for a microfluidic chamber of a rectangular cross-section, whose illustration is shown in **Figure 1** (left))

$$\frac{\partial C}{\partial t} = -v\frac{\partial C}{\partial x} + D\left(\frac{\partial^2 C}{\partial x^2} + \frac{\partial^2 C}{\partial y^2} + \frac{\partial^2 C}{\partial z^2}\right) \tag{1}$$

Here, D is the diffusion coefficient of analyte particles, and v is the flow velocity of the sample. The remaining n equations pertain to the processes of reversible binding of particles to adsorption sites of different types. Each of these processes, which are coupled in a general case, can be regarded as one of n components of a complex AD process. It is known that the Langmuir adsorption model assumes the uniformity of adsorption sites. In the case of heterogeneous surface sites, it can be assumed that the adsorbent surface consists of a collection of locally homogeneous surfaces, and that the adsorption on each of them can be considered as Langmuir adsorption. All the parts of the sensing surface S with the adsorption sites of the type i, constitute the surface S_i of area A_i. The above-mentioned set of n equations can thus be written as

$$\begin{array}{ll} \dfrac{\partial \eta_i}{\partial t} = k_{ai} C_S(\eta_{\max,i} - \eta_i) - k_{di}\eta_i, & (x,0,z) \in S_i \\ \eta_i = 0 & ,\ (x,0,z) \notin S_i \end{array} ,i = 1,2 \dots n \tag{2}$$

Here η_i is the surface density of the analyte particles adsorbed on sites of the ith type, $\eta_{max,i}$ is the surface density of adsorption sites of the matching kind, and C_s is the analyte concentration adjacent to the sensing surface. It is assumed that the adsorption sites are uniformly distributed across the surface S_i, so $\eta_{max,i}$ does not depend on the coordinates x and z.

The boundary and initial conditions are as follows: 1. at the entrance of the chamber ($x = 0$) the concentration is equal to that in the analyzed sample: $C(t,0,y,z) = C_0$; 2. at the exit from the chamber the continuity condition assumes free convection: $\partial C/\partial x = 0$ for $x = L_c$; 3. the initial adsorbate particle distribution in the chamber is uniform: $C(0,x,y,z) = C_0$, 4. in the zone of the sensing element, which is defined by the coordinates $y = 0$, $x_1 \le x \le x_1 + L_s$, $z_1 \le z \le z_1 + w_s$ (L_s is the adsorption zone length, and w_s is its width), there is a balance between the diffusion flux in the direction perpendicular to the surface, and the net adsorption rate per unit surface

$$D\frac{\partial C}{\partial y}\bigg|_{(t,x,0,z)} = k_{ai} C_s(\eta_{\max,i} - \eta_i) - k_{di}\eta_i, i = 1, 2, \dots, n \tag{3}$$

The ith Eq. (3) is valid on the parts of adsorbing surface with the adsorption sites of the ith type; on the remaining part of the chamber's surface where $y = 0$, and on the whole chamber's surface where $y = h_c$, the zero flux condition is valid; 5. on the edges of every adsorption zone the flux equals zero (the adsorbed particles leave the adsorbing zone only by desorption); 6. the adsorption begins at the moment $t = 0$: $\eta(0,x,z) = 0$.

For the determination of $C(t,x,y,z)$ and $\eta_i(t,x,z)$, it is necessary to solve Eqs. (1) and (2) with the mentioned initial and boundary conditions, by using numerical methods. The number of adsorbed particles on the sites of the ith type, $N_i(t)$, can be determined by integration of $\eta_i(t,x,z)$ over the sensing element surface. If the contribution of a particle adsorption to the senor signal does not depend on the place on the sensing surface where the particle is bound, but only on the type of the adsorption site, the sensor response will depend on the numbers of adsorbed particles per each site type.

When the total sensor response is the sum of contributions of n components, of which each is the product of the number of adsorbed particles of a given component, $N_i(t)$, and the corresponding weight factor w_i (i = 1, 2, ... , n), the temporal response is

$$R = w_1 N_1 + w_2 N_2 + \ldots + w_n N_n \quad (4)$$

The weight factor w_i equals the average contribution of a single adsorbed particle of the ith component to the sensor response. However, for some types of adsorption-based sensors, the response can be represented by the simpler expression

$$R = w \sum_{i=1}^{n} N_i \quad (5)$$

For instance, in the case of resonant micro/nanocantilevers and acoustic wave mechanical sensors, particle adsorption changes the mass of the mechanical sensing structure, so that w is determined by the mass of a single analyte particle, thus it is independent on the type of the site where the particle was adsorbed. Also, in the case of plasmonic sensors, it is reasonable to assume that the mean refractive index change when an analyte particle is adsorbed is $w = (n_a - n_e)/N_{max}$, where n_a is the refractive index value of the analyte, n_e is the refractive index of the surrounding medium, and N_{max} is the total number of adsorption sites on the surface [42]. In these cases, it is justified to use Eq. (5).

Numerical solving of Eqs. (1) and (2) requires the surface distributions of different adsorption sites to be known, which is rarely the case. Instead of that, approximations can be introduced in order to simplify the equations, which can even enable obtaining of the analytical solution valid for the transient regime and/or the steady state. The approximations are introduced based on the comparison of adsorption, convection and diffusion time scales.

2.2 Adsorption limited response kinetics

A significant reduction of mathematical complexity of the problem is possible when it is justified to assume that the concentration of the analyte in the reaction chamber is spatially uniform, constant in time, and equal to the concentration in the sample injected in the chamber. Eq. (3) is then reduced to $C(t,x,y,z) = C_0$ = const. The spatial independence of the concentration Co and $\eta_{max,i}$ implies the uniformity of the surface density of adsorbed particles η_i on the surface S_i, so the number of particles adsorbed on sites of the ith type is $N_i = \eta_i A_i$. The number of adsorption sites of that type is $N_{max,i} = \eta_{max,i} A_i = \nu_i N_{max}$, where ν_i is introduced as a measure of abundance of these sites in the total number of sites on the sensing surface, N_{max}. The model of the multicomponent AD process of a single analyte on the surface with n types of adsorption sites, derived from Eqs. (2), is therefore represented by the set of n mutually independent equations

$$\frac{dN_i}{dt} = k_{ai} C_o (N_{\max,i} - N_i) - k_{di} N_i = a_i - d_i, i = 1, 2, \ldots, n \quad (6)$$

The analytical solution of each of Eqs. (6), with the initial condition $N_i(0) = 0$, is

$$N_i(t) = \frac{k_{ai}C_0}{k_{di} + k_{ai}C_0} N_{\max,i}\left(1 - e^{-(k_{di}+k_{ai}C_0)t}\right) = N_{ie}\left(1 - e^{-t/\tau_{AL,i}}\right) \tag{7}$$

where N_{ie} is the number of adsorbed particles in the steady state, which establishes with the time constant of the AD process, $\tau_{AL,i}$. For the steady state $dN_i/dt = 0$, i.e. $a_i = d_i$. The sensor response is determined by Eq. (4) or Eq. (5).

This model is applicable in the cases where the transfer flux toward the sites of each type is sufficiently greater than the adsorption flux, so that the binding kinetics is adsorption limited [31, 32, 37]. This means that the number of adsorbed particles on the given surface and at the given analyte concentration is determined only by the AD process parameters at any given time. This is the ideal case for obtaining the data about the AD process and its kinetics from the measured time response of the sensor. The transport-adsorption regime of this kind is typical for fast diffusing particles (such as gas molecules and certain biomolecules of small mass).

2.3 Mass transfer influenced response kinetics

When the transport flux of analyte particles is lower than the adsorption flux, or comparable with it, the time evolution of the numbers of adsorbed particles is affected by mass transfer processes [31, 32, 37]. The temporal and spatial change of the analyte concentration in the sensor chamber depends on the parameters of AD and mass transfer processes in the system of a given geometry. As the adsorption flux becomes more dominant, the change of the analyte concentration in the chamber becomes more pronounced due to the slow compensating influx of particles carried by transport processes in the space that is being depleted of particles due to their fast binding to the adsorbing surface. Here, the analysis will be focused on the situation in which a thin depleted layer is formed adjacent to the sensing surface, because it is common in many types of microfluidic sensors (especially those whose reaction chamber height is of the order of ≥10 μm [43]). It also enables approximations to be used, which lead to the simplified time response mathematical model, and also yield the analytical expression for the AD noise spectral density.

When the diffusion time scale is greater than the convection time scale (expressed by $h_c^2/D > L_c/v_m$, where v_{m} is the mean convection velocity), not all the particles from the chamber volume can participate in the adsorption process, but only those from the layer of a certain thickness adjacent to the adsorbing surface. If the thickness of that layer is small compared to the chamber height and the length of the adsorbing zone, the temporally and spatially variable analyte concentration in the chamber can be approximated by the two-compartment model (TCM), whose applicability is experimentally confirmed [31, 44, 45]. According to that model, the chamber can be divided into two parts (compartments). One of them is the inner compartment, which is adjacent to the adsorbing surface, and contains a variable analyte concentration due to the depletion of analyte particles. The other, outer compartment, contains the analyte at the same concentration as it is in the sample injected in the chamber, C_0. Also, according to the model, all quantities are averaged over the adsorbing surface, and the transport between the two compartments is described by the mass transfer coefficient, k_m. It is assumed that the zones S_i (with binding sites of the type i) consist of a multitude of smaller areas scattered over the sensing surface (as illustrated in **Figure 1** (right)), so that different adsorption sites are mixed. The averaging of quantities over the sensing surface can thus approximate the actual conditions with sufficient accuracy, making the use of TCM justified. Furthermore, the model equates the rate of change of the total number of adsorbed particles with the net number of particles that enter the inner compartment in unit time, i.e.

$$\frac{dN}{dt} = k_m A (C_0 - C_{s,TCM}) \tag{8}$$

where the mass transfer coefficient is given as $k_m = 1.467(D^2 v_m/(L_s h_c))^{1/3}$ [31]. Since the total number of particles adsorbed on the entire sensing surface equals

$$N = \sum_{i=1}^{n} N_i, \tag{9}$$

and Eqs. (2) after averaging of the quantities over the surface yield

$$\frac{dN_i}{dt} = k_{ai} C_{s,TCM} (N_{\max,i} - N_i) - k_{di} N_i = a_{eff,i} - d_{eff,i} \ (i = 1, 2, \ldots, n), \tag{10}$$

Eqs. (8)–(10) imply that the analyte concentration adjacent to the adsorbing surface is determined by the expression

$$C_{s,TCM} = \frac{C_0 + \sum_{k=1}^{n} k_{dk} N_k / (k_m A)}{1 + \sum_{k=1}^{n} k_{ak} (N_{\max,k} - N_k)/(k_m A)} \tag{11}$$

The time evolution of the numbers of adsorbed particles on different types of sites is determined by Eqs. (10) and (11), i.e. by $n + 1$ coupled equations. This system of equations is significantly simpler than the starting system (Eqs. (1) and (2)), and can be efficiently solved by using numerical methods for the given initial conditions. The sensor response is then determined by Eq. (4) or (5). The steady-state values of the numbers of adsorbed particles are obtained from Eqs. (10) for $dN_i/dt = 0$, and they are the same as in the case of adsorption-limited regime

$$N_{ie} = \frac{k_{ai} C_0}{k_{di} + k_{ai} C_0} N_{\max,i}, i = 1, 2, \ldots, n. \tag{12}$$

The presented mathematical model is applicable for the thin depleted zone adjacent to the sensing surface, which is more likely to exist at lower D values, higher h_c, and faster convection. The analysis of Eq. (11) shows that at

$$k_m A >> \sum_{k=1}^{n} k_{ak} N_{\max,k} \tag{13}$$

$C_{s,TCM} \approx C_0$, so the model given by Eq. (10) reduces to the model that is valid in the case of adsorption-limited binding (Eq. (6)). Therefore, Eq. (13) is the condition for the transfer flux to dominate over the adsorption flux (while the diffusion is slow compared to the convection). When the condition (13) is not satisfied, it is necessary to use the mathematical model given by Eqs. (10) and (11) for the response analysis of sensors in which a thin depleted zone is formed. Based on these considerations, it can be concluded that the equations obtained by using TCM have broader applicability than expected: they are valid both for mass-transfer influenced and for adsorption-limited (the case of sufficiently high k_m, according to Eq. (13)) binding kinetics.

The simplest heterogeneous sensing surface contains two types of adsorption sites. The corresponding equations are

$$\begin{aligned}\frac{dN_i}{dt} &= k_{ai}\frac{C_0 + (k_{d1}N_1 + k_{d2}N_2)/k_mA}{1 + [k_{a1}(N_{m1} - N_1) + k_{a2}(N_{m2} - N_2)]/k_mA}(N_{mi} - N_i) - k_{di}N_i \\ &= a_{eff,i} - d_{eff,i}\end{aligned} \tag{14}$$

where i equals 1 or 2.

3. Mathematical models of adsorption-desorption noise

Due to the inherently stochastic nature of processes involved in the analyte particle binding-unbinding events on the sensing surface, the number of adsorbed particles randomly fluctuates, even after reaching the steady state, so it can be expressed as

$$N = N_e + \Delta N \tag{15}$$

where ΔN denotes fluctuations. The fluctuations of the number of adsorbed particles, $\Delta N(t)$, result in the fluctuations of the sensor's time response, $\Delta R(t)$, which constitute the inevitable adsorption–desorption (AD) noise. Based on Eq. (4), these fluctuations are related as

$$\Delta R = \sum_{i=1}^{n} w_i \Delta N_i, \tag{16}$$

assuming n AD processes on the sensing surface, where ΔN_i denote the fluctuations of the number of particles that participate in the ith AD process.

Here, the goal is to obtain the analytical expression for the spectral density of sensor AD noise, when all the transient processes are finished, i.e. when an steady state is established. According to Eq. (16), the basis of this analysis is the analysis of fluctuations of the number of adsorbed particles around the steady-state values. Before presenting the theoretical models of AD noise of sensors with heterogeneous sensing surface, a short overview will be given of the already published results that include mathematical modeling of AD noise of sensors and other micro/nanodevices.

An insight into the existing literature shows that AD noise analyses have been usually limited to the consideration of individual phenomena pertinent to fluctuations of the number of adsorbed particles – e.g. fluctuations originating from a stochastic single-analyte AD process [46] or fluctuations due to surface diffusion of adsorbed particles [47].

First papers on AD noise in micro/nanodevices were focused on resonant mechanical structures [12, 48, 49]. Dating from the same period is the first paper on AD fluctuations in micro-biosensors [13]. In subsequent publications, the analysis of AD fluctuations was performed for various types of sensors (mass sensors with micro/nanocantilevers [15, 16, 50], semiconductor resistive gas sensors [51], plasmonic sensors [52], quartz crystal microbalance gas sensors [19]), which operate in a single-gas environment, assuming Langmuir adsorption. In [53] a theoretical AD noise model is presented for the Wolkenstein adsorption of particles of a single gas, applicable in the case of chemical adsorption in semiconductor resistive sensors.

In real situations, certain processes (e.g. various cases of non-specific adsorption, or mass transfer processes), which are coupled with the AD process of target particles, affect the sensor response, and thus influence the response fluctuations. Therefore, it is necessary for the AD noise analysis to include the coupling of multiple processes, depending on the considered practical case. In [54] the expression is derived for the PSD of adsorbed mass fluctuations due to the coupled AD processes of an arbitrary number of gases, by using the Langevin approach. The AD noise model in the case of multilayer adsorption according to the BET model is presented in [55, 56]. Analyte diffusion within the sensor chamber is considered together with the binding of particles to the surface sites, in order to analyze the fluctuations and noise figures of merit of biosensors in [14, 57] assuming the adsorption surface of infinite capacity. The coupling of mass transfer (convection and diffusion) and AD processes of one or multiple substances on the sensing surface is taken into account in the development of the AD noise model of microfluidic sensors, which is presented in [58–60]. The combined effect of the AD process, the mass transfer in the sensor chamber and the surface diffusion on the fluctuations of the number of adsorbed particles is analyzed in [61], and a good match is shown between the derived PSD of AD noise and the experimental results obtained by using a graphene gas sensor [62]. The influence of the analyte depletion from the sample on the AD noise is modeled and analyzed in [63]. In [64] the analysis is presented of the signal-to-noise ratio of a nanowire biosensor, based on stochastic simulations of the AD process coupled with diffusion.

According to the current trends in micro- and nanosensor development (the decrease of the sensing surface area, and the decrease of detectable concentrations), the analysis of AD fluctuations becomes increasingly significant for the estimation of limiting performances of such devices, and for optimization of sensor design and experimental methods. In spite of that, the topic of AD noise is scarce in the literature, compared to the total number of papers on chemical and biological sensors. Also, the published experimental results pertinent to AD noise are very scarce, and can be found for gas sensors [17–20].

In the following part of this Section, mathematical models will be presented that take into account the existence of different types of adsorption sites on the sensing surface.

3.1 Langevin method for multicomponent stochastic processes

There are two approaches that are commonly used for the analysis of the fluctuations of the number of adsorbed particles: the first is based on the master equation, and the second on the Langevin equation, with the use of Wiener-Khinchin theorem. Both the approaches are described in detail in Supplementary data of Ref. [59] for a competitive AD process of two analytes, and all the given expressions can be generalized in a simple manner in order to be valid for n-component AD processes, where $n \geq 2$. Here, the Langevin method will be presented, which enables efficient determination of the analytical expression for the power spectral density (PSD) of the sensor response fluctuation, starting from the kinetic macroscopic equations that describe a multicomponent stochastic process.

When adsorption and desorption processes occur on the heterogeneous active surface of a sensor, the number of particles adsorbed on each type of adsorption sites stochastically fluctuates in time. The fluctuations of the number of particles adsorbed on sites belonging to the ith type are denoted with ΔN_i ($i = 1, 2 \ldots n$). All these fluctuating processes, when observed together, constitute a single complex random process, which belongs to the class of multicomponent Markov "gain and loss" processes [65]. Fluctuations on one type of sites (ΔN_i) are a single component of that process. A complex process that has n ($n \geq 2$) components can be represented by an n-dimensional column vector $\mathbf{\Delta N} = [\Delta N_1 \Delta N_2 \ldots \Delta N_n]^{\mathbf{T}}$

(the superscript "T" denotes matrix transposition). The Langevin equation expressed in the matrix form is then (Supplementary data of Ref. [59])

$$\frac{d(\Delta\mathbf{N}(t))}{dt} = -\mathbf{K}\cdot\Delta\mathbf{N}(t) + \boldsymbol{\xi}(t) \tag{17}$$

where $\boldsymbol{\xi}(t) = [\xi_1(t)\xi_2(t)\ \dots\ \xi_n(t)]^{\mathbf{T}}$ is the vector of the Langevin source functions, and $\mathbf{K}$ is the square $n \times n$ matrix whose elements are determined by the process parameters that influence the dynamics of analyte particles binding-unbinding random events. Elements of this matrix will later be derived for each of the analyzed cases of adsorption on heterogeneous surfaces. The symbol "·" is the matrix multiplication operator.

The Langevin equation in the complex domain ($\omega = 2\pi f$, f being the Fourier frequency) yields

$$\Delta\mathbf{N}(\mathrm{j}\omega) = (\mathbf{K} + \mathrm{j}\omega\mathbf{I})^{-1}\cdot\boldsymbol{\xi}(\mathrm{j}\omega) \tag{18}$$

(where $\Delta\mathbf{N}(\mathrm{j}\omega) = [\Delta N_1(\mathrm{j}\omega)\ \Delta N_2(\mathrm{j}\omega)\ \dots\ \Delta N_n(\mathrm{j}\omega)]^{\mathbf{T}}$, $\boldsymbol{\xi}(\mathrm{j}\omega) = [\xi_1(\mathrm{j}\omega)\xi_2(\mathrm{j}\omega)\ \dots\ \xi_n(\mathrm{j}\omega)]^{\mathbf{T}}$, and $\mathbf{I}$ is the $n \times n$ unity matrix), and then the $n \times n$ matrix of single-sided power spectral and cross-spectral densities of the numbers of adsorbed particles, $\mathbf{S}^2{}_{\Delta\mathbf{N}}(\omega)$, whose elements are determined by the expression

$$\begin{aligned}\mathbf{S}^2_{\Delta\mathbf{N}}(\omega) &= <\Delta\mathbf{N}(\mathrm{j}\omega)\Delta\mathbf{N}^{\mathbf{T}}(-\mathrm{j}\omega)> \\ &= (\mathbf{K}+\mathrm{j}\omega\mathbf{I})^{-1}\cdot<\boldsymbol{\xi}(\mathrm{j}\omega)\cdot\boldsymbol{\xi}^{\mathbf{T}}(-\mathrm{j}\omega)>\cdot\left((\mathbf{K}-\mathrm{j}\omega\mathbf{I})^{-1}\right)^{\mathbf{T}} \\ &= (\mathbf{K}+j\omega\mathbf{I})^{-1}\cdot\mathbf{S}^2_{\boldsymbol{\xi}}\cdot\left(\mathbf{K}^{\mathbf{T}}-j\omega\mathbf{I}\right)^{-1}\end{aligned} \tag{19}$$

The expressions for the elements of the matrix $\mathrm{S}_{\xi}{}^2$ can be derived by using the formal statistical approach, as presented in [66]. Here only the final result is shown (d_{ie} are the effective probabilities of increase or decrease of the number of adsorbed particles at sites of the ith type in unit time)

$$S^2_{\xi,il} = \begin{cases} 4d_{ie}, & i = l \\ 0, & i \neq l \end{cases} \tag{20}$$

By using the Wiener-Khinchin theorem [67] and Eqs. (16) and (19) the expression is obtained for the PSD of the sensor response fluctuations [59], i.e. for the PSD of AD noise

$$\begin{aligned}S^2_{\Delta R}(\omega) &= \sum_{i=1}^{n}\sum_{k=1}^{n}\left(w_i w_k S^2_{\Delta N,ik}(\omega)\right) \\ &= \mathbf{W}\cdot\mathbf{S}^2_{\Delta\mathbf{N}}(\omega)\cdot\mathbf{W}^{\mathbf{T}} \\ &= \mathbf{W}\cdot(\mathbf{K}+j\omega\mathbf{I})^{-1}\cdot\mathbf{S}^2_{\boldsymbol{\xi}}\cdot\left(\mathbf{K}^{\mathbf{T}}-j\omega\mathbf{I}\right)^{-1}\cdot\mathbf{W}^{\mathbf{T}}\end{aligned} \tag{21}$$

where the row vector of weight factors $\mathbf{W} = [w_1\, w_2\ \dots\ w_{\mathrm{n}}]$ is introduced.

3.2 Adsorption limited binding

In the case of the transport-adsorption regime, known as the rapid mixing regime, the transfer flux toward the adsorption sites dominates over the adsorption flux, so the dependence of the concentration on the spatial coordinates is negligible, and it results in adsorption-limited response kinetics, determined by the kinetic Eqs. (6). These equations are mutually independent, and show the change of the number of adsorbed particles on any of n sites, in the form of the difference of the actual adsorption and desorption rates, a_i and d_i, which are linear functions of the number of adsorbed particles N_i (i = 1,2 … n). The fluctuations can then be analyzed by directly applying the Langevin method. This approach is usually applicable in the case of AD process of gas particles. In other cases (e.g. in biological sensors, where the analyte particles are typically large macromolecules with slow diffusion in liquid samples) it is necessary to take into account the influence of transfer processes on the fluctuations of the number of adsorbed particles.

Eqs. (6) and (15) directly yield the system of n independent Langevin equations

$$\frac{d\Delta N_i}{dt} = -(k_{ai}C_o + k_{di})\Delta N_i + \xi_i, i = 1, 2, \ldots, n \tag{22}$$

after a random source function is added on the right side of each equation.

When this system of equations is written in the matrix form, as shown in SubSection 3.1, the quadratic diagonal matrix **K** is obtained, and its elements are

$$K_{il} = \begin{cases} k_{ai}C_o + k_{di}, & i = l \\ 0, & i \neq l \end{cases}, i = 1, 2, \ldots, n, l = 1, 2, \ldots, n \tag{23}$$

The elements of the matrix $\mathbf{S}^2_\xi$ are (Eq. (20))

$$S^2_{\xi,il} = \begin{cases} 4k_{di}N_{ie}, & i = l \\ 0, & i \neq l \end{cases}, i = 1, 2, \ldots, n, l = 1, 2, \ldots, n \tag{24}$$

where N_{ie} is given by Eq. (7).

Since all the quadratic matrices on the right side of Eq. (19) are diagonal, the matrix $\mathbf{S}^2_{\Delta\mathrm{N}}(\omega)$ is also diagonal, i.e. the cross-spectral densities $S^2_{\Delta\mathrm{N},il}$ are equal to zero (the random processes ΔN_i and ΔN_l are statistically independent for every pair of i and l, $i \neq l$). The spectral densitities of fluctuations of the numbers of adsorbed particles are of the Lorenzian type

$$S^2_{\Delta N,ii}(f) = \frac{4k_{di}N_{ie}\tau^2_{AL,i}}{1 + (2\pi f)^2\tau^2_{AL,i}} \tag{25}$$

with the characteristic frequency $f_{c,AL,i} = 1/(2\pi\tau_{AL,i})$, where $\tau_{AL,i} = k_{ai}C_O + k_{di}$, and the AD noise PSD of a sensor with n types of adsorption sites is determined by the sum of Lorenzians

$$S^2_{\Delta R}(f) = \sum_{i=1}^{n} w_i^2 S^2_{\Delta N,ii}(f) = \sum_{i=1}^{n} w_i^2 \frac{4k_{di}N_{ie}\tau^2_{AL,i}}{1 + (2\pi f)^2\tau^2_{AL,i}} \tag{26}$$

3.3 Mass transfer influenced binding

The use of TCM for approximation of spatially and temporally dependent analyte concentration in a sensor chamber (see SubSection 2.3) has enabled the presentation of the macroscopic kinetic equations (Eqs. (10), (11) and (14)) in the form in which the change of the number of adsorbed particles in unit time equals the difference between the instantaneous effective rates of adsorption and desorption, $a_{eff,i}$ and $d_{eff,i}$, which are explicitely dependent only on the instantaneous numbers of adsorbed particles on adsorption sites of all types. Such form of the equations is suitable for fluctuation analysis. In order for the Langevin method to be applicable for obtaining the PSD of fluctuations of a sensor response when coupling of complex (n-component) AD process and mass transfer is considered, a linear approximation of the functions $a_{eff,i}$ and $d_{eff,i}$ around the equilibrium values of the numbers of adsorbed particles is used (assuming small fluctuations relative to the equilibrium values, $\Delta N_i << N_{ie}$) [59, 66]

$$a_{eff,i} \approx a_{eff,i}(N_{1e}, N_{2e} \dots N_{ne}) + \sum_{k=1}^{n} \left(\left. \frac{\partial a_{eff,i}}{\partial N_k} \right|_e \cdot \Delta N_k \right) \tag{27}$$

$$d_{eff,i} \approx d_{eff,i}(N_{ie}) + \left. \frac{\partial d_{eff,i}}{\partial N_i} \right|_e \cdot \Delta N_i \tag{28}$$

All the derivatives are calculated for $N_1 = N_{1e}, N_2 = N_{2e} \dots N_n = N_{ne}$ (the equilibrium values are determined by Eq. (12)), which is in the above expressions denoted with the subscript "e" within the derivatives. It can be noticed that $a_{eff,i}(N_{1e}, N_{2e} \dots N_{ne}) = d_{eff,i}(N_{ie})$, since the adsorption and desorption rates are pertinent to the equilibrium state, according to the condition $dN_i/dt = 0$. By substituting Eqs. (27) and (28) into Eqs. (10), linearized kinetic equations are obtained, which, after the addition of Langevin source functions on their right side assume the form of Langevin equations, shown by the matrix Eq. (17). The obtained expressions imply that the elements of the quadratic matrix **K** are

$$K_{il} = \begin{cases} -\left(\left. \frac{\partial a_{eff,i}}{\partial N_i} \right|_e - \left. \frac{\partial d_{eff,i}}{\partial N_i} \right|_e \right), & i = l \\ -\left. \frac{\partial a_{eff,i}}{\partial N_l} \right|_e, & i \neq l \end{cases}, i = 1, 2, \dots, n, l = 1, 2, \dots, n \tag{29}$$

and after differentiation

$$K_{ii} = \frac{k_{ai}C_0 + k_{di} + \left(k_{ai} \sum\limits_{\substack{k=1 \\ k \neq i}}^{n} k_{dk}N_{ek} + k_{di} \sum\limits_{\substack{k=1 \\ k \neq i}}^{n} k_{ak}(N_{\max,k} - N_{ek}) \right) / (k_m A)}{1 + \sum\limits_{k=1}^{n} k_{ak}(N_{\max,k} - N_{ek})/(k_m A)} \tag{30}$$

$$K_{ij} = -\frac{k_{ai}}{k_m A} \frac{k_{aj}C_0 + k_{dj} + \left(k_{aj} \sum\limits_{k=1}^{n} k_{dk}N_{ek} + k_{dj} \sum\limits_{k=1}^{n} k_{ak}(N_{\max,k} - N_{ek}) \right) / (k_m A)}{\left(1 + \sum\limits_{k=1}^{n} k_{ak}(N_{\max,k} - N_{ek})/(k_m A) \right)^2} (N_{\max,i} - N_{ei}) \tag{31}$$

Based on Eq. (20)

$$S^2_{\xi,il} = \begin{cases} 4k_{di}N_{ie}, & i = l \\ 0, & i \neq l \end{cases}, i = 1, 2, \dots, n, l = 1, 2, \dots, n \tag{32}$$

Now, all the quantities are known that enable the determination of the spectral and cross-spectral densities of fluctuations of the numbers of adsorbed particles on different types of adsorption sites, according to Eq. (19), as well as the spectral density of the sensor response fluctuations, based on Eq. (21)

When there are two types of adsorption sites on the sensing surface, the elements of the matrices **K** and $\mathbf{S}^2_\xi$ are, according to Eqs. (30)–(32)

$$K_{ii} = \frac{k_{ai}C_0 + k_{di} + (k_{ai}k_{dj}N_{ej} + k_{di}k_{aj}(N_{\max,j} - N_{ej}))/(k_m A)}{1 + (k_{a1}(N_{\max,1} - N_{e1}) + k_{a2}(N_{\max,2} - N_{e2}))/(k_m A)}, i = 1,2, j = 1,2.$$

$$K_{ij} = -\frac{k_{ai}}{k_m A}\frac{k_{aj}C_0 + k_{dj} + (k_{aj}k_{dj}N_{\max,j} + k_{aj}k_{di}N_{ei} + k_{dj}k_{ai}(N_{\max,i} - N_{ei}))/(k_m A)}{\left(1 + \sum_{k=1}^{n} k_{ak}(N_{\max,k} - N_{ek})/(k_m A)\right)^2}(N_{\max,i} - N_{ei})$$

$$\mathbf{S}^2_\xi = \begin{bmatrix} 4k_{d1}N_{e1} & 0 \\ 0 & 4k_{d2}N_{e2} \end{bmatrix}$$

so the PSD of the AD noise, calculated based on Eq. (21), is

$$S^2_{\Delta R}(f) = 4\left(w_1^2 k_{d1}N_{e1} + w_2^2 k_{d2}N_{e2}\right)\frac{\tau^2_{MT,1}\tau^2_{MT,2}}{\tau^2_{Mt,3}}\frac{1 + (2\pi f)^2\tau^2_{MT,3}}{\left(1 + (2\pi f)^2\tau^2_{MT,1}\right)\left(1 + (2\pi f)^2\tau^2_{MT,2}\right)} \tag{33}$$

where

$$\tau_{MT,1,2} = 2\left[K_{11} + K_{22} \pm \sqrt{(K_{11} - K_{22})^2 + 4K_{12}K_{21}}\right]^{-1} \tag{34}$$

$$\tau_{MT,3} = \sqrt{\left(w_1^2 d_{1e} + w_2^2 d_{2e}\right)\left[(w_1K_{22} - w_2K_{21})^2 d_{1e} + (w_2K_{11} - w_1K_{12})^2 d_{2e}\right]^{-1}} \tag{35}$$

The characteristic frequencies of the AD noise spectrum are $f_{c,\mathrm{MT},i} = 1/(2\pi\tau_{MT,i})$, where i is 1, 2 or 3.

The expressions for K_{ii} and K_{ij} for a fast mass transfer (at suffuciently high k_m) become approximately equal to the expressions given by Eq. (23), which are valid for the case of adsorption-limited binding. Also, in that case, Eq. (33) reduces to Eq. (26) for $n = 2$. This demonstrates a wider applicability of the expressions derived by using TCM. Namely, when the zone adjacent to the sensing surface, which contains the analyte particles that can participate in the adsorption is narrow, the expressions derived by using TCM for mass transfer influenced binding are valid even in the case of high k_m values, when the binding is adsorption limited.

4. Results and discussion

In order to analyze the effects of mass transfer and surface heterogeneity on the sensor temporal response and AD noise, numerical calculations are performed for the case of protein biosensor, on whose active surface two types of adsorption sites exist with different affinities toward the target analyte. The results are presented in terms of the adsorbed mass on the sensing surface, assuming the values of adsorption and desorption rate constants from the ranges corresponding to biomolecules and biosensors [68]: $k_{a1} = 1.3 \cdot 10^{-18}$ m^3/s, $k_{d1} = 0.4$ 1/s, $k_{a2} = 1.3 \cdot 10^{-20}$ m^3/s and $k_{d2} = 0.02$ 1/s, the mass of a single analyte particle $w = 20$ kDa, and the total of $N_{max} = 10^8$ adsorption sites on the sensing surface of area $A = 10^{-9}$ m^2. The analyte concentration is $C_0 = 5 \cdot 10^{17}$ 1/m^3.

Figure 2 shows the temporal change of adsorbed mass, representing the temporal response of the sensor whose measured parameter is a function of the total bound mass of the target protein. The total mass adsorbed on the sensing surface is

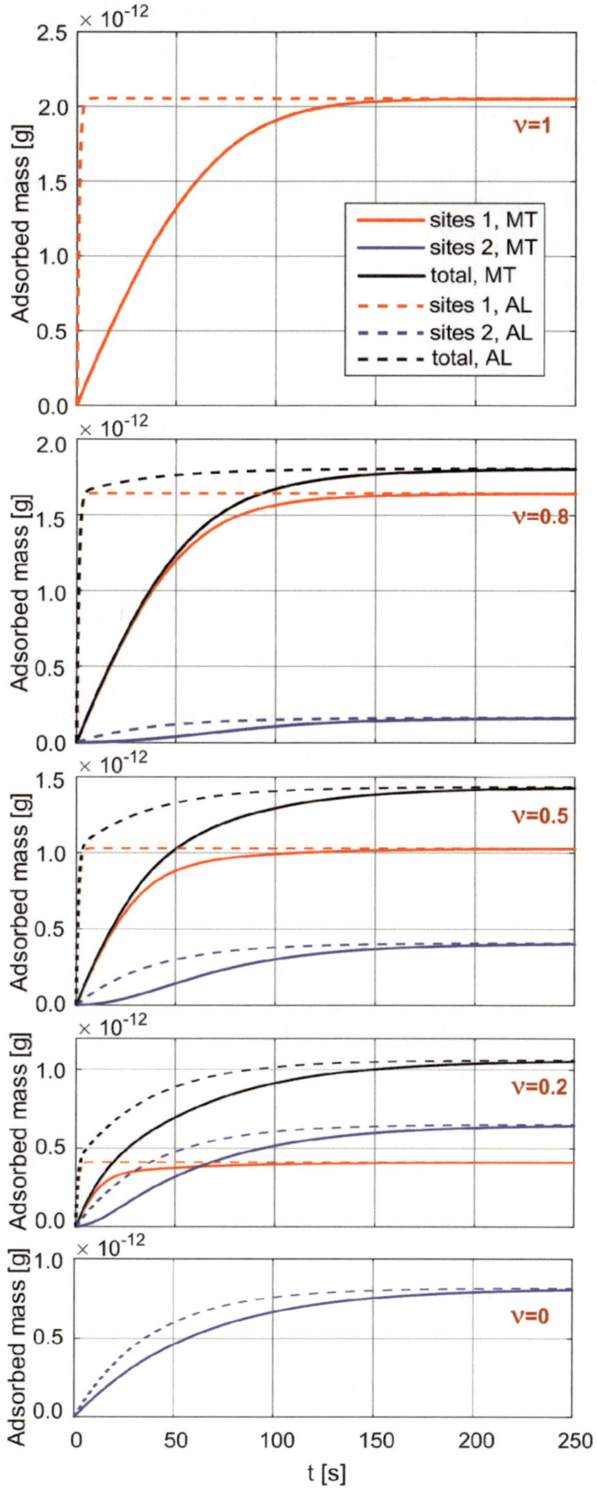

Figure 2.
The temporal change of the total adsorbed mass (black lines) on the heterogeneous surface of a biosensor. The adsorbed mass on each type of adsorption sites are also shown (red and blue lines). The five diagrams correspond to different shares of the types of adsorption sites in the overall number of sites, which is expressed by different values of the parameter ν*, where* $N_{max,1} = \nu N_{max}$ *and* $N_{max,2} = (1-\nu)N_{max}$*. The solid-line curves represent "slow" mass transfer (denoted as "MT"), and the dashed-line curves represent adsorption- limited kinetics (denoted as "AL").*

shown (black lines), as well as the adsorbed amounts on each of the two types of adsorption sites (red lines for the type 1 sites, blue lines for the type 2 sites). The five diagrams correspond to different shares of the types of adsorption sites in the overall number of sites, which is expressed by different values of the parameter ν (1; 0.8; 0.5; 0.2, 0), where $N_{max,1} = \nu N_{max}$ and $N_{max,2} = (1\text{-}\nu)N_{max}$. Different cases are illustrated: from the presence of only the high-affinity sites (type 1 sites), to various ratios of the numbers of sites belonging to the two types ($N_{max,1}$:$N_{max,2}$ that equals 4:1, 1:1 and 1:4), and, finally, to the presence of only the low-affinity sites (type 2 sites) on the sensing surface. As the measure of the affinity, the affinity constant is used, which is defined by the ratio k_{ai}/k_{di}. The curves are obtained by computer simulation, based on the model that takes into account the mass transfer effects (Eqs. (14)), for two values of the mass transfer coefficient: $k_{mI} = 2{\cdot}10^{-3}$ m/s (solid line) and $k_{mII} = 9{\cdot}10^{-1}$ m/s (dashed line). For $k_m > k_{mII}$, the obtained curves overlap with those for k_{mII}, and they also overlap with the curves obtained by the use of the model that neglects mass transfer (Eqs. (6) and (7)). This means that the value of k_{mII} is high enough for the influence of mass transfer on the sensor's temporal response to be considered as negligible, so that conclusions about the mass transfer influence can be made by comparing the responses for k_{mI} and k_{mII}.

In the absence of the mass transfer influence (dashed-line curves shown in the diagram), the existence of two types of adsorption sites is clearly noticeable based on the sharp transition from fast to slow transient regime (for ν equal to 0.8, 0.5 or 0.2). The time evolution of the total adsorbed mass is rapid at first, as it is dominantly determined by adsorption on the higher affinity sites, with the time constant of approximately 1 s, but it then slowly approaches the steady state, with the time constant of approximately 38 s (AD process on sites of lower affinity). Even with a lower share of low affinity sites, the AD process occurring on them determines the sensor response rate. Different shares of the two types of adsorption sites influence the sensor response value in the steady state.

When the mass transfer is characterized by k_{mI}, a pronounced MT influence on the sensor response kinetics is evident at all values of ν. Such results are in accord with Eq. (13) by which the analytic criterion is defined for a negligible influence of MT on the response. For two types of adsorption sites, that criterion is $k_m >> k_{mg}$, where $k_{mg} = (k_{a1}{\cdot}\nu + k_{a2}{\cdot}(1\text{-}\nu)){\cdot}N_{max}/A$, and for the given parameters k_{mg} equals $1.3{\cdot}10^{-1}$ m/s, $1{\cdot}10^{-1}$ m/s, $6.6{\cdot}10^{-2}$ m/s, $2.7{\cdot}10^{-2}$ m/s, and $1.3{\cdot}10^{-3}$ m/s for ν equal to 1, 0.8, 0.5, 0.2 and 0, respectively. Hence, when $k_m = k_{mI}$, the above-mentioned condition is not satisfied for any ν. It can be seen that the minimal MT coefficient value at which the response kinetics can be considered as adsorption limited increases with the increase of the type 1 sites share. The influence of mass transfer characterized by the parameter k_{mI} on the time evolution of the number of adsorbed particles is more pronounced for the sites with a higher adsorption rate constant. Thus, the initial evolution of the total number of adsorbed particles is much slower compared to the case of adsorption limited binding.

Figure 3 shows the spectral density (SD) of adsorbed mass fluctuations, $(S_{\Delta R}{}^2(f))^{1/2}$, i.e. the spectral density of sensor AD noise, for the same parameter values for which the response shown in **Figure 2** was obtained. It is obtained as a square root of the PSD, given by Eq. (33), which, apart from surface heterogeneity, takes into account mass transfer. SDs of the total adsorbed mass are shown for two values of the MT coefficient: $k_{mI} = 2{\cdot}10^{-3}$ m/s (solid red lines) and $k_{mII} = 9{\cdot}10^{-1}$ m/s (solid blue lines), for each of five values of ν. As in the case of response, the curves obtained for $k_m > k_{mII}$ match those for k_{mII}. Also matching with them are the curves obtained by using Eq. (26), i.e. the model that neglects mass transfer. According to that model, PSD of AD noise equals the sum of PSDs of fluctuations of adsorbed masses on two types of sites. The SDs corresponding to these components are also

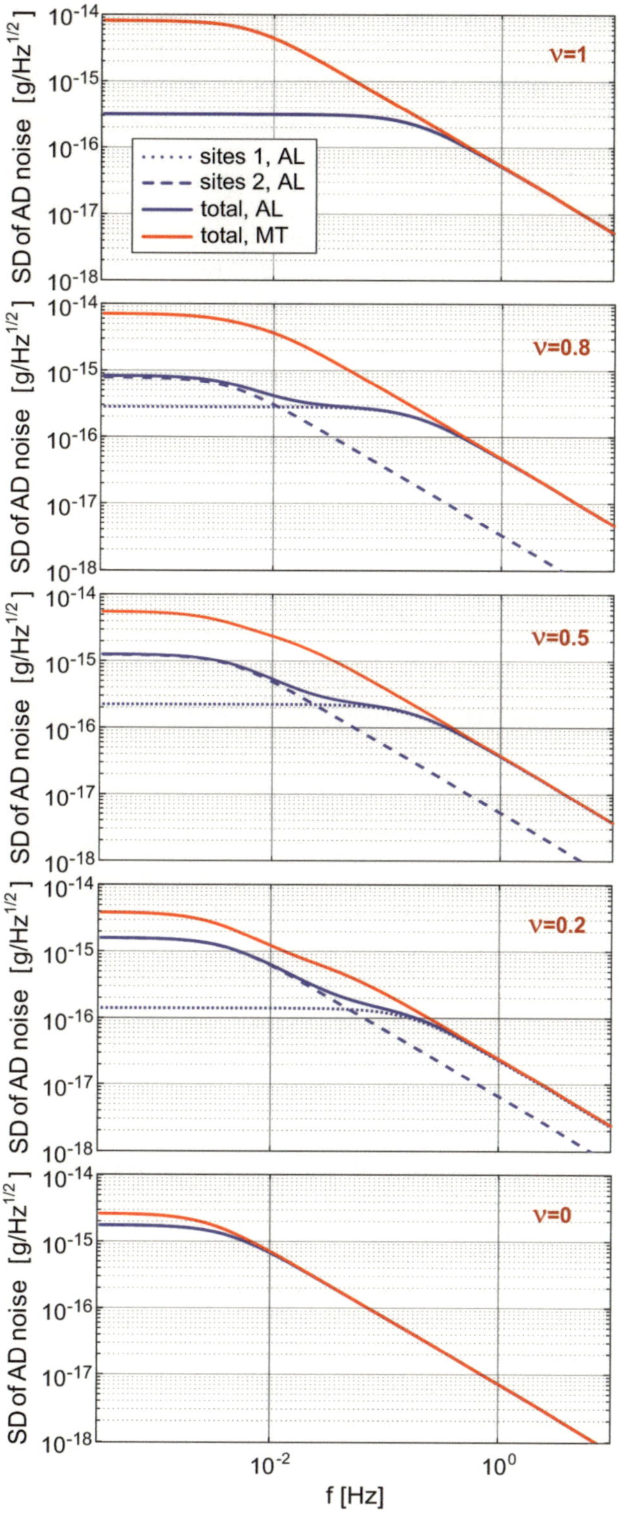

Figure 3.
The spectral density (SD) of adsorbed mass fluctuations, i.e. the spectral density of biosensor AD noise, for the same parameter values for which the response shown in ***Figure 2*** *was calculated. The total adsorbed mass SDs are shown for the cases when the mass transfer influence is pronounced (solid red lines), and when it is negligible (solid blue lines), for each of the five values of ν. Also shown are SDs of fluctuations of adsorbed masses on two types of sites (dotted lines denote type 1 sites, and dashed lines denote type 2 sites) in the absence of the mass transfer influence.*

shown in the diagrams (dotted lines denote type 1 sites, and dashed lines denote type 2 sites). Hence, the influence of mass transfer on the AD noise is negligible for $k_m = k_{mII}$, and the comparison of the results for the shown SDs of total fluctuations for a given ν enables making conclusions on the influence of mass transfer on the sensor AD noise.

It can be noticed that at all the values of ν, mass transfer leads to the increase of the AD noise magnitude in the part of the spectrum where the characteristic frequencies belong. It also increases the AD noise (obtained by integration of the AD noise SD in the frequency range of interest), and thus influences the fundamental detection and quantification limits of a biosensor. For a given ν, mass transfer also causes a shift of the characteristic frequencies of the AD noise spectrum. Thus, the AD noise spectral analysis can yield information not only on adsorption and desorption rate constants and analyte concentration, but also on mass transfer parameters.

By comparing the diagrams for the case of a surface containing a single type of adsorption sites (i.e. for $\nu = 1$ or $\nu = 0$) with the diagrams for the sensors with a heterogeneous adsorbing surface (i.e. when ν equals 0.8, 0.5 or 0.2), it is obvious that the latter diagrams may exhibit a greater number of characteristic frequencies (three in the case of two type of adsorption sites), which can indicate the existence of different types of adsorption sites.

The diagrams also show that when the mass transfer influence is negligible, the two characteristic frequencies of the AD spectrum do not change at different shares of adsorption site types on the sensing surface. They are determined by the characteristic frequencies that correspond to the fluctuation spectra of adsorbed masses on each of site types, which are given by expressions $f_{c,AL,i} = 1/(2\pi\tau_{AL,i})$, where $\tau_{AL,i} = k_{ai}C_0 + k_{di}$, as given in Section 3.2. Contrary to that, when the mass transfer influence is pronounced, all the three AD noise spectrum characteristic frequencies change with ν, so that their values also contain the data on the share of a specific site type on the sensing surface. Therefore, as the parameters of all the processes and effects that influence the sensor temporal response are contained in the characteristic features of the AD noise spectrum, noise spectrum analysis can be used as an additional source of data in biosensing.

5. Conclusions

In this chapter, the mathematical modeling has been performed of time response and adsorption–desorption (AD) noise in microfluidic adsorption-based biosensors whose active surface is heterogeneous in the sense that it contains adsorption sites of different affinity toward the target analyte. The adsorption–desorption processes of analyte particles on different types of adsorption sites, as well as mass transfer in a microfluidic chamber, have been taken into account as the coupled processes that generate the sensor signal. The devised model of AD noise is the first that simultaneously takes into account surface heterogeneity and mass transfer through both the convection and diffusion of analyte particles. The analytical expression of the spectral density of AD noise has been derived. The models of the time response and AD noise of a sensor with heterogeneous adsorbing surface in the case of negligible mass transfer influence have also been presented. The criterion is given based on which it can be discerned whether the mass transfer influence is significant or negligible, so that the appropriate mathematical model of the response and noise can be chosen.

The derived mathematical models have been used for the analysis of the response and AD noise of protein biosensors that have two types of adsorption sites on the sensing surface. The comparison of the results obtained by the use of the models that take into account mass transfer effects, and those that neglect them, for different shares of two types of binding sites, has enabled drawing conclusions on both separate and coupled influences of surface heterogeneity and transport processes on the sensor response and noise.

While a slow mass transfer increases the sensor response time, the existence of different adsorption site types affects both the transient regime and the sensor response magnitude in the steady state. The minimal mass transfer coefficient value at which the response kinetics can be considered as adsorption limited increases with the increase of the share of high affinity binding sites. The influence of mass transfer (of given parameters) on the time evolution of the number of adsorbed particles is more pronounced on sites with a higher adsorption rate constant.

At any share of the two types of binding sites on the sensing surface, mass transfer causes the increase of the AD noise, and thus increases the sensor's fundamental limits of analyte detection and quantification. For a given ratio of the numbers of adsorption sites of the two types, mass transfer causes a shift of the characteristic frequencies in the AD noise spectrum. When the mass transfer influence is pronounced, the characteristic frequencies shift with the change of the ratio of the numbers of sites of different types. Therefore, the AD noise spectrum analysis can yield information not only on adsorption and desorption rate constants and analyte concentration, but also on mass transfer parameters and on the share of a certain type of binding sites on the sensing surface. It can be used as an additional source of data in biosensing.

As the results of the performed analysis have shown a potentially significant influence of sensing surface heterogeneity and mass transfer processes on the sensor temporal response, as well as on AD noise, which is inevitable in adsorption-based sensors and determines their ultimate sensing performance, the presented mathematical models can enable better interpretation of measurement results, and give guidelines for ensuring lower noise levels and improved detection limits in microfluidic biosensors.

Acknowledgements

This research was funded by the Ministry of Education, Science and Technological Development of the Republic of Serbia, grant number 451-03-9/2021-2114/200026. It was also supported by the Science Fund of the Republic of Serbia, PROMIS, #6057070, Gramulsen.

Author details

Ivana Jokić
University of Belgrade – Institute of Chemistry, Technology and Metallurgy – National Institute of the Republic of Serbia, Belgrade, Serbia

*Address all correspondence to: ijokic@nanosys.ihtm.bg.ac.rs

References

[1] Sackmann EK , Fulton AL, Beebe DJ. The present and future role of microfluidics in biomedical research. Nature. 2014;507: 181–189.

[2] Luka G, Ahmadi A, Najjaran H, Alocilja E, DeRosa M, Wolthers K, Malki A, Aziz H, Althani A, Hoorfar M. Microfluidics integrated biosensors: A leading technology towards lab-on-a-chip and sensing applications. Sensors. 2015;15: 30011–30031.

[3] Liu K-K, Wu R-G, Chuang Y-J, Khoo HS, Huang S-H, Tseng F-G. Microfluidic systems for biosensing. Sensors. 2010;10:6623–6661.

[4] Xua D, Huangc X, Guod J, Ma X. Automatic smartphone-based microfluidic biosensor system at the point of care. Biosensors and Bioelectronics. 2018;10:78–88.

[5] Srinivasan B, Tung S. Development and Applications of Portable Biosensors. Journal of Laboratory Automation. 2015; 20:365–389. doi.org/10.1177/2211068215581349

[6] Zu, Z.-H. Wang, N.-K. Chou, S. S. Lu, "A Wireless Bio-MEMS Sensor for C-Reactive Protein Detection Based on Nanomechanics", IEEE Internat. Conf. on Solid-State Circuits ISSCC 2006, San Francisco 2006, pp. 2298–2307.

[7] Padash M, Enz C, Carrara S. Microfluidics by Additive Manufacturing for Wearable Biosensors: A Review. Sensors. 2020;20:4236. doi: 10.3390/s20154236

[8] Nightingale AM, Leong CL, Burnish RA et al. Monitoring biomolecule concentrations in tissue using a wearable droplet microfluidic-based sensor. Nat. Commun. 2019;10:2741. https://doi.org/10.1038/s41467-019-10401-y

[9] Mejía-Salazar JR, Cruz KR, Vásques EMM, de Oliveira Jr. ON. Microfluidic Point-of-Care Devices: New Trends and Future Prospects for eHealth Diagnostics. Sensors. 2020,20: 1951. doi:10.3390/s20071951

[10] Mohd-Yasin F, Nagel DJ, Korman CE. Noise in MEMS. Meas. Sci. Technol. 2010;21:012001 1–22.

[11] Palasantzas G. Adsorption-desorption noise influence on mass sensitivity and dynamic range of nanoresonators with rough surfaces. J. Appl. Phys. 2007;101:076103 1–3.

[12] Djurić Z. Noise in Microsystems and Semiconductor Photodetectors. In: Proc. of the XLIV Conference ETRAN; 2000; Sokobanja. Serbia. 2000. p. 9–16.

[13] Arakelian VB, Wildt JR, Simonian AL. Investigation of stochastic fluctuations in the signal formation of microbiosensors. Biosensors and Bioelectronics. 1998.13:55–59.

[14] Hassibi A, Zahedi S, Navid R, Dutton RW, Lee TH. Biological shot-noise and quantum-limited signal-to-noise ratio in affinity-based biosensors. J. Appl. Phys. 2005.97:084701 1–10.

[15] Djurić Z, Jokić I, Frantlović M, Jakšić O. Influence of Adsorption-Desorption Process on Resonant Frequency and Noise of Micro- and Nanocantilevers. In: Proc. 23rd Internatinal Conference on Microelectronics (MIEL); 12–15 May 2002; Niš. Serbia. 2002. Vol. 2: p. 243–246.

[16] Kim S-J, Ono T, Esashi M. Study on the noise of silicon capacitive resonant mass sensors in ambient atmosphere. J. Appl. Phys. 2007;102:104304 1–6.

[17] Amin KR, Bid A. Effect of ambient on the resistance fluctuations of graphene. Appl. Phys. Lett. 2015;106:183105 1–5.

[18] Contaret T, Florido T, Seguin J-L, Aguir K. A Physics-Based Noise Model

for Metallic Oxide Gas Sensors Characterization. Procedia Engineering. 2011;25:375–378.

[19] Sedlak P, Sikula J, Majzner J, Vrnata M, Fitl P, Kopecky D, Vyslouzil F, Handel PH. Adsorption–desorption noise in QCM gas sensors. Sens. Actuators B: Chemical. 2012;166–167:264–268.

[20] Contaret T, Seguin J-L, Menini P, Aguir K. Physical-Based Characterization of Noise Responses in Metal-Oxide Gas Sensors. IEEE Sensors Journal. 2013;13:980–986. 10.1109/JSEN.2012.2227707

[21] Wang DS, Fan SK. Microfluidic Surface Plasmon Resonance Sensors: From Principles to Point-of-Care Applications. Sensors. 2016;16:1175. doi: 10.3390/s16081175

[22] Peña-Bahamonde J, Nguyen HN, Fanourakis SK, et al. Recent advances in graphene-based biosensor technology with applications in life sciences. J. Nanobiotechnol. 2018;16:75.

[23] Ambhorkar P, Wang Z, Ko H, Lee S, Koo K-in, Kim K, Cho D-il. Nanowire-Based Biosensors: From Growth to Applications. Micromachines. 2018;9: 679. doi:10.3390/mi9120679

[24] Liu S, Guo X. Carbon nanomaterials field-effect-transistor-based biosensors. NPG Asia Mater. 2012;4:e23.

[25] Voiculescu I, Nordin AN. Acoustic wave based MEMS devices for biosensing applications. Biosensors and Bioelectronics. 2012;33:1–9.

[26] Zhang Y, LuoJ, Flewitt AJ, Cai Z, Zhao X. Film bulk acoustic resonators (FBARs) as biosensors: A review. Biosensors and Bioelectronics. 2018;116: 1–15.

[27] Arlett JL, Myers EB, Roukes ML, Comparative advantages of mechanical biosensors. Nature Nanotechnology. 2011;6:203–215.

[28] Zheng F, Wang P, Du Q, Chen Y, Liu N. Simultaneous and Ultrasensitive Detection of Foodborne Bacteria by Gold Nanoparticles-Amplified Microcantilever Array Biosensor. Front. Chem. 2019;7:232.

[29] Mehand M, Srinivasan B, De Crescenzo G. Optimizing Multiple Analyte Injections in Surface Plasmon Resonance Biosensors with Analytes having Different Refractive Index Increments. Sci. Rep. 2015;5:15855. https://doi.org/10.1038/srep15855

[30] Schuck P, Zhao H. The role of mass transport limitation and surface heterogeneity in the biophysical characterization of macromolecular binding processes by SPR biosensing. Methods Mol. Biol. 2010;627:15–54. doi: 10.1007/978-1-60761-670-2_2.

[31] Myszka DG, He X, Dembo M, Morton TA, Goldstein B. Extending the Range of Rate Constants Available from BIACORE: Interpreting Mass Transport-Influenced Binding Data. Biophys. J. 1998;75:583–594.

[32] Gervais T, Jensen KF. Mass transport and surface reactions in microfluidic systems. Chem. Eng. Sci. 2006;61:1102–1121.

[33] Squires TM, Messinger RJ, Manalis SR. Making it stick: convection, reaction and diffusion in surface-based biosensors. Nature Biotechnology. 2008; 26:417–426.

[34] Bishop J, Chagovetz AM, Blair S. Competitive displacement: A sensitive and selective method for the detection of unlabeled molecules. Optics Express. 2007;15:4390–4397.

[35] Karlsson R. Real-time competitive kinetic analysis of interactions between low-molecular-weight ligands in

solution and surface-immobilized receptors. Analytical Biochemistry. 1994;221:142–151.

[36] Tripathi S, Tabor RF. Modeling two-rate adsorption kinetics: Two-site, two-species, bilayer and rearrangement adsorption processes. Journal of Colloid and Interface Science. 2016;476:119–131.

[37] Jokić I, Radulović K, Frantlović M, Đurić Z, Vasiljević-Radović D. Combined influence of competitive binding and mass transfer on response of affinity-based biosensors. In: Proc. Regional Biophysics Conference; 3.-7 September 2012; Kladovo. Serbia. 2012. p. 45–47.

[38] Ding YX, Hlady V. Competitive Adsorption of Three Human Plasma Proteins onto Sulfhydryl-to-sulfonate Gradient Surfaces. Croat. Chem. Acta. 2011;84:193–202.

[39] Svitel J, Boukari H, Van Ryk D, Willson RC, Schuck P. Probing the Functional Heterogeneity of Surface Binding Sites by Analysis of Experimental Binding Traces and the Effect of Mass Transport Limitation. Biophysical Journal. 2007;92:1742–1758.

[40] Kumar KV, Gadipelli S, Wood B, Ramisetty KA, Stewart AA, Howard CA, Brett DJL, Rodriguez-Reinoso F. Characterization of the adsorption site energies and heterogeneous surfaces of porous materials. J. Mater. Chem. A. 2019;7:10101–10137.

[41] Andrić S, Tomašević-Ilić T, Bošković MV, Sarajlić M, Vasiljević-Radović D, Smiljanić MM, Spasenović M. Ultrafast humidity sensor based on liquid phase exfoliated graphene. Nanotechnology. 2020;32: 025505: 1–8.

[42] Choy TC. Effective Medium Theory: Principles and Applications. Oxford: Oxford University Press; 2015. https://doi.org/10.1093/acprof:oso/9780198705093.001.0001

[43] Gervais T. Mass transfer and structural analysis of microfluidic sensors [thesis]. Massachusetts Institute of Technology; 2006.

[44] Anderson H, Wingqvist G, Weissbach T, Wallinder D, Katardjiev I, Ingemarsson B. Systematic investigation of biomolecular interactions using combined frequency and motional resistance measurements. Sens. Actuators B: Chemical. 2011;153:135–144.

[45] Kusnezow W, Syagailo YV, Rüffer S, Klenin K, Sebald W, Hoheisel JD, Gauer C, Goychuk I. Kinetics of antigen binding to antibody microspots: Strong limitation by mass transport to the surface. Proteomics. 2006;6:794–803.

[46] Djurić Z. Mechanisms of noise sources in microelectromechanical systems. Microelectronics Reliability. 2000;40:919–932.

[47] Schmera G, Kish LB. Fluctuation-enhanced gas sensing by surface acoustic wave devices. Fluctuation and Noise Letters. 2002;2:L117–L123.

[48] Nguyen CT-C. Micromechanical resonators for oscillators and filters. In: Proc. IEEE Int. Ultrasonics Symposium; 7–10 November 1995; Seattle. WA. 1995. p. 489–499.

[49] Vig JR, Kim Y. Noise in microelectromechanical system resonators. IEEE Trans. Ultrason. Ferroelectr. Freq. Control. 1999;46: 1558–1565.

[50] Ekinci KL, Yang YT, Roukes ML. Ultimate limits to inertial mass sensing based upon nanoelectromechanical systems. J. Appl. Phys. 2004;95:2682–2689.

[51] Gomri S, Seguin J-L, Aguir K. Modelling on oxygen chemisorption induced noise in metallic oxide gas

sensors. Sens. Actuators B. 2005;107: 722–729.

[52] Jakšić Z , Đurić Z, Jakšić O, Jokić I, Frantlović M. Adsorption-desorption noise in surface plasmon resonance sensors. In: Proc. 8th International Conference on Fundamental and Applied Aspects of Physical Chemistry; 26–29 September 2006; Belgrade. Serbia. 2006. Vol. II: p. 671–673.

[53] Gomri S, Seguin J-L, Guerin J, Aguir K. Adsorption–desorption noise in gas sensors: Modelling using Langmuir and Wolkenstein models for adsorption. Sens. Actuators B: Chemical. 2006;114: 451–459.

[54] Djurić Z, Jokić I, Frantlović M, Jakšić O. Fluctuations of the number of particles and mass adsorbed on the sensor surface surrounded by a mixture of an arbitrary number of gases. Sensors and Actuators B: Chemical. 2007;127: 625–631. DOI: 10.1016/j.snb.2007.05.025

[55] Djurić ZG, Jokić IM, Frantlović MP, Radulović KT. Two-layer adsorption and adsorbed mass fluctuations on micro/nanostructures. Microelectronic Engineering. 2009;86:1278–1281.

[56] Djurić Z, Jokić I, Djukić I, Frantlović M. Fluctuations of the adsorbed mass and the resonant frequency of vibrating MEMS/NEMS structures due to multilayer adsorption. Microelectronic Engineering. 2010;87: 1181–1184.

[57] Hassibi A, Vikalo H, Hajimiri A. On noise processes and limits of performance in biosensors. J. Appl. Phys. 2007;102:014909 1–12.

[58] Jokić I, Djurić Z, Frantlović M, Radulović K, Krstajić P, Jokić Z. Fluctuations of the number of adsorbed molecules in biosensors due to stochastic adsorption-desorption processes coupled with mass transfer. Sensors and Actuators B: Chemical. 2012;166–167:535–543. http://dx.doi.org/10.1016/j.snb.2012.03.004

[59] Frantlović M, Jokić I, Djurić Z, Radulović K. Analysis of the Competitive Adsorption and Mass Transfer Influence on Equilibrium Mass Fluctuations in Affinity-Based Biosensors. Sensors and Actuators B: Chemical. 2013;189:71–79. doi:10.1016/j.snb.2012.12.080

[60] Jokić I, Frantlović M, Djurić Z, Radulović K, Jokić Z. Adsorption–desorption noise in microfluidic biosensors operating in multianalyte environments. Microelectronic Engineering. 2015;144:32–36. dx.doi.org/10.1016/j.mee.2015.02.032

[61] Djurić Z, Jokić I, Peleš A. Fluctuations of the number of adsorbed molecules due to adsorption-desorption processes coupled with mass transfer and surface diffusion in bio/chemical MEMS sensors. Microelectronic Engineering. 2014;124:81–85. http://dx.doi.org/10.1016/j.mee.2014.06.001

[62] Rumyantsev S, Liu G, Shur MS, Potyrailo RA, Balandin AA. Selective gas sensing with a single pristine graphene transistor. NanoLetters. 2012;12:2294–2295.

[63] Jokić I, Jakšić O. A second-order nonlinear model of monolayer adsorption in refractometric chemical sensors and biosensors: case of equilibrium fluctuations. Optical and Quantum Electronics. 2016;48:1–7. DOI: 10.1007/s11082-016-0620-0

[64] Tulzer G, Heitzinger C. Fluctuations due to association and dissociation processes at nanowire biosensor surfaces and their optimal design. Nanotechnology. 2015;26:025502 1–9.

[65] Van Kampen NG. Stochastic processes in physics and chemistry. Amsterdam: Elsevier BV; 1981–2007.

[66] Van Vliet CM. Macroscopic and microscopic methods for noise in devices. IEEE Trans. Electr. Dev. 1994; 41:1902–1915.

[67] Van der Ziel A. Fluctuation Phenomena in Semi-Conductors. London: Butterwrths; 1959.

[68] Canziani G, Zhang W, Cines D, Rux A, Willis S, Cohen G, Eisenberg R, Chaiken I. Exploring Biomolecular Recognition Using Optical Biosensors. Methods. 1999;19(2):253–269.

Chapter 8

Hybrid Heterostructures for SPR Biosensor

Md. Shamim Anower, Md. Mahabubur Rahman and M. Saifur Rahman

Abstract

Surface plasmon resonance (SPR) based biosensors have been enormously studied in the last decade for their better sensitivity. In recent years hybrid heterostructures are getting popularity to implement these SPR biosensors for their superior sensing capability. This chapter demonstrates the details of SPR technology with two recently studied prism-based hybrid heterostructures. These heterostructures are made up of conventional SPR biosensors with two additional layers of recently invented transition metal dichalcogenides, platinum di-selenide ($PtSe_2$), and highly sensitive 2D material, tungsten di-sulfide (WS_2). Angular interrogation method is discussed to investigate the sensing capabilities of the sensors which prove the superiority of the Ag-$PtSe_2$-WS_2 structure. The sensing capability of this structure has been found at least 1.67 times higher than that of the conventional non-hybrid structures, respectively, with comparable FOM and QF. A comparison table has been provided at the end of this chapter which also shows the impressive performance of the hybrid heterostructures for SPR biosensors. Proper demonstration with a suitable example of this chapter will emphasize the potential use of hybrid heterostructure based SPR biosensors in prospective medical diagnostics and biomedical detection applications.

Keywords: biosensor, hybrid heterostructure, sensitivity, surface plasmon resonance

1. Introduction

Surface plasmon resonance (SPR) biosensors have become one of the most promising, standard, and affordable technology due to prompt research and expansion of SPR phenomenon in the last two decades. Nowadays, SPR sensors are broadly implemented for numerous biological and biochemical analytes identification and characterization due to its high sensitivity, real-time monitoring, level free detection assay, small sample size, and reusable sensor chip [1–5]. To be detailed, the SPR biosensors are adopted to agriculture and food quality monitoring [6], security and safely analysis [7], in need of medical diagnostics, environmental monitoring, bio-imaging [8–10], cancer detection [11, 12], DNA hybridization [13, 14], enzyme detection [15], protein-protein, protein-DNA, and protein-virus hybridization [16, 17], microorganisms identifying [18], industrial appliance's condition monitoring, temperature monitoring [19], gas sensing [20, 21], chemical and biochemical analysis [22, 23], pharmaceutical and biological molecule analysis [24, 25], oil condition monitoring [26], and so on. In the year 1902, Wood [27] first

observed unexpected optical power attenuation characteristic at the time of measuring the reflection of light from metallic gratings. This phenomenon occurs due to absorbance and conversion of photon energy to surface plasma wave (SPW) which is the result of combined oscillation of excited electrons called surface plasmon polaritons (SPPs). This oscillating electron consumes maximum energy at a certain wavelength for a specific angle of incidence of light which is called resonance condition. That is why this phenomenon is named surface plasmon resonance (SPR).
In 1968, Otto [28] and Kretschmann [29] introduced attenuated total internal reflection (ATR), which encouraged scientists and researchers to concentrate on the implementation of SPR sensing technology practically. In 1982, the SPR sensing technique was first demonstrated by Nylander and Liedberg [4, 30] for the practical application of gas sensing. After that, SPR sensing technology has been getting ceaselessly developing consideration from the scientific and academic network. In 1990, the SPR sensing instrument was first commercially produced and introduced to the market by Biacore AB. Since then a considerable number of manufacturers e.g. IBIS Technologies B.V., Graffinity pharmaceuticals, GWC Technologies, Bio-Red, AutoLab, Farfield Sensors, Genoptics Bio Interactions, Microvaccum, Biosensing Instrument, and SPR Navi have launched their SPR instruments to the market [17, 31].

Different optical techniques are currently proposed for sensing purposes, including Ramman scattering based sensors [32, 33], grating coupled sensors [34, 35], prism coupled sensors [36, 37], optical fiber-based sensors [38, 39], planner waveguide-based sensors [40, 41] etc. The optical biosensors basically work with the measurement of change in input incident light and detected light at the output terminal. To be specific, the change in phase, amplitude, wavelength, frequency, or polarization of light is measured at the output terminal of the sensors and the changes in these parameters are observed. Among them, the commonly used technique is observing the reflected light angle where maximum light is attenuated. This method is called angular interrogation approach with attenuated total internal reflection (ATR) that is applied usually in prism coupled devices. The performance of an optical sensor is basically measured in terms of its sensitivity, detection accuracy or detection limit, the figure of merits (FOM) and quality factor (QF), etc. The researchers and scientists are continuously working for the improvement of the performances of the SPR sensors [31, 42–44].

In SPR biosensors, the most crucial parameters determining the characteristics of the sensors are plasmonic materials. Materials with adequate free electrons at their valance bands can be used as plasmonic materials. To be specific, metals e.g. gold (Au), aluminum (Al), silver (Ag), copper (Cu), etc. are a good candidate to be used as a plasmonic material [45, 46]. Al and Cu have not gained much interest to be used because of their high damping nature, prone to oxidation, corrosion, and interband transition characteristics. But Silver (Ag) can be nominated as a potential candidate for SPR sensors as it attributes outstanding optical properties, such as no interband transfer at the visible light frequency, small optical damping, and sharper resonance peak [46–48], etc. Using Ag in SPR sensors, better sensitivity can be captured, but it shows poor chemical stability as it creates brittle oxide layers with liquid analyte [49]. Some researchers have reported that applying bimetallic layer on the Ag surface can resolve this problem [50, 51]. On the other hand, Au is more chemically stable compared to Ag and free of corrosion and oxidation problems. But, gold offers a slightly higher damping loss and widen SPR curve that restricts the detection accuracy and figure of merits (FOM) of the sensors [52]. The sensitivity of Au-based sensors is also slightly lower because of the low biomolecular adsorption characteristics of the gold surface. In order to improve the sensitivity of the sensors, researchers recommended various approaches in which the application

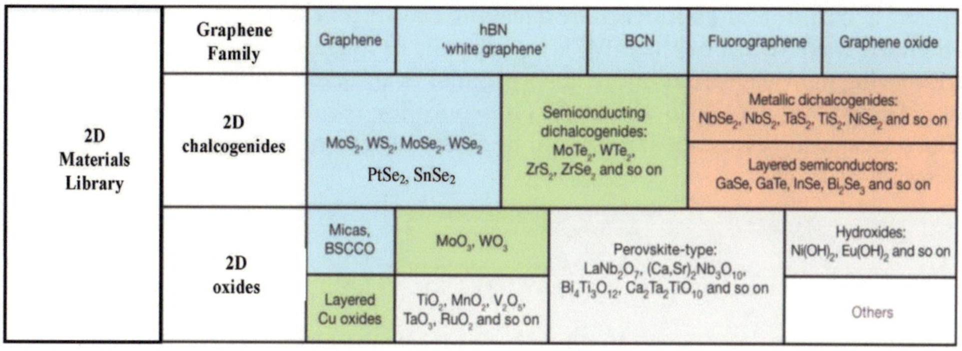

Figure 1.
2D materials library where blue shaded materials are stable at ambient condition, green-shaded are probably stable, pink shaded are unstable at ambient condition but stable at inert condition. The gray shaded mistrials are 3D but can be exfoliated down to monolayers [60, 61].

of hybrid structures (multilayer structures) are widely used [53–56]. Various 2D materials are used in the hybrid configuration of SPR based sensors. A single atom thick carbon nanostructure (graphene) is often applied on the top of the plasmonic materials to avoid oxidation problems and increase the performance of the sensors because of its chemical inertness and high adsorption characteristics [57, 58]. There are also some other nanomaterials e.g. graphene oxides, graphene carbon nitrite (g-C_3N_4), transition metal dichalcogenides (TMDCs: MoS_2, $MoSe_2$, WS_2, WSe_2, $PtSe_2$, $SnSe_2$, etc.), transition metal chalcogenides ($NbSe_3$, $TaSe_3$), transition metal oxides (TMOs: $LaVO_3$, $LaMnO_3$), Black phosphorene (BP), hexagonal boron nitride (hBN), group IV elements [59, 60] and so on which are summarized in the **Figure 1**.

This chapter mainly focuses on the recent trends applied for enhancing the performance of the Kretschmann configuration based prism coupled SPR sensors and their potential applications. The fundamental theory of SPR phenomena is presented first. Then, the method of angular interrogation utilizing attenuated total internal reflection and the performance measuring parameters of the SPR sensors are narrated. Finally, with their compressive architectures, recent developments of the prism coupled SPR sensors are discussed.

2. Principle of SPR phenomena

Metals are composed of positively charged nuclei with a lot of free electrons in their conduction band (surface of the metal). If an external electric field is applied close to the metal surface, free electrons are dislocated, resulting in an electric dipole [61]. A longitudinal oscillation has resulted from such electron transportation in a metal surface known as surface plasmons (SPs) [49]. To support the generated SPs a metal and dielectric interface is needed [46] whereas excitation of these SPs leads to an enhanced electromagnetic field resulting in a collective oscillation of free electrons or electron plasma [46, 61, 62]. The basic principle of the construction of SPR based sensors lies in the generation and propagation of electromagnetic waves called surface plasmon wave (SPW) due to the interaction of irradiating electric fields and the generated fields for dislocation of the electrons between the metal-dielectric interface [4]. The SPWs can only be produced by the incidence of a transverse magnetic (TM-) or plane (p-) polarized field as Maxwell's equations supports no solution for transverse electric (TE-) polarized case [46]. Furthermore, the fact that electron oscillation means resistive losses. Thus, when an optical field appears at the metal-dielectric boundary, the SPW produces due to optical absorption of exponentially decaying evanescent waves. Mathematically, when the wave vector of the SPW is equal to the propagation constant of the irradiating lightwave, maximum absorption of evanescent field is observed leading to a strong SPW generation [63, 64]. This condition is called resonance condition. The propagating evanescent wave can be characterized by propagation constant β_{ev} as follows [10, 65]:

$$\beta_{ev} = \frac{2\pi}{\lambda} n \times \sin\theta \tag{1}$$

Where λ, n, θ indicate the incident light wavelength, refractive index of the medium, and angle of incident of light at the metal surface, respectively. The equation as follows characterizes the SPW [66]:

$$\beta_{SPW} = \beta_f \sqrt{\frac{\varepsilon_m \varepsilon_d}{\varepsilon_m + \varepsilon_d}} \tag{2}$$

Where $\beta_f = \frac{2\pi}{\lambda}$, is the wave vector of light at free space. Also, ε_m and ε_d indicate the dielectric constants of plasmonic material and dielectric medium, respectively. Eq. (2) can also be rewritten in terms of the refractive index as follows [31]:

$$\beta_{SPW} = \frac{2\pi}{\lambda} \sqrt{\frac{n_m^2 n_d^2}{n_m^2 + n_d^2}} \tag{3}$$

Where the RI of plasmonic material (n_m) and sensing medium (n_d) are related to the dielectric constants as $n_m^2 = \epsilon_m$ and $n_d^2 = \epsilon_d$, respectively. The resonance condition is located in SPR based sensor, where the propagation constant of incident light (β_{ev}) is matched with the SPW's wave vector β_{SPW} [67]. From Eqs. (1) and (3), it can be related that by controlling the incident angle for a particular frequency of light, the resonance condition can be achieved. This method is called the angular interrogation method. Similarly, the light wavelength can be modified to achieve the SPR condition for a particular angle of incident light for the wavelength interrogation method [68]. At this condition, the electrons start to resonate triggering the generation of SPW on the metal-dielectric interface where a sharp loss peak called the SPR point appears. The SPR point is extremely responsive to the refractive index (RI) of the surrounding medium where a minor change in RI of the dielectric (sensing) medium shifts the SPR point to a new state [69].

3. Angular interrogation approach and performance parameters of the sensor

Due to its outstanding performance characteristics, commercial standardization, and ease of manufacturing technology, the angular interrogation method using ATR has become more popular today among various SPR based sensors. When light is directly coupled to the metal-dielectric interface, due to a mismatch of momentum, the SPs are not sufficiently excited to generate SPWs [70]. Researchers have suggested several special arrangements called Otto configuration [71], Kretschmann configuration [72, 73] as visualized in **Figure 2** to alter the momentum of the photon to couple with the SPPs leading to propagation of SPW. In prism

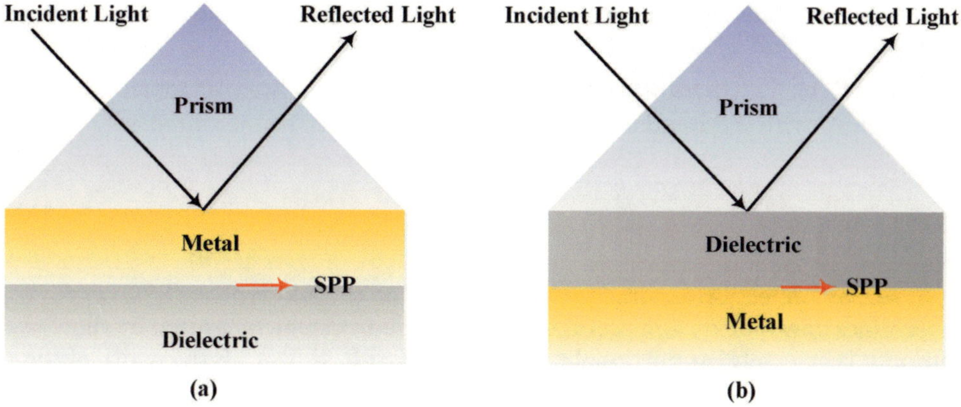

Figure 2.
Special Arrangements [74] e.g. (a) Kretschmann configuration, and (b) Otto configuration to match the momentum of incident photon and SPW.

based Otto configuration, there is a distance where a dielectric layer with a smaller RI is used between the prism and metal sheet on which the light is employed. On contrary, Kretschmann configuration the metallic layer is in direct contact with the prism. Among them, the Kretschmann configuration is the most popular solution to ensure the coupling of the strongest evanescent wave passing through the metal and generate SPW [53, 74–76]. In the Kretschmann configuration, the light is incident at the metal-dielectric interface through a high index prism [77].

Usually, the incident light bounces back from the interface while the evanescent field is induced by a portion of light penetrating through the metal. For a particular sensor configuration and light frequency, the momentum of the evanescent field is aligned with the wave vector of SPW at a specific angle called resonance angle [76]. Maximum light is coupled to the oscillating electrons at this resonance condition, leading to minimum reflection. If the reflected light is plotted concerning the incident angle, then a resonance dip of reflection spectrum is observed called SPR point which is highly responsive to the RI of the sensing medium. By interrogating this SPR point the analyte can be detected easily. The performance measuring parameters e.g. sensitivity, detection accuracy, FOM, and QF should be as high as possible to eliminate false positive detection. The sensitivity of the sensor operating on the angular interrogation approach depends on the change in the SPR point or resonance angle with a change in RI of the sensing medium. **Figure 3** illustrates the

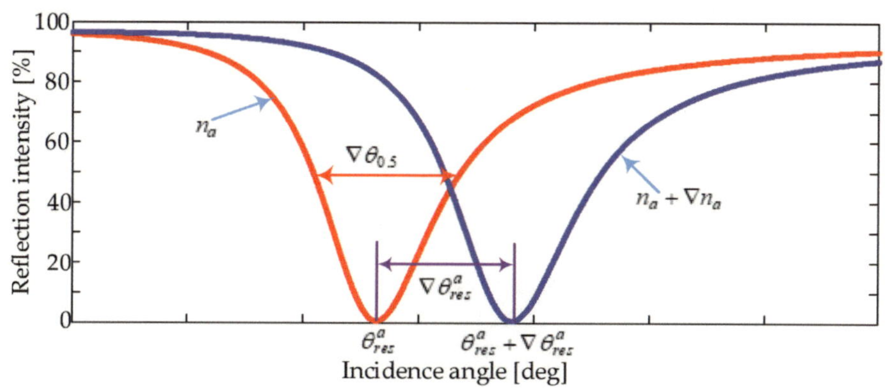

Figure 3.
Illustration of the SPR curve variation due to change in sensing medium RI.

SPR curve variation due to change in sensing medium RI where the resonance point is found at θ^a_{res} and $\theta^a_{res} + \nabla\theta^a_{res}$ for sensing medium RI of n_a and $n_a + \nabla n_a$. Due to change in RI of ∇n_a the shift in SPR is observed as $\nabla\theta^a_{res}$. Thus, the sensitivity (S_a) of the sensor with the angular interrogation approach can be measured as [78]:

$$S_a = \frac{\nabla\theta^a_{res}}{\nabla n_a} \tag{4}$$

A sensor's detection accuracy, which depends on the width of the SPR curve, determines how quickly and accurately the SPR point can be measured by the sensor. It is inversely proportional to the width of SPR. If $\nabla\theta_{0.5}$ is the width of the SPR curve corresponding to 50% reflection then the detection accuracy (D.A.), FOM, and QF can be defined as [15, 79, 80]:

$$D.A. = \frac{1}{\nabla\theta_{0.5}} \tag{5}$$

$$FOM = \frac{\nabla\theta^a_{res}/\nabla n_{\mathbf{a}}}{\nabla\theta_{0.5}} = S_a \times D.A. \tag{6}$$

$$QF = \frac{\nabla\theta^a_{res}}{\nabla\theta_{0.5}} \times S_a \tag{7}$$

4. Recent trends to enhance the performance of the SPR sensors

Nowadays, the prime concern of scientists, researchers, and academicians are to enhance the performance of the SPR based sensor. To date, several attempts have

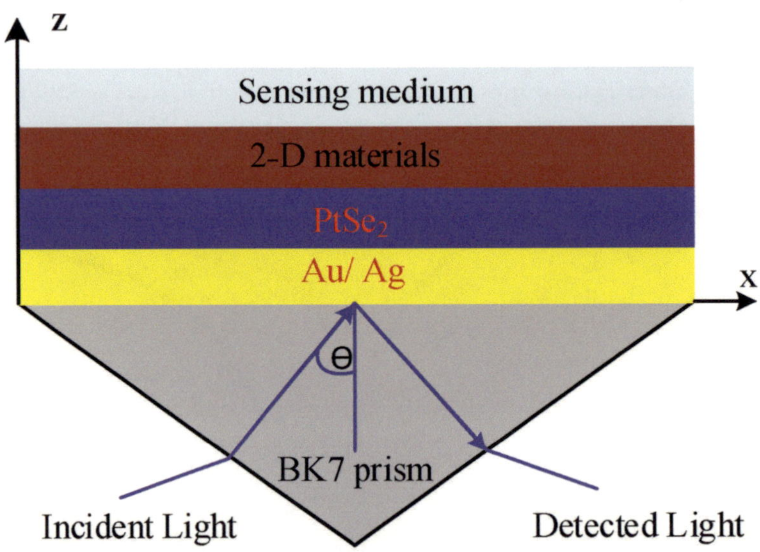

Figure 4.
Schematic Illustration of SPR biosensor employing hybridization of 2D materials with Ag/Au [86].

been reported to attain highly sensitive sensors where the use of bimetallic coating and hybridization of numerous 2D materials along with plasmonic materials are the most popular approach to accommodate the angular interrogation approach. Benaziez S. et al. [81] reported a sensor where Ag is considered as an SPR active material. They showed that the addition of mostly used 2D material graphene on Ag surface enables to reduce the oxidation problem as well as increase the sensitivity up to 9.3%. Yet, the detection accuracy of the sensor is slightly reduced. Also, Rouf H. K. and Haque A. [82] proposed a hybrid structure using InP and Ti with the Ag-Au bimetallic configuration. Their sensor shows maximum sensitivity of 70.90 deg/RIU. Similarly, Mishra S. K. and their team [83] have demonstrated a configuration with excellent sensor sensitivity of 229 deg/RIU. They used a rarely used material

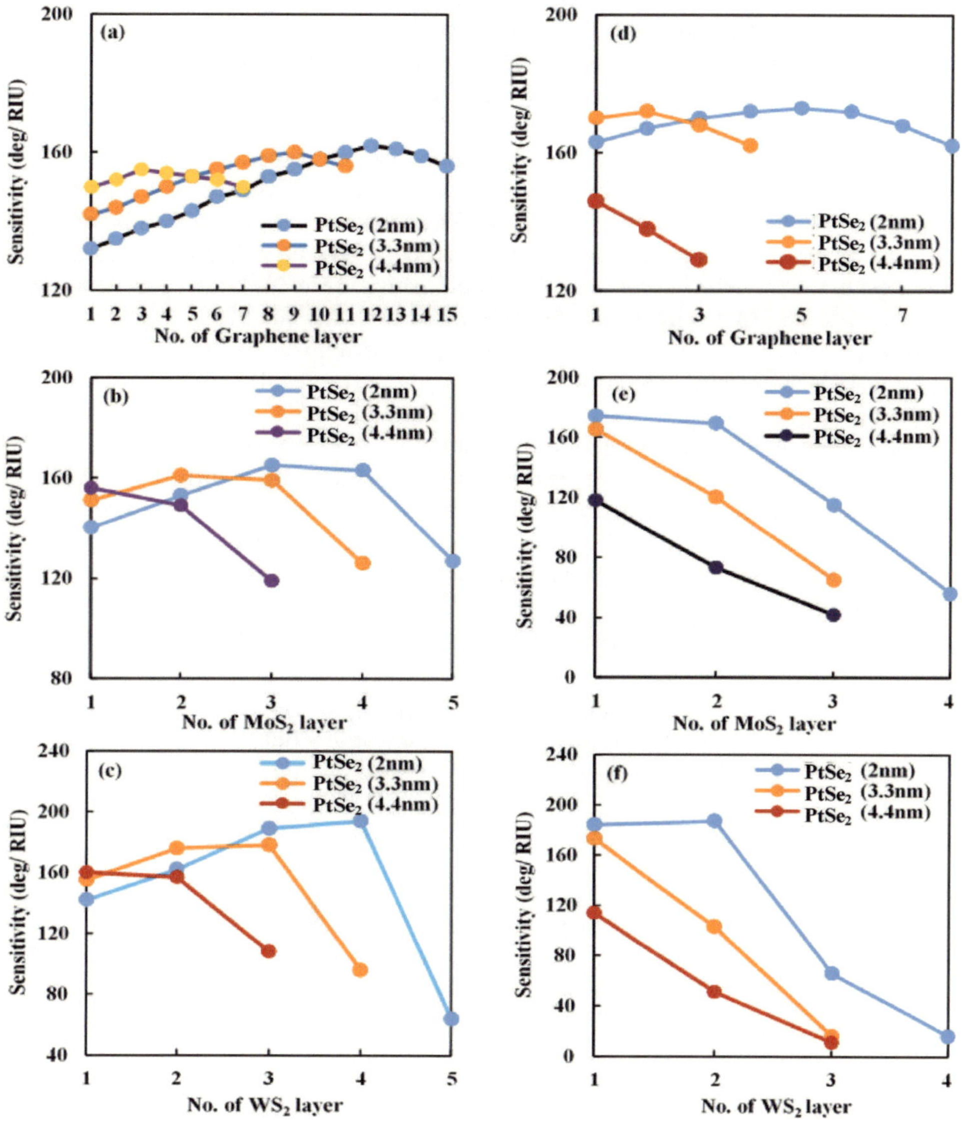

Figure 5.
Sensitivity variation due to change in the thickness of $PtSe_2$, and number of (a) Graphene layer (b) MoS_2 layer, (c) WS_2 layer for BK7/Ag (50 nm)/$PtSe_2$/2D materials (Graphene/MoS_2/WS_2) hybrid structure; and number of (d) Graphene layer, (e) MoS_2 layer, and (f) WS_2 layer for BK7/Au (50 nm)/$PtSe_2$/2D materials (Graphene/MoS_2/WS_2) hybrid structure [86].

Rhodium (Rh) with Ag to realize bimetallic configuration. Also, they used a silicon layer on the bimetallic layer to lessen the limitations of Ag. Likewise, N. Mudgal et al. [3] proposed a four-layer hybrid structure that consists of Au, molybdenum disulfide (MoS_2), h-BN (hexagonal boron nitride), and graphene to detect urine glucose. The structure can enhance the sensor sensitivity up to 194.12 deg/RIU with the detection accuracy of 16.04/RIU. In the same way, Hailin Xu et al. [84] proposed an optical sensor with the graphene-Al-graphene sandwich structure where graphene prevents the oxidation issue of Al as well as enhances the sensor sensitivity 3.4 times more than only Al-based sensor. Besides, Wang M. et al. [85] suggested a sensor consisting of graphene, Tungsten disulfide (WS_2), and Au-Ag bimetallic film. They observed that hybridization of single layer graphene and WS_2 with Au-Ag bimetallic nanostructure leads to sensitivity up to 182.5 deg/RIU which is superior to Au-only based sensor. Incorporating the advantages of hybrid structure and bimetallic configuration, very recently Rahman M. et al. [86] also proposed a new configuration of SPR biosensors utilizing the newly emerged TMDC ($PtSe_2$) embedded 2D materials as illustrated in **Figure 4**.

In this configuration, a heterostructure of $PtSe_2$/2D material (e.g., graphene, MoS_2, WS_2) has been employed to realize the hybrid configuration whereas BK7 prism is used as a coupler that increases the momentum of the evanescent wave to match with the wave vector of the SPW. The sensor comprises a thin layer (50 nm) of Au or Ag as an SPR active material between the prism coupler and $PtSe_2$/2D material heterostructure. A monochromatic He-Ne laser source having a wavelength of 633 nm have been incorporated to excite the SPPs. The sensor parameters are altered and optimized varying the thickness of $PtSe_2$ and number 2D material's layer to get better performance where the results are revealed in **Figure 5**.

The effects of alteration of different parameters of $PtSe_2$, and 2D materials have been analyzed comprehensively and two new sensors have been introduced with excellent performance characteristics. The details of optimized design parameters and performances are listed in **Table 1**. As well, **Table 2** shows the performance comparison of different SPR biosensors based on Kretschmann configuration with a hybrid structure.

Sl. no.	Proposed SPR sensors with optimized structural parameters			Operating range of sensing medium RI	FOM [RIU^{-1}]	QF [deg/RIU]	Sensitivity [deg/RIU]
01.	$Ag/PtSe_2/WS_2$	Thickness of Ag (nm)	50	1.33-1.38	17.64	34.22	194
		Thickness of $PtSe_2$ (nm)	02				
		Number of WS_2 Layers	04				
02.	$Au/PtSe_2/WS_2$	Thickness of Au (nm)	50	1.33-1.38	15.72	29.39	187
		Thickness of $PtSe_2$ (nm)	02				
		Number of WS_2 Layers	02				

Table 1.
Details of optimized design parameters and results of the proposed SPR biosensors [86].

Ref.	Configuration of the sensors	Sensitivity (deg/RIU)
[83]	Prism/Air/Titanium (Ti)/Ag/Au/InP	70.90
[84]	Prism/Rh/Ag/Si	229
[3]	Prism/MoS_2/h-BN/graphene	194.12
[85]	Prism/Ag/Au/WS_2/graphene	182.5
[86]	Prism/Ag/$PtSe_2$/WS_2	194
[86]	Prism/Au/$PtSe_2$/WS_2	187
[87]	Prism/Au/Black Phosphorous (BP)	180
[2]	Prism/Au/Graphene/MoS_2	89.29
[1]	Prism/Au/MoS_2	75.34
[88]	Prism/ZnO/Ag/Au/graphene	66
[89]	Prism/Au/MoS_2/WS_2/WSe_2	142
[90]	Prism/Au/MoS_2/Au film/graphene	182
[55]	Prism/MoS_2/aluminum (Al) film/MoS_2/ graphene	190.83
[91]	Prism/Ag/$PtSe_2$	162
[91]	Prism/Au/$PtSe_2$	165

Table 2.
Sensitivity comparison of Kretschmann configuration based SPR biosensors comprising hybrid structures.

5. Conclusion

This chapter provides a detailed description of the surface plasmon resonance phenomenon with the recent trends that are being applied in the advancement of SPR based sensors where the application of hybrid structures as well as bimetallic configurations are found to be potential techniques to enhance the sensor performances. Besides, it demonstrates different 2D materials applied for sensing capability enhancement of the hybrid SPR biosensors. Also, two 5 layer prism based hybrid heterostructures (Prism-Au-$PtSe_2$-WS_2 and Prism-Ag-$PtSe_2$-WS_2) have been comprehensively discussed here to show the effectiveness of hybrid technology.

Author details

Md. Shamim Anower[1*], Md. Mahabubur Rahman[2] and M. Saifur Rahman[1]

1 Department of Electrical and Electronic Engineering, Rajshahi University of Engineering and Technology, Rajshahi-6204, Bangladesh

2 Department of Electrical and Computer Engineering, Rajshahi University of Engineering and Technology, Rajshahi-6204, Bangladesh

*Address all correspondence to: md.shamimanower@yahoo.com

References

[1] Q. Ouyang, S. Zeng, X.-Q. Dinh, P. Coquet, and K.-T. Yong, "Sensitivity enhancement of MoS_2 nanosheet based surface plasmon resonance biosensor," *Procedia engineering,* vol. 140, pp. 134-139, 2016.

[2] M. S. Rahman, M. S. Anower, M. R. Hasan, M. B. Hossain, and M. I. Haque, "Design and numerical analysis of highly sensitive Au-MoS2-graphene based hybrid surface plasmon resonance biosensor," *Optics Communications,* vol. 396, pp. 36-43, 2017.

[3] N. Mudgal, A. Saharia, A. Agarwal, J. Ali, P. Yupapin, and G. Singh, "Modeling of highly sensitive surface plasmon resonance (SPR) sensor for urine glucose detection," *Optical and Quantum Electronics,* vol. 52, p. 307, 2020.

[4] C. Basak, M. K. Hosain, and A. A. Sazzad, "Design and Simulation of a High Sensitive Surface Plasmon Resonance Biosensor for Detection of Biomolecules," *Sensing and Imaging,* vol. 21, no. 1, p. 2, 2020.

[5] B. A. Prabowo, A. Purwidyantri, and K.-C. Liu, "Surface plasmon resonance optical sensor: A review on light source technology," *Biosensors,* vol. 8, no. 3, p. 80, 2018.

[6] M. Hossain and M. Rana, "Graphene coated high sensitive surface plasmon resonance biosensor for sensing DNA hybridization," *Sensor Letters,* vol. 14, no. 2, pp. 145-152, 2016.

[7] M. B. Hossain, M. M. Rana, L. F. Abdulrazak, S. Mitra, and M. Rahman, "Graphene-MoS_2 with TiO_2/SiO_2 layers based surface plasmon resonance biosensor: Numerical development for formalin detection," *Biochemistry and biophysics reports,* vol. 18, p. 100639, 2019.

[8] K. Narsaiah, S. N. Jha, R. Bhardwaj, R. Sharma, and R. Kumar, "Optical biosensors for food quality and safety assurance—a review," *Journal of food science and technology,* vol. 49, no. 4, pp. 383-406, 2012.

[9] M. Piliarik, L. Párová, and J. Homola, "High-throughput SPR sensor for food safety," *Biosensors and Bioelectronics,* vol. 24, no. 5, pp. 1399-1404, 2009.

[10] H. Šípová and J. Homola, "Surface plasmon resonance sensing of nucleic acids: a review," *Analytica chimica acta,* vol. 773, pp. 9-23, 2013.

[11] J. Homola, "Surface plasmon resonance sensors for detection of chemical and biological species," *Chemical reviews,* vol. 108, no. 2, pp. 462-493, 2008.

[12] M. B. Hossain, T. B. A. Akib, L. F. Abdulrazak, and M. M. Rana, "Numerical modeling of graphene-coated fiber optic surface plasmon resonance biosensor for BRCA1 and BRCA2 genetic breast cancer detection," *Optical Engineering,* vol. 58, no. 3, p. 037104, 2019.

[13] M. B. Hossain, M. M. Islam, L. F. Abdulrazak, M. M. Rana, T. B. A. Akib, and M. Hassan, "Graphene-coated optical fiber SPR biosensor for BRCA1 and BRCA2 breast cancer biomarker detection: a numerical design-based analysis," *Photonic Sensors,* vol. 10, no. 1, pp. 67-79, 2020.

[14] M. S. Rahman, M. Anower, M. K. Rahman, M. R. Hasan, M. B. Hossain, and M. I. Haque, "Modeling of a highly sensitive MoS_2-Graphene hybrid based fiber optic SPR biosensor for sensing DNA hybridization," *Optik,* vol. 140, pp. 989-997, 2017.

[15] B. Meshginqalam and J. Barvestani, "Performance enhancement of SPR

biosensor based on phosphorene and transition metal dichalcogenides for sensing DNA hybridization," *IEEE Sensors Journal,* vol. 18, no. 18, pp. 7537-7543, 2018.

[16] Y. Iwasaki, T. Horiuchi, and O. Niwa, "Detection of electrochemical enzymatic reactions by surface plasmon resonance measurement," *Analytical chemistry,* vol. 73, no. 7, pp. 1595-1598, 2001.

[17] J. Pollet *et al.*, "Fiber optic SPR biosensing of DNA hybridization and DNA–protein interactions," *Biosensors and Bioelectronics,* vol. 25, no. 4, pp. 864-869, 2009.

[18] J. Lee *et al.*, "Top publications by reads," *Journal of Stroke and Cerebrovascular Diseases,* vol. 27, no. 12, 2018.

[19] N. Mudgal, P. Yupapin, J. Ali, and G. Singh, "$BaTiO_3$-Graphene-Affinity Layer–Based Surface Plasmon Resonance (SPR) Biosensor for Pseudomonas Bacterial Detection," *Plasmonics,* pp. 1-9, 2020.

[20] J. S. Velázquez-González, D. Monzón-Hernández, D. Moreno-Hernández, F. Martínez-Piñón, and I. Hernández-Romano, "Simultaneous measurement of refractive index and temperature using a SPR-based fiber optic sensor," *Sensors and Actuators B: Chemical,* vol. 242, pp. 912-920, 2017.

[21] E. Della Gaspera *et al.*, "Au nanoparticles in nanocrystalline TiO_2–NiO films for SPR-based, selective H_2S gas sensing," *Chemistry of Materials,* vol. 22, no. 11, pp. 3407-3417, 2010.

[22] M. G. Manera *et al.*, "Enhanced gas sensing performance of TiO_2 functionalized magneto-optical SPR sensors," *Journal of Materials Chemistry,* vol. 21, no. 40, pp. 16049-16056, 2011.

[23] F. Baldini, M. Brenci, F. Chiavaioli, A. Giannetti, and C. Trono, "Optical fibre gratings as tools for chemical and biochemical sensing," *Analytical and bioanalytical chemistry,* vol. 402, no. 1, pp. 109-116, 2012.

[24] R. Gordont and D. Sinton, "KL kavanagh and AG Brolo," *Accounts of Chemical Research,* vol. 41, pp. 1049-1057, 2008.

[25] J. M. McDonnell, "Surface plasmon resonance: towards an understanding of the mechanisms of biological molecular recognition," *Current opinion in chemical biology,* vol. 5, no. 5, pp. 572-577, 2001.

[26] A. Olaru, C. Bala, N. Jaffrezic-Renault, and H. Y. Aboul-Enein, "Surface plasmon resonance (SPR) biosensors in pharmaceutical analysis," *Critical reviews in analytical chemistry,* vol. 45, no. 2, pp. 97-105, 2015.

[27] A. K. Paul, "Design and analysis of photonic crystal fiber plasmonic refractive Index sensor for condition monitoring of transformer oil," *OSA Continuum,* vol. 3, no. 8, pp. 2253-2263, 2020.

[28] R. W. Wood, "XLII. On a remarkable case of uneven distribution of light in a diffraction grating spectrum," *The London, Edinburgh, and Dublin Philosophical Magazine and Journal of Science,* vol. 4, no. 21, pp. 396-402, 1902.

[29] A. Otto, "Excitation of nonradiative surface plasma waves in silver by the method of frustrated total reflection," *Zeitschrift für Physik A Hadrons and nuclei,* vol. 216, no. 4, pp. 398-410, 1968.

[30] E. Kretschmann and H. Raether, "Radiative decay of non-radiative surface plasmons excited by light," *Z. Naturforsch. a,* vol. 23, no. 12, pp. 2135-2136, 1968.

[31] B. Liedberg, C. Nylander, and I. Lunström, "Surface plasmon resonance for gas detection and biosensing," *Sensors and actuators,* vol. 4, pp. 299-304, 1983.

[32] A. H.-P. Ho, S.-Y. Wu, S.-K. Kong, S. Zeng, and K.-T. Yong, "SPR Biosensors 5," *channels,* vol. 15, p. 37, 2017.

[33] K. L. Lee, C. Y. Hung, M. Y. Pan, T. Y. Wu, S. Y. Yang, and P. K. Wei, "Dual Sensing Arrays for Surface Plasmon Resonance (SPR) and Surface-Enhanced Raman Scattering (SERS) Based on Nanowire/Nanorod Hybrid Nanostructures," *Advanced Materials Interfaces,* vol. 5, no. 21, p. 1801064, 2018.

[34] F. Wang, S. Cao, R. Yan, Z. Wang, D. Wang, and H. Yang, "Selectivity/specificity improvement strategies in surface-enhanced Raman spectroscopy analysis," *Sensors,* vol. 17, no. 11, p. 2689, 2017.

[35] K. M. Byun, S. J. Kim, and D. Kim, "Grating-coupled transmission-type surface plasmon resonance sensors based on dielectric and metallic gratings," *Applied optics,* vol. 46, no. 23, pp. 5703-5708, 2007.

[36] K. Lin, Y. Lu, J. Chen, R. Zheng, P. Wang, and H. Ming, "Surface plasmon resonance hydrogen sensor based on metallic grating with high sensitivity," *Optics express,* vol. 16, no. 23, pp. 18599-18604, 2008.

[37] Y. Dai, H. Xu, H. Wang, Y. Lu, and P. Wang, "Experimental demonstration of high sensitivity for silver rectangular grating-coupled surface plasmon resonance (SPR) sensing," *Optics Communications,* vol. 416, pp. 66-70, 2018.

[38] H. R. Gwon and S. H. Lee, "Spectral and angular responses of surface plasmon resonance based on the Kretschmann prism configuration," *Materials transactions,* vol. 51, no. 6, pp. 1150-1155, 2010.

[39] M. M. Rahman, M. M. Rana, M. Anower, M. S. Rahman, and A. K. Paul, "Design and analysis of photonic crystal fiber-based plasmonic microbiosensor: an external sensing scheme," *SN Applied Sciences,* vol. 2, no. 7, pp. 1-11, 2020.

[40] M. M. Rahman, M. A. Molla, A. K. Paul, M. A. Based, M. M. Rana, and M. Anower, "Numerical investigation of a highly sensitive plasmonic refractive index sensor utilizing hexagonal lattice of photonic crystal fiber," *Results in Physics,* vol. 18, p. 103313, 2020.

[41] R. Kashyap and G. Nemova, "Surface plasmon resonance-based fiber and planar waveguide sensors," *Journal of Sensors,* vol. 2009, 2009.

[42] J. Dostalek *et al.*, "Surface plasmon resonance biosensor based on integrated optical waveguide," *Sensors and actuators B: Chemical,* vol. 76, no. 1-3, pp. 8-12, 2001.

[43] W.-C. Kuo, C. Chou, and H.-T. Wu, "Optical heterodyne surface-plasmon resonance biosensor," *Optics letters,* vol. 28, no. 15, pp. 1329-1331, 2003.

[44] C. Chou, H.-T. Wu, Y.-C. Huang, Y.-L. Chen, and W.-C. Kuo, "Characteristics of a paired surface plasma waves biosensor," *Optics Express,* vol. 14, no. 10, pp. 4307-4315, 2006.

[45] J.-Y. Lee, L.-W. Mai, C.-C. Hsu, and Y.-Y. Sung, "Enhanced sensitivity to surface plasmon resonance phase in wavelength-modulated heterodyne interferometry," *Optics Communications,* vol. 289, pp. 28-32, 2013.

[46] K. M. McPeak *et al.*, "Plasmonic films can easily be better: rules and recipes," *ACS photonics,* vol. 2, no. 3, pp. 326-333, 2015.

[47] A. A. Rifat, M. R. Hasan, R. Ahmed, and A. E. Miroshnichenko, "Microstructured optical fiber-based plasmonic sensors," in *Computational Photonic Sensors*: Springer, 2019, pp. 203-232.

[48] M. A. Ordal, R. J. Bell, R. W. Alexander, L. L. Long, and M. R. Querry, "Optical properties of fourteen metals in the infrared and far infrared: Al, Co, Cu, Au, Fe, Pb, Mo, Ni, Pd, Pt, Ag, Ti, V, and W," *Applied optics,* vol. 24, no. 24, pp. 4493-4499, 1985.

[49] P. R. West, S. Ishii, G. V. Naik, N. K. Emani, V. M. Shalaev, and A. Boltasseva, "Searching for better plasmonic materials," *Laser & Photonics Reviews,* vol. 4, no. 6, pp. 795-808, 2010.

[50] J. Homola, "Present and future of surface plasmon resonance biosensors," *Analytical and bioanalytical chemistry,* vol. 377, no. 3, pp. 528-539, 2003.

[51] S. Bharadwaj, P. K. Maharana, R. Das, and R. Jha, "Effect of chalcogenide glass and plasmonic metal on electric field enhancement in surface plasmon resonance sensor," in *International Conference on Fibre Optics and Photonics*, 2012: Optical Society of America, p. TPo. 19.

[52] B. Gupta and A. K. Sharma, "Sensitivity evaluation of a multi-layered surface plasmon resonance-based fiber optic sensor: a theoretical study," *Sensors and Actuators B: Chemical,* vol. 107, no. 1, pp. 40-46, 2005.

[53] H. R. Gwon and S. H. Lee, "Spectral and angular responses of surface plasmon resonance based on the Kretschmann prism configuration," *Materials transactions,* vol. 51, no. 6, pp. 1150-1155, 2010.

[54] J. Maurya, Y. Prajapati, V. Singh, and J. Saini, "Sensitivity enhancement of surface plasmon resonance sensor based on graphene–MoS 2 hybrid structure with TiO_2–SiO_2 composite layer," *Applied Physics A,* vol. 121, no. 2, pp. 525-533, 2015.

[55] L. Wu *et al.*, "Sensitivity improved SPR biosensor based on the MoS2/ graphene–aluminum hybrid structure," *Journal of Lightwave Technology,* vol. 35, no. 1, pp. 82-87, 2016.

[56] L. Wu, J. Guo, X. Dai, Y. Xiang, and D. Fan, "Sensitivity enhanced by MoS_2–graphene hybrid structure in guided-wave surface plasmon resonance biosensor," *Plasmonics,* vol. 13, no. 1, pp. 281-285, 2018.

[57] L. Han and C. Wu, "A Phase Sensitivity-Enhanced Surface Plasmon Resonance Biosensor Based on ITO-Graphene Hybrid Structure," *Plasmonics,* vol. 14, no. 4, pp. 901-906, 2019.

[58] Y. Zhao and Y. Zhu, "Graphene-based hybrid films for plasmonic sensing," *Nanoscale,* vol. 7, no. 35, pp. 14561-14576, 2015.

[59] P. O. Patil *et al.*, "Graphene-based nanocomposites for sensitivity enhancement of surface plasmon resonance sensor for biological and chemical sensing: A review," *Biosensors and Bioelectronics,* vol. 139, p. 111324, 2019.

[60] X. Gan, H. Zhao, and X. Quan, "Two-dimensional MoS_2: A promising building block for biosensors," *Biosensors and Bioelectronics,* vol. 89, pp. 56-71, 2017.

[61] K. Shavanova *et al.*, "Application of 2D non-graphene materials and 2D oxide nanostructures for biosensing technology," *Sensors,* vol. 16, no. 2, p. 223, 2016.

[62] J. Krajczewski, K. Kołątaj, and A. Kudelski, "Plasmonic nanoparticles in chemical analysis," *RSC advances,* vol. 7, no. 28, pp. 17559-17576, 2017.

[63] M. Pelton and G. W. Bryant, *Introduction to metal-nanoparticle plasmonics*. John Wiley & Sons, 2013.

[64] N. Mudgal, M. K. Falaswal, T. Ismail, I. Fahim, M. Tiwari, and G. Singh, "Study of Approaches to

Implement the Prism-Based Surface Plasmon Resonance Sensors," in *Optical and Wireless Technologies*: Springer, 2020, pp. 353-362.

[65] C. T. Wittek *et al.*, "Prevalence and predictors of video game addiction: A study based on a national representative sample of gamers," *International journal of mental health and addiction,* vol. 14, no. 5, pp. 672-686, 2016.

[66] M. B. Hossain and M. M. Rana, "Graphene coated high sensitive surface plasmon resonance biosensor for sensing DNA hybridization," *Sens. Lett.,* vol. 13, pp. 1-8, 2015.

[67] J. Homola, "Electromagnetic theory of surface plasmons," in *Surface plasmon resonance based sensors*: Springer, 2006, pp. 3-44.

[68] L. E. Ronald, Jr., Multiwavelength Surface Plasmon Resonance Sensor Designs for Chemical and Biochemical Detection, Ph.D. thesis, Dept. of Chemistry, Virginia Polytechnic Institute and State University, 1998.

[69] G. S. Mei, P. S. Menon, and G. Hegde, "ZnO for performance enhancement of surface plasmon resonance biosensor: a review," *Materials Research Express,* vol. 7, no. 1, p. 012003, 2020.

[70] A. A. Rifat *et al.*, "Photonic crystal fiber based plasmonic sensors," *Sensors and Actuators B: Chemical,* vol. 243, pp. 311-325, 2017.

[71] D. Zhang, L. Men, and Q. Chen, "Microfabrication and applications of opto-microfluidic sensors," *Sensors,* vol. 11, no. 5, pp. 5360-5382, 2011.

[72] E. K. Akowuah, T. Gorman, and S. Haxha, "Design and optimization of a novel surface plasmon resonance biosensor based on Otto configuration," *Optics express,* vol. 17, no. 26, pp. 23511-23521, 2009.

[73] H.-S. Leong, J. Guo, R. G. Lindquist, and Q. H. Liu, "Surface plasmon resonance in nanostructured metal films under the Kretschmann configuration," *Journal of applied physics,* vol. 106, no. 12, p. 124314, 2009.

[74] V. G. Achanta, "Surface waves at metal-dielectric interfaces: Material science perspective," Reviews in Physics, p. 100041, 2020.

[75] S. Deng, P. Wang, and X. Yu, "Phase-sensitive surface plasmon resonance sensors: Recent progress and future prospects," *Sensors,* vol. 17, no. 12, p. 2819, 2017.

[76] D. Barchiesi and A. Otto, "Excitations of surface plasmon polaritons by attenuated total reflection, revisited," *La Rivista del Nuovo Cimento,* vol. 36, pp. 173-209, 2013.

[77] B. D. Gupta and R. K. Verma, "Surface plasmon resonance-based fiber optic sensors: principle, probe designs, and some applications," *Journal of sensors,* vol. 2009, 2009.

[78] F. Liu, J. Zhang, Y. Deng, D. Wang, Y. Lu, and X. Yu, "Detection of EGFR on living human gastric cancer BGC823 cells using surface plasmon resonance phase sensing," *Sensors and Actuators B: Chemical,* vol. 153, no. 2, pp. 398-403, 2011.

[79] A. K. Mishra, S. K. Mishra, and R. K. Verma, "Graphene and beyond graphene MoS_2: a new window in surface-plasmon-resonance-based fiber optic sensing," *The Journal of Physical Chemistry C,* vol. 120, no. 5, pp. 2893-2900, 2016.

[80] S. A. Zynio, A. V. Samoylov, E. R. Surovtseva, V. M. Mirsky, and Y. M. Shirshov, "Bimetallic layers increase sensitivity of affinity sensors based on surface plasmon resonance," *Sensors,* vol. 2, no. 2, pp. 62-70, 2002.

[81] S. Benaziez, Z. Dibi, and N. Benaziez, "Reflectivity optimization of the SPR graphene sensor," *Nanopages,* vol. 13, no. 1, pp. 5-17, 2018.

[82] H. K. Rouf and T. Haque, "Performance enhancement of Ag-Au bimetallic surface plasmon resonance biosensor using InP," *Progress In Electromagnetics Research*, vol. 76, pp. 31-42, 2018.

[83] S. K. Mishra, K. D. Malviya, and A. K. Mishra, "Highly sensitive bimetallic plasmonic sensing probe for aqueous samples."

[84] H. Xu, L. Wu, X. Dai, Y. Gao, and Y. Xiang, "An ultra-high sensitivity surface plasmon resonance sensor based on graphene-aluminum-graphene sandwich-like structure," *Journal of Applied Physics,* vol. 120, no. 5, p. 053101, 2016.

[85] M. Wang *et al.*, "Theoretical design of a surface plasmon resonance sensor with high sensitivity and high resolution based on graphene–WS_2 hybrid nanostructures and Au–Ag bimetallic film," *RSC advances,* vol. 7, no. 75, pp. 47177-47182, 2017.

[86] M. M. Rahman, M. M. Rana, M. S. Rahman, M. Anower, M. A. Mollah, and A. K. Paul, "Sensitivity enhancement of SPR biosensors employing heterostructure of $PtSe_2$ and 2D materials," *Optical Materials,* vol. 107, p. 110123, 2020.

[87] S. Pal, A. Verma, Y. Prajapati, and J. Saini, "Influence of black phosphorous on performance of surface plasmon resonance biosensor," *Optical and Quantum Electronics,* vol. 49, no. 12, p. 403, 2017.

[88] R. Kumar, A. S. Kushwaha, M. Srivastava, H. Mishra, and S. Srivastava, "Enhancement in sensitivity of graphene-based zinc oxide assisted bimetallic surface plasmon resonance (SPR) biosensor," *Applied Physics A,* vol. 124, no. 3, p. 235, 2018.

[89] Z. Lin, S. Chen, and C. Lin, "Sensitivity Improvement of a Surface Plasmon Resonance Sensor Based on Two-Dimensional Materials Hybrid Structure in Visible Region: A Theoretical Study," *Sensors,* vol. 20, no. 9, p. 2445, 2020.

[90] Z. Lin et al., "Tuning and sensitivity enhancement of surface plasmon resonance biosensor with graphene covered Au–MoS2–Au films," IEEE Photonics Journal, vol. 8, no. 6, pp. 1-8, 2016.

[91] Y. Jia, Z. Li, H. Wang, M. Saeed, and H. Cai, "Sensitivity Enhancement of a Surface Plasmon Resonance Sensor with Platinum Diselenide," *Sensors,* vol. 20, no. 1, p. 131, 2020.

Section 4

Biological Monitoring with Biosensors

Chapter 9

Advanced Biosensing towards Real-Time Imaging of Protein Secretion from Single Cells

Lang Zhou, Pengyu Chen and Aleksandr Simonian

Abstract

Protein secretion of cells plays a vital role in intercellular communication. The abnormality and dysfunction of cellular protein secretion are associated with various physiological disorders, such as malignant proliferation of cells, aberrant immune function, and bone marrow failure. The heterogeneity of protein secretion exists not only between varying populations of cells, but also in the same phenotype of cells. Therefore, characterization of protein secretion from single cell contributes not only to the understanding of intercellular communication in immune effector, carcinogenesis and metastasis, but also to the development and improvement of diagnosis and therapy of relative diseases. In spite of abundant highly sensitive methods that have been developed for the detection of secreted proteins, majority of them fall short in providing sufficient spatial and temporal resolution for comprehensive profiling of protein secretion from single cells. The real-time imaging techniques allow rapid acquisition and manipulation of analyte information on a 2D plane, providing high spatiotemporal resolution. Here, we summarize recent advances in real-time imaging of secretory proteins from single cell, including label-free and labelling techniques, shedding light on the development of simple yet powerful methodology for real-time imaging of single-cell protein secretion.

Keywords: cytokines, growth factors, SPR imaging, nanoplasmonic, interferometric scattering microscopy, Photonic Crystal Resonator, fluorescence, total internal reflection fluorescence

1. Introduction

Cells secrete proteins into the extracellular environment to achieve important physiological processes, such as transportation of nutrients, digestion of food, regulation of metabolic processes, etc [1–5]. Cell secretion can be classified into the constitutive and regulated secretory pathway [6–8]. The constitutive secretory pathway is associated with transportation of secretory vesicles to the cell surface and their release independently of stimulus [9–11]. The regulated secretory pathway produces secretory granules, stores them in the cytoplasm, and secretes them into the extracellular environment only upon receiving stimuli [12]. In human, more than 15% of the genome encoded proteins are associated with the secretion process [13]. These released proteins include neurotransmitters, protein hormones, growth factors, cytokines, enzymes, antibodies, etc [14]. They play a vital role in intercellular communication [15], which further regulates cell functions in immunology [16–18], neurobiology [19–21], endocrinology [22–24], etc. For instance, as the immune cells are stimulated, they undergo dynamic alternation and secrete various types of cytokines in a heterogenous manner. These secreted cytokines regulate the maturation and growth of immune cells, and activate the immune effector and memory immune responses.

The heterogeneity of cellular protein secretion has been found in various human diseases, including malignant proliferation of cells, aberrant immune function, bone marrow failure, etc [25–27]. This heterogeneity is present between distinct cell populations such as normal and pathological cells, as well as the same phenotype of cells [28–30]. This secretome heterogeneity creates diverse microenvironment for cells. The proliferation and metastasis of tumor cells can be prohibited or promoted upon the discrepancy of microenvironment, in spite of within the same tumor [31]. Meanwhile, the secretome change is frequently associated with atypical cellular phenotypes [32], which are indicative of diseases such as cancers, thus can be used as significant markers for tumorigenic process at single cell level. Therefore, characterization of protein secretion from single cell play a vital role in not only understanding the intercellular communication in immune effector, carcinogenesis and metastasis, but also developing and improving the current diagnosis and therapy of relative diseases [33–35]. In spite of abundant highly sensitive methods that have been developed for the detection of secreted proteins, majority of them have insufficient resolution in space and time, thus are not capable of providing deep insight into the behavior of protein secretion from single cells. Ideally, a detection method is supposed to be equipped with a high spatial resolution that enables differentiation of single cells from each other, and visualization of the spatial distribution of secreted proteins among multiple single cells, as well as a high temporal resolution that can recognize the dynamic alteration of secretion in a quantitative manner. The real-time imaging techniques feature rapid acquisition of analyte information on a 2D plane, and high spatial and temporal resolution, thus attract considerable attention in recent years, for its high potential to realize the deep exploration of single cellular protein secretion. Here, we review the involved works towards real-time imaging of single cell's protein secretion, including the detection of single or multiplex protein secretion, from group cells or single cells, in a real-time or near real-time manner, analyze their advantages and limitations, and discuss their major challenges.

2. Label-free techniques

In previous works, the real-time monitoring of cell secretion was achieved by label-free techniques such as plasmonic sensors, or label-required techniques such as fluorescence microscopy. The principles for all these methods are demonstrated in **Figure 1**. The representative works are summarized as shown in **Table 1**.

2.1 Plasmonic sensors

Plasmonic sensors have received tremendous attention owing to the label-free process, high sensitivity and fast response [36–38]. Plasmonic sensors generate surface plasmons and evanescence field that is sensitive to the changes of refractive index on sensing interfaces [39, 40]. By functionalization of the sensing interfaces, the change of refractive index upon specific binding of target molecules can be recognized. The plasmonic sensing could be implemented on varying materials, geometries and structures, such as flat metal films (surface plasmon resonance)

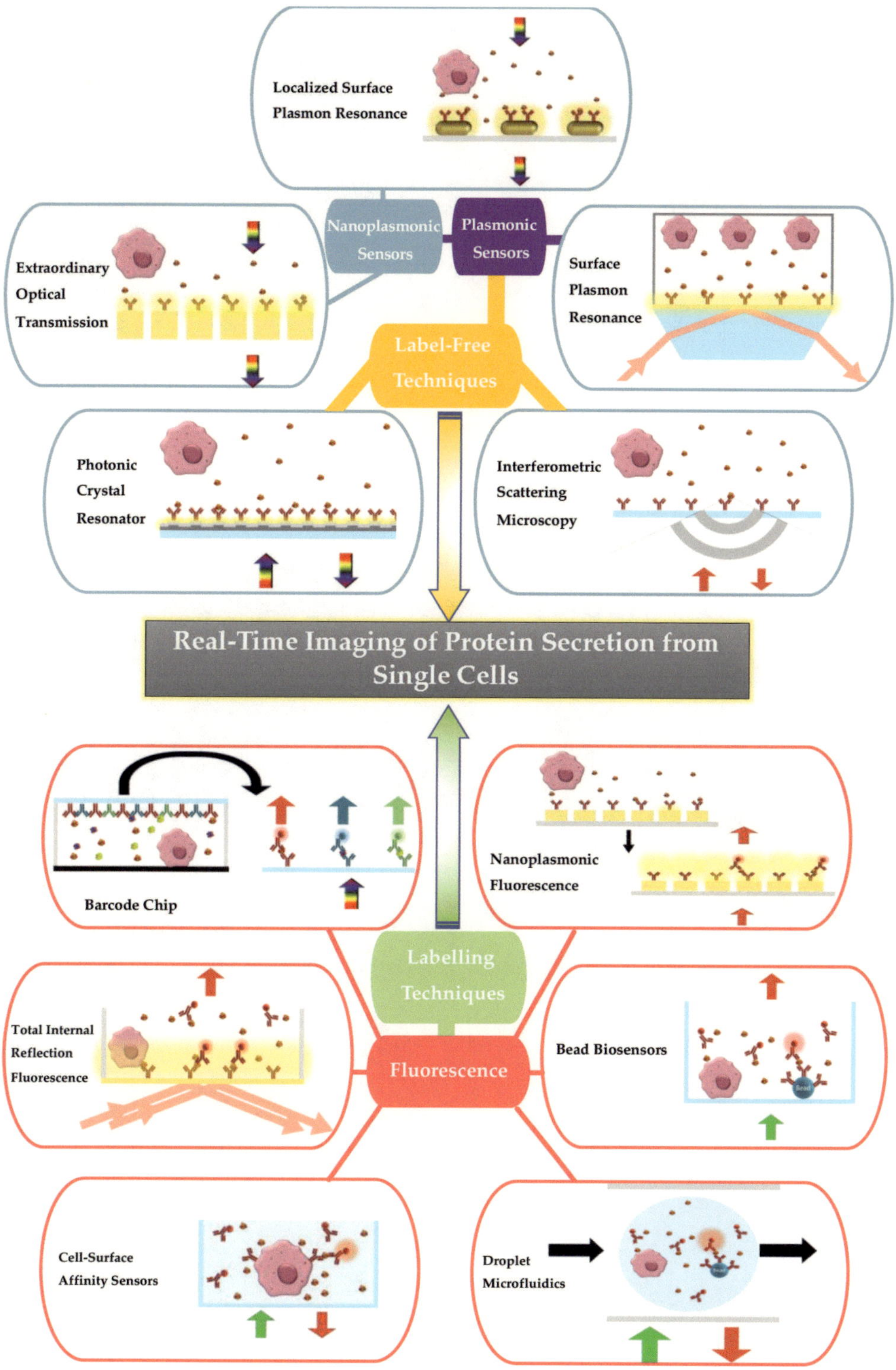

Figure 1.
Demonstration of methodology towards the real-time imaging of protein secretion from single cells.

[41, 42], nanoparticles (localized surface plasmon resonance) [43, 44] and nanoholes (extraordinary optical transmission) [45, 46]. These differences result in diverse applications and sensor performances.

Detection method	Cell	Stimuli	Secretion molecule	Cell confinement	Surface functionalization	Multiplex detection	Real-time imaging	LOD	Ref.
SPR	Human ovarian carcinoma SKOV-3	Ca^{2+} ionophore	VEGF	Attached on the ceiling of a flow cell chamber by gelatin	Gold/MUA/protein G/antibody	No	No	<100 ng/mL	[48]
SPR imaging	Murine B cell hybridoma	No	HEL-specific antibodies	Suspended in medium for sedimentation	Gold/electro-copolymerization of pyrrole and pyrrole-modified antigen	No	Yes (for group cells)	<50 ng/mL	[49]
SPR imaging	Human $CD4^{+}$T-cells	TB-specific proteins, ESAT-6, CFP-10	IFN-γ	Captured on poly(OEGMA-co-HEMA) / anti-$CD4^{+}$ antibody	Poly(OEGMA-co-HEMA) brush/ antibody	No	Yes (for group cells)	50 ng/mL	[50]
SPR imaging	EpCAM hybridoma	No	Anti-EpCAM antibodies	Suspended in medium for sedimentation	Gold/hydrogel/ EpCAM	No	Yes (for single cells)	N.A.	[51]
LSPR	Jurkat T cells	No	IL-6	Enclosed in a microwell	Gold-capped nanopillar-structured cyclo-olefin-polymer film/ MUA/antibody	No	No	10 ng/mL	[62]
LSPR	Jurkat T cells	Ionomycine, phorbol myristal acetate (PMA)	IL-2, IL-10, IFN-γ, TNF-α	Separate operation for cell secretion and detection	CTAB-coated AuNRs/ /MUA/ antibodies	Yes	No	20–30 pg/mL	[63]
LSPR	Jurkat T cells	Oligomeric and amyloid fibrils	IL-6 ,TNF	Separate operation for cell secretion and detection	CTAB-coated AuNRs/ /MUA/ antibodies	Yes	No	N.A.	[64]

Detection method	Cell	Stimuli	Secretion molecule	Cell confinement	Surface functionalization	Multiplex detection	Real-time imaging	LOD	Ref.
LSPR	Neutrophils	PMA	Fibrils, neutrophil extracellular traps	Enclosed in a microwell	Gold-capped nanopillar-structured cyclo-olefin polymer	No	No	N.A.	[65]
LSPR	9E10 Hybridoma cells	No	Anti-c-myc antibodies	Suspended in medium for sedimentation	Au nanostructure/c-myc peptide	No	Yes (for single cell)	100 pM (~4.88 ng/mL)	[66]
Extraordinary Optical Transmission	Hela cells	Ca^{2+} ionophore A23187	VEGF	Cells grow in a cell module, the secreted cytokines are delivered to the adjacent detection module.	Gold nanohole/PEG-ylated Alkanethiol/ streptavidin/ biotinylated antibodies	No	No	145 pg/mL	[68]
Extraordinary Optical Transmission	EL4 lymphoma cells	Ionomycin and PMA	IL-2	Enclosed in a small-volume microchamb-er with valve gates and hydraulic regulat-ion channel	Gold nanohole/ PEGylated alkanethiols/ streptavidin/ biotinylated antibody	No	Yes (for single cell)	39 pg/mL	[69]
Photonic crystal resonant	HepG2 liver cells, baby hamster kidney cells	No	Thrombopoietin	Suspended in medium for sedimentation	Si_3N_4/oxidized dextran/antibodies	No	Yes (for single cell)	<125 ng/mL	[72]
Interferometric scattering	Epstein–Barr virus-transformed B cell line, Laz 388	No	IgG antibodies	Suspended in medium for sedimentation	NHS coated glass/ anti-IgG antibodies	Yes	Yes (for single cell)	N.A.	[75]

Detection method	Cell	Stimuli	Secretion molecule	Cell confinement	Surface functionalization	Multiplex detection	Real-time imaging	LOD	Ref.
Microengraving	Human peripheral blood mononuclear cells	B cell receptor crosslinking antibody and CD40L	IFN-γ, IL-6, proinsulin-reactive antibodies	Enclosed in a microwell	Epoxy coated glass slide/ antibodies or antigens	Yes	No	N.A.	[79]
Barcode chip	U937-derived macrophages	Lipopolysaccharide	42 types of immune effector proteins	Enclosed in a microwell	Glass slide/ poly-L-lysine/ antibodies	Yes	No	N.A.	[81]
Total Internal Reflection Fluorescence	Human peripheral blood $CD14^+$ monocytes	Lipopolysaccharide, ATP	IL-6, IL-1b	Enclosed in a microwell	Aminated glass slide/ antibodies	No	Yes (for single cell)	2000 molecules	[82]
Nanoplasmonic resonator	Jurkat T cells	Ionomycin and PMA	IL-2	Suspended in medium for sedimentation	Gold nanostructure array/ poly-D-lysine/ antibody	No	Yes (for single cell)	<100 ng/mL	[83]
Bead	Human peripheral blood $CD4^+$ T cells	Ionomycin and PMA	IFN-γ	Enclosed in a microwell	Streptavidin-coated microbeads/ biotinylated antibodies	No	No	21.4 ng/mL	[86]
Bead	Human peripheral blood $CD56^{dim}CD16^+$ NK cells	Ionomycin and PMA	IFN-γ	Enclosed in a microwell	Anti- IgG-Fc beads/ antibodies	No	No	2.5 ng/ml	[87]
Bead	Human peripheral blood mononuclear cells	Phytohaemagglutinin	IL-6, IL-8, TNF	Cells grow in a culture chamber, the secreted cytokines are delivered a the adjacent detection unit.	Commercial bead detection kit	Yes	No	20 pg/ml	[88]

Detection method	Cell	Stimuli	Secretion molecule	Cell confinement	Surface functionalization	Multiplex detection	Real-time imaging	LOD	Ref.
Cell-surface affinity	BV2 microglial cells	Lipopolysaccharide	IL-6	Suspended in medium for sedimentation	Biotinylated cell surface/neutravidin/ biotinylated antibody	No	No	0.1 pg/ml	[96]
Droplet microfluidics	Human peripheral blood mononuclear T cells	Ionomycin and PMA	IFN-γ	Encapsulated in a droplet	Cell surface/ cholesterol/aptamer	No	No	14.5 ng/mL	[94]
Droplet microfluidics	Jurkat T cells	Ionomycin and PMA	IL-2, IFN-γ, TNF-α	Encapsulated in a droplet	Commercial bead detection kit	Yes	No	N.A.	[99]
Droplet microfluidics +LSPR	MDA-MB-213 breast cancer cells, HL-60 leukemia cells	TNF-α	VEGF, IL-8	Encapsulated in a droplet	Gold nanorod/ PEGylated alkanethiols/ antibody	Yes	No	6–7 ng/mL	[100]

N.A., not applicable; MUA, 11-Mercaptoundecanoic acid or 10-carboxy-1-decanethiol; AuNR, gold nanoparticle.

Table 1.
Summery for detection methodology of real-time monitoring of cell secretion.

2.1.1 Surface plasmon resonance (SPR)

SPR is a sensitive label-free technique for characterization of molecular interaction and detection of molecules through the affinity recognition. Due to surface plasmons excited on the surface of a thin metal film and an evanescence field created on surface, the refractive index change in the vicinity of the sensor surface (within ~200 nm) can be detected. This relatively large sensing depth allows SPR to monitor the changes occurred not only on surfaces, but also in the bulk. SPR has been applied in various studies for molecules with molecular weight between 1000 Da~500 kDa [47]. Liu et al. [48] attached human ovarian carcinoma SKOV-3 cells on the ceiling of a flow cell chamber, and detected their vascular endothelial growth factor (VEGF) secretion by monitoring the SPR signal of the antibodies-immobilized gold chip at the bottom of the flow cell. This SPR sensor has a linear dynamic range of 0.1–2.5 μg mL^{-1}. Of note, even though SPR features label-free measurement and high sensitivity, the lack of spatial resolution restricts its application in the mapping of protein secretion. In the meantime, SPR imaging is suitable to achieve this goal. Instead of measurement of the SPR angle shifts in SPR spectroscopy, plenty of SPR imaging systems use fixed angle and wavelength of incident light for the excitation of SPR so that the reflection intensities of multiple spots within imaging area are obtained simultaneous.

Milgram et al. [49] took advantage of SPR imaging to real-time monitor the secretion of immunoglobulins from B-cells hybridoma. They assembled an antigen microarray using electro-copolymerization of free pyrrole and pyrrole-modified antigen on a gold chip. The secreted immunoglobulins were captured by the antigen proteins, triggering the refractive index changes. The SPR intensity changes were consequently observed at a fixed angle using a 12-bit CCD. A sharp SPR kinetic curve was observed after several minutes of incubation, indicating fast and sensitive detection of immunoglobulins. Wu et al. [50] used anti-CD4 antibody to capture and immobilize human $CD4^{+}$T-cells on a sensing chip, and detected their in-situ secretion of Interferon gamma (IFN-γ) through functionalized anti-IFN-γ antibody located at the neighboring sites. The detection limit for IFN-γ was ~50 ng/mL. Stojanović et al. [51] applied SPR imaging to quantify the antibody production from single EpCAM hybridoma cells. Based on the measured SPR signal alteration, the overall secretion antibody amount from a single cell was calculated as 0.02 to 1.19 pg per cell per hour. However, this estimation is questionable because not all the antibodies secreted from cell were captured. To solve this problem, they performed simulation using COMSOL Multiphysics and found the captured antibodies by sensors accounts for 99% of the excreted antibodies, only 1% excreted antibodies are not detected [52].

A major limitation of intensity-based SPR imaging is its relatively low sensitivity. Compared to SPR of high sensitivity, intensity-based SPR imaging suffers from one order of magnitude lower of sensitivity [53]. This relatively low sensitivity is dominantly contributed by the fluctuations of the incident light intensity, photon statistics associated shot noise, and detector noise [54]. This issue could be improved by performing optical multilayer structured long-rang surface plasmons [55], angle-resolved or spectral SPR imaging [56], NIR light source [57], etc.

2.1.2 Nanoplasmonic biosensors

Different from SPR sensors utilizing propagating surface plasmons generated on flat metal film, nanoplasmonic sensors generate and manipulate localized surface plasmons on nanostructures [58]. Conventionally, nanoapertures or nanoparticles are fabricated to interact with light, leading to localized surface plasmon resonance

(LSPR) or extraordinary optical transmission (EOT). As nanoplasmonic biosensors combine with cell imaging, a powerful tool is created for protein secretion imaging. Nanoplasmonic biosensors generate strong evanescence field in the vicinity of less than 30 nm, thus are highly sensitive to the local refractive index changes, allowing the detection of target molecules captured on surfaces. Since the excitation of these nanostructures did not require complex optical devices, the instrumentation can be simple and straightforward. By tracing the dynamic alteration of reflection or transmission spectra, these changes can be recorded in a simple and real-time manner. Therefore, this feature allows a simple-but-sensitive label-free detection.

2.1.2.1 Localized surface plasmon resonance (LSRP)

LSRP generated on nanostructures results in the collective oscillation of electrons at the interface of metallic structures. A localized electromagnetic field is sensitive to the nanostructure shape and changes of refractive index at the distance of 10–30 nm [59, 60]. A molecular binding event on these nanostructures, causes a red shift in SPR peak, and gives rise to the scattering intensity of light at the same time. Due to a short electromagnetic field decay length, LSPR is insensitive to the changes of the refractive index in bulk, therefore the bulk effect can be minimized. This feature allows LSPR to measure temperature-dependent binding process, and investigate the effects of various environment factors on molecular interactions, such as solution pH and ionic strength [61].

LSPR measurement can be implemented by recording either SPR peak shift or scattering intensity changes. In the SPR peak shift based detection, Zhu et al. [62] combined microwell technique with LSPR to monitor Interleukin 6 (IL-6) secretion in the single cell level. The microwells were adapted to trap cells, a gold-capped nanopillar-structured cyclo-olefin-polymer film was covered on the top of microwells. The transmittance spectrum of the gold nanostructured surface provides real-time information on the absorption peak shift of nanogold during cell secretion. This nanostructured film further fabricated with Anti-IL-6 antibody realized a detection limitation of 10 ng/mL for IL-6.

In the scattering intensity based detection, Oh et al. [63] developed a multiplexed LSPR system for simultaneous measurements of pro-inflammatory cytokines (IL-2, IFN-γ, and TNF-α) and anti-inflammatory cytokines (IL-10) secreted by T cells. The cell culture and cytokine detection were conducted in independent steps. The sensitivity reached 20–30 pg/mL. Faridi et al. [64] applied similar system to characterize the secretion of IL-6 and tumor necrosis factor alpha (TNF), secreted from human monocytes and lymphocytes. The same principle has been applied to monitor neutrophil extracellular traps (NETs) and fibril released from single neutrophils [65]. Raphael et al. [66] achieved the real-time imaging of anti-c-myc antibodies secreted from single hybridoma cells with gold nanostructured arrays. The electron beam lithography was implemented to fabricate the square arrays of gold nanostructure on glass coverslips. The gold nanostructure arrays have a diameter of 70 nm, a height of 75 nm and a separation distance of 300 nm. The differing distances between the position of the settled single cell and the centers of arrays provide spatial resolution to observe the protein secretion. The c-myc peptides conjugated to plasmonic gold nanostructures captured the secreted anti-c-myc antibodies in a real-time manner. The caused binding displayed an increase in scattering intensity due to LSPR effect, which is measured through changes of light reflection. In parallel with reflected light based LSPR characterization, the transmitted light and fluorescence microscopy were integrated for live cell imaging. The transmitted light imaging enables observation of the position of single cell and its morphological change. The fluorescence microscopy allows the monitoring of membrane dynamics through a cell plasma membrane label-dye rhodamine DHPE, which distinguishes the signal due to occasional outward protrusions of lamellipodia from protein secretion signal. To model the singular cell secretion, the cell was assumed a spherical emitter producing a propagating pulse of antibodies with a Gaussian concentration profile, where the diffusion constant $D = r^2/6 \cdot t$. This method provides a sensitivity of 100 pM (~4.88 ng/mL) for the detection of anti-c-myc antibodies.

2.1.2.2 Extraordinary optical transmission (EOT)

In EOT biosensor, regularly periodic nanohole structure of subwavelength in a metallic film results in significant enhancement of light transmission through the nanoholes. This phenomenon is associated with both localized and propagating surface plasmons on the nanohole structures. By collecting and analyzing the transmission spectra, the light frequency-dependent transmission enhancement could be easily recognized. The molecular binding event on surface is corresponding to the transmission spectral shift. Consequently, the binding event can be visualized in a real-time manner through tracking the changes of transmission spectra. Combining localized and propagating surface plasmons, the spectra of EOT provide a wealth of information with varying sensitivities at different regions of nanoholes. In addition, the nanohole structures allows the flow-through design, which changes the manner of the mass transfer of analytes, and increases delivering rate of analytes from bulk to the sensing surface [67].

To achieve real-time imaging of cell secretion, Li et al. [68] first developed a microfluidic device that separated a cell culture module and an EOT sensing module. The nanohole array sensor has a hole diameter of 200 nm and a periodicity of 600 nm, and was fabricated by deep-UV lithography and functionalized by biotinylated antibodies. This detection module is directly connected with an adjacent cell culture module made of a zigzag single-channel PDMS unit. This biosensor system achieved a detection limit of 145 pg/mL for VEGF. In this study, the VEGF secretion was detected from the media containing a group of cancer cells, and the mapping of secretion was disabled due to the separated configuration of detection and cell culture modules. Subsequently, they developed a microfluidic system suitable for the secretion imaging of a single cell [69]. Enclosed in a microchamber, a single cell was attached to nanohole arrays, functionalized by antibodies. To achieve the function of real-time imaging, spectrum profiles on a perpendicular 1D line was collected, and the selected positions of the region-of-interest were analyzed. This sensor achieved a detection limit of 39 pg/mL for interleukin-2 (IL-2) in complex media.

2.2 Photonic Crystal Resonator (PCR)

Similar with plasmonic sensors, Photonic Crystal Resonator (PCR) exploits an evanescence field to interact with and sense the surrounding medium, i.e. the changes of its refractive index. PCR is created by Photonic Crystals (PCs) that own periodically varied refractive indices, which forbid the light propagation of certain wavelength of light in certain directions inside the material. This causes constructive or destructive interference of the light, and therefore a minimum in the transmission spectrum and a maximum in the reflection spectrum could be observed. Dependent on material, geometry and the index contrast, the decay length of PCs ranges from dozens of nanometers to the order of a few microns [70]. PCs composed of silicon nitride (Si_3N_4) or titanium dioxide (TiO_2) have been proved able to achieve cellular imaging with resolution 2–6 μm [71].

Juan-Colás et al. [72] monitored the secretion of thrombopoietin at single cell level using photonic crystal resonant imaging (**Figure 2**). The PCR surface microfabricated by electron beam lithography, consists of a grating with period of 555 nm on a 150-nm-thick Si_3N_4 film. It displayed a penetration depth of ~200 nm. To realize hyperspectral resonance image, reflection spectra was taken in a sequence of illumination wavelengths with 0.25-nm wavelength step. Under each wavelength, the intensity value of each pixel was analyzed and fit into a Fano resonance curve to accurately obtain the resonance wavelength for each pixel. To create a sensitive surface for analyte capture, antibodies were functionalized on a 3D matrix consisting of branched glucan dextran, which increased the density of antibodies on the surface. This sensor was demonstrated to detect lower than 125 ng/mL of suspended recombinant Human thrombopoietin. The interaction of antibody-antigen was treated as a single adsorption process, and the protein secretion was modeled as a Langmuir adsorption distribution. By quantifying the total secretion area in a timely manner, the single-cell secretion rate was calculated as 22 μm2/h. In addition, the wide field of view allows parallel imaging of 30 cells on an area of 500 × 500 μm, so that their dynamics and the kinetics could be characterized simultaneously.

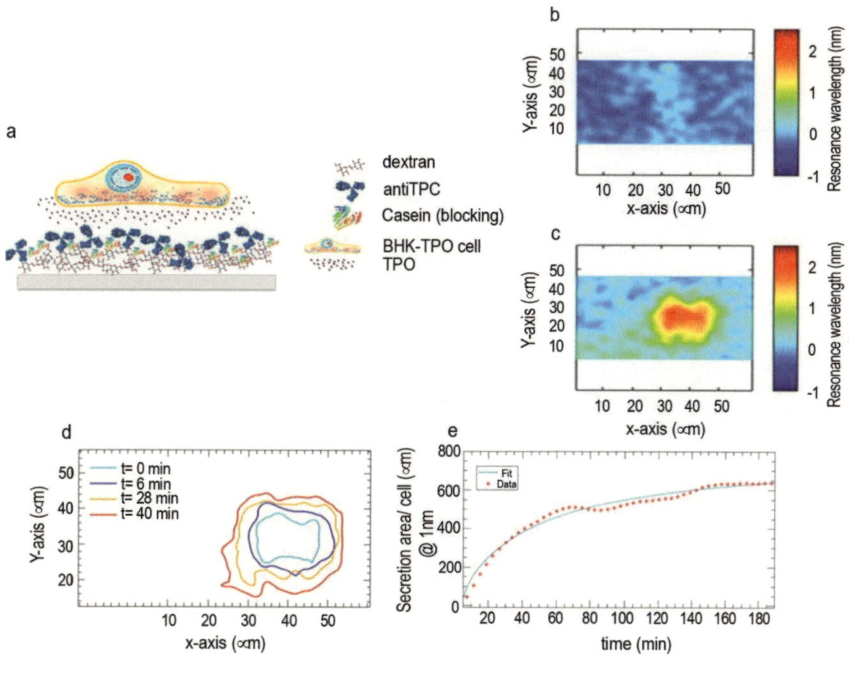

Figure 2.
Photonic crystal resonant imaging protocol for monitoring TPO secretion from a single BHK-TPO cell. (a) Dextran molecules are employed to create a 3D network of antibodies. Casein protein is employed as a blocking agent to prevent nonspecific binding from other proteins expressed by the cells. The secreted cytokines (i.e., TPO) from attached cells diffuse through the 3D network to specifically bind to the antibodies immobilized throughout the dextran network. The amount of deposited casein protein is optimized to maximize the signal-to-noise ratio of the detection system. (b) The region of interest (55 × 40 μm), with a wavelength uniformity of Δλ ± 0.5 nm. (c) A hyperspectral PCRS image reveals the adhesion of a -BHK-TPO cell to the PCRS, whose high concentration of cell adhesion molecules located in the inner region is translated into a higher refractive index content area. (d) Over time, this secretion area increases as TPO molecules are secreted from the cell and bind to the surface-immobilized antibodies, therefore locally increasing the refractive index around the BHK- TPO area. (e) The secretion of TPO is then monitored over time, and a Langmuir adsorption distribution is fitted to the data to model the secretion from the BHK-TPO cell accounting for the area covered by the adhered cell. Reprint (adapted) with permission from Ref. [27] under the terms of the Creative Commons Attribution License. Copyright 2018 Juan-Colás et al.

2.3 Interferometric Scattering Microscopy (iSCAT)

Interferometric Scattering Microscopy (iSCAT) is a single-molecule detection based approach. It relies on the light scattered by subwavelength objects. The signals come from the interference between the scattered light by the detected object and a reference light (**Figure 3d**). With the capability of single-molecule detection, iSCAT has shown its remarkably high sensitivity in cell imaging, single-particle tracking, label-free imaging of nanoscopic (dis)assembly, and quantitative single-molecule characterization [73]. Meanwhile, iSCAT microscopy itself does not provide adequate chemical or biological specificity due to its nature in collection of scattered light from all small objects [74].

McDonald et al. [75] reported an iSCAT contrast method to distinguish proteins secreted from an Epstein–Barr virus (EBV)-transformed B cell line (**Figure 3a**). The observed contrast on an iSCAT image reflects the amplitude of the electromagnetic field scattered by proteins, which is directedly correlated with the scattering cross-sections of detected molecules (**Figure 3c**). Here, the iSCAT demonstrated its capability of monitoring secreted proteins with varying molecular

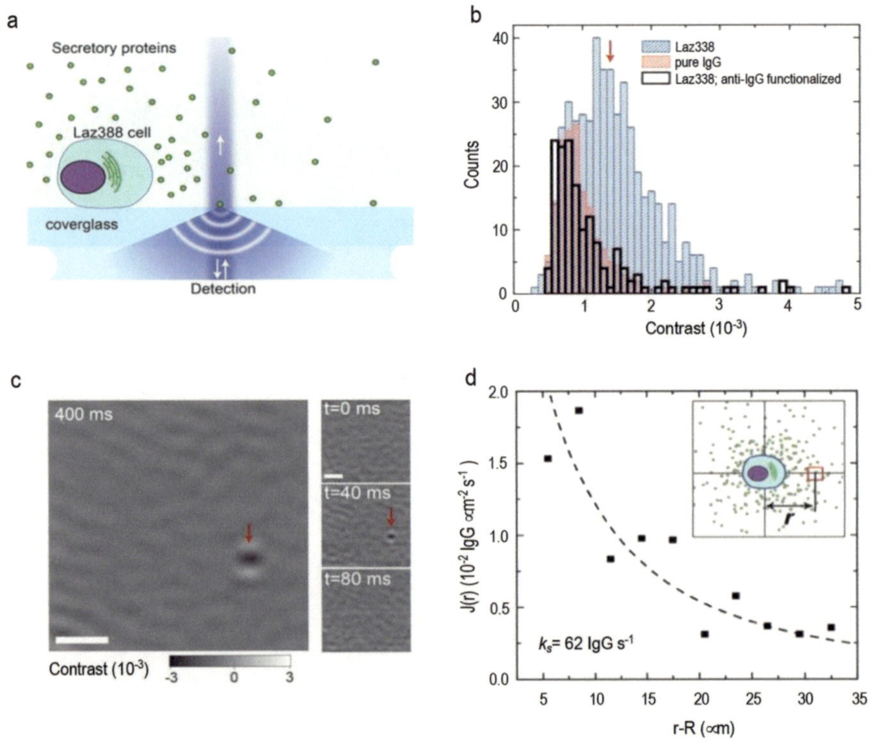

Figure 3.
Secretome quantification and identification. (a) Cartoon of the detection region. (b) Histogram of detected proteins during a 125 s long measurement period in which detected contrasts are counted in bins of 1×10^{-4} contrast (diagonal-hatched blue bars). 503 distinct proteins were counted in this period. The red arrow indicates the expected contrast corresponding to an IgG dimer. Superimposed over the cell secretion data is the contrast distribution of a purified IgG solution injected into the iSCAT FOV with a micropipette (diagonal-hatched rose bars, normalized for clarity). The detected secretion events from a single Laz388 cell on an anti-human IgG-functionalized coverglass are also shown (125 s integration, hollow black bars). The anti-human IgG surface selectively binds all four IgG antibody subtypes and resists the adsorption of other proteins. (c) Comparison of 2.5 fps (400 ms) and 25 fps (40 ms) image acquisitions of a single Laz388 cell's secretions. The right column shows three sequential 40 ms images, while the left displays the 400 ms image composed of 10 total images, including the three shown on the right. Scale bar: 1 μm. (d) IgG secretion rates and secretion heterogeneity. Reprinted (adapted) with permission from Ref. [28]. Copyright 2018 American Chemical Society.

weight 100 kDa–1 MDa. To provide iSCAT the detection specificity for human Immunoglobulin G(IgG), the sensing surface was functionalized with anti-human IgG, which showed high specificity on the adsorption event of IgG (**Figure 3b, d**). The quantification of IgG was realized by counting over certain integration period. It was found that the secretion of IgG antibodies in single Laz388 cells proceeded at a rate of 100 molecules per second.

One of the challenges in iSCAT for cell secretion is that, the recognition of small molecules is difficult due to their limited iSCAT contrast. In above work, the minimum protein molecular weight from iSCAT was approximately 100 kDa. Most cytokines have molecular weight range from approximately 6 to 70 kD, which fall out of the iSCAT's detection range.

3. Labelling techniques

3.1 Fluorescence

Fluorescence based detection provides superb sensitivity of detection, and flexibility in labeling. Fluorescence microscopy features high spatial and temporal resolution, and capability of tracking multiple cells simultaneously [14]. Therefore, fluorescence based detection has been widely used for tracking protein secretion.

3.1.1 FLUOROSpot

A simple and widely used method of single cell secretion analysis is the enzyme-linked immune absorbent spot (ELISpot) that utilizes the immunosandwich-based assay for the measurement of footprint of cells [76]. Cells are loaded into wells precoated with primary antibody. Secreted proteins are captured, and further bound with labeled secondary antibodies. The addition of substrate gives rise to the spots indicative of secretion footprint. Based on similar principle, FLUOROSpot was developed which uses fluorescent dyes to replace the enzyme labels. In this way, more than one protein could be analyzed at the same time [77]. In spite that ELISpot and FlUOROSpot have been used as common methods for the detection of cell secretion, several drawbacks hinder its applications in the real-time imaging of protein secretion, including spectral overlap, varied individual spots, limited temporal resolution caused by long incubation time (12–48 h), limited number of simultaneously tracked proteins, and cell lost during the process [78].

3.1.2 Microengraving

Inspired by the principle of FLUOROSpot, the microengraving method was developed to isolate and confine single cells in a planar array of microwells. The protein secretion of segregated cells can be tracked as protein detection microarrays are integrated with the microwells, which are conventionally made of elastomeric polymers such as polydimethylsiloxane (PDMS). These microfabricated wells have subnanoliter volumes. A glass side fabricated with antibodies is covered to the array of microwells, to capture the proteins secreted by confined cells. Subsequently, the slide is removed and incubated with fluorescently labelled secondary antibodies. The single-cell cytokine secretion analysis is implemented by fluorescence imaging. Bradshaw et al. [79] showed that the same cells in the microwell can be applied on two detection microarrays successively, allowing monitoring the secretion of four types of cytokines and antibodies. In the meantime, the segregated cells in the wells can also be directly stained by immunofluorescence to determine their lineages.

A drawback in this method is that, the tracked number of proteins is limited by the capability of differentiation of multiple fluorophores within a single spectrum.

3.1.3 Barcode chip

The number of secretion protein types from above methods is limited due to the spectral overlap as multiple fluorescence labels employed on the same detection chip. This spectral overlap was overcome by separating functionalized antibodies into different lines, using a barcode design. With a proper distance between, up to 15 parallel antibody lines can be contained within a nanoliter cell-trapping chamber. This improved spatial resolution results in an enhanced its capability of simultaneous multiplex detection [28, 29, 80]. Lu et al. [81] further extended the multiplexing capacity by further improving the spectral encoding, namely, in each isolated line, three antibodies with distinct fluorescent labels are contained. This strategy enables simultaneous analysis of 42 types of proteins secreted from a single cell.

Barcode chips provide valuable information for accumulated cell secretion over a period of time. However, the underlying limitations restrict its applications on the real-time monitoring of protein secretion. For instance, the lag between cell secretion and protein detection is inevitable since capture antibody and detection antibody have to play their part in distinct steps. Given their coexistence during cell secretion, strong background fluorescence signal is expected from the unbound labeled antibodies, thus secreted proteins are difficult to be distinguished from the background noise. In addition, to remove excess probes and avoid non-specific bindings, the sensor surface after incubation with cells requires intensive wash steps, which inhibits the shortening of analysis duration into a few hours.

3.1.4 Total internal reflection fluorescence microscopy (TIRFM)

Shiraskaki et al. [82] proposed a solution for the challenge mentioned above using total internal reflection fluorescence microscopy (TIRFM) combined with microengraving method. They deposited single cells on microwells, on the bottom of which anti-cytokine capture antibodies were fabricated. Instead of separate incubation of a sensor chip with a cell and the detection antibody, the fluorescent detection antibody is present in the cell culture medium, so the cytokine capture is in step with the binding of detection antibody. An objective lens of high numerical aperture was used to achieve high incidence angles, generating evanescence field. The near-field excitation by total internal refection enhances the fluorescence signal from the detection antibody in the sandwich immunocomplex, and reduces the background signal from the unbound detection antibodies in the culture medium (**Figure 4a**). With these features, imaging of cytokine secretion was achieved within a single step (**Figure 4b**). Meanwhile, the cell staining (calcein and SYTOX) was applied to investigate the membrane integrity during IL-1b secretion (**Figure 4c**). It was found the onset of IL-1b secretion was consistent with the onset of calcein disappearance and the second protein SYTOX influx (**Figure 4d**). This phenomenon indicated the loss of membrane during IL-1b secretion. The limit of detection of this approach reached down to 2000 cytokine molecules.

3.1.5 Nanoplasmonic fluorescence

The near-field excited fluorescence can also be realized by nanoplasmonic resonator. Wang et al. [83] developed a tunable nanoplasmonic resonator (TNPR) enhanced fluorescence immunoassay for imaging of IL-2 secretion in

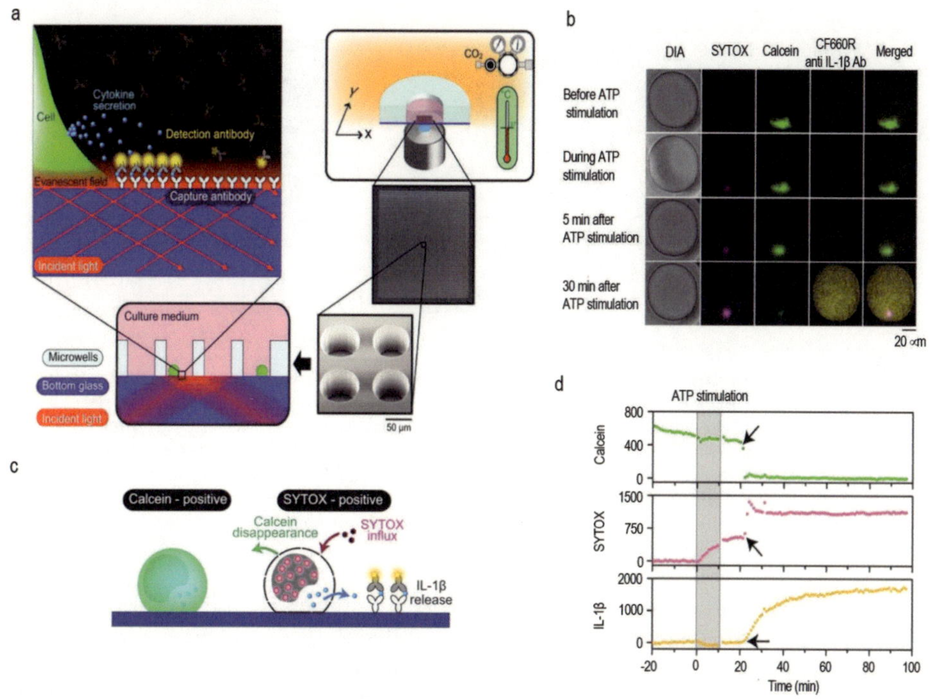

Figure 4.
Time-resolved monitoring of IL-1β secretion on the PDMS MWA chip. (a) Concept of the real-time single cell secretion assay platform. The platform works with micro-fabricated well-array chip on a fully automated fluorescence microscopy. The platform maintains the environment (temperature, concentration of CO_2 and humidity) of the chip. The chip has an array of nanolitre-sized microwells with a glass bottom, into which individual cells were introduced separately. The well has open-ended structure; therefore, culture medium was exchanged constantly during the observation. The anti-cytokine capture antibody was immobilized on the well bottom, onto which secreted cytokine and fluorescently labelled detection antibody were bound to form a sandwich immunocomplex. Near-field excitation by total internal reflection enabled selective detection of the cytokine sandwich immunocomplex immediately following secretion without the requirement for wash steps. (b) Representative images of multichannel microscopy. Morphological features of a human monocyte were monitored under diascopic illumination (DIA). The fluorescence signal of SYTOX-stained nuclei was magenta (SYTOX), that of a calcein-stained cell bodies was green (Calcein) and that of secreted IL-1β was yellow (CF660R anti IL-1β Ab). Merged images of these three fluorescence signals are also displayed (Merged). Each image was obtained at the described period. Scale bar, 20 µm. (c) Schematic of simultaneous monitoring of IL-1β secretion and cell membrane integrity using calcein and SYTOX staining. SYTOX influx and fluorescent calcein disappearance was observed due to compromised plasma membrane integrity. (d) Example of the signal time course during time-resolved monitoring. Grey bands represent the period when the monocytes were exposed to ATP. Arrows represent the transition time of the respective signals. Reprinted (adapted) with permission from Ref. [31]. Copyright 2014, Springer Nature.

submicrometer resolution (**Figure 5**). In this study, the fluorescent secondary antibody was not present while the cytokine secretion was in progress. Instead, cytokine capture and detection step was separated by washing step. With a TNPR structure of 100 nm in diameter, and an optimized fluorescence enhancement at ~10 nm from a gold surface, the fluorescence signal was enhanced 117-fold in the TNPR area. The limit of detection was lower than 100 ng/mL.

3.1.6 Bead biosensors

Another fluorescence based strategy is associated with bead-based biosensors. The cells are confined in microwells, along with antibody-labeled microbeads, and fluorescently-labeled secondary antibody. The capture of secreted proteins on beads was accompanied by the increasing density of secondary antibody, and increasing fluorescence intensity of microbeads. A key advantage of bead biosensors is that,

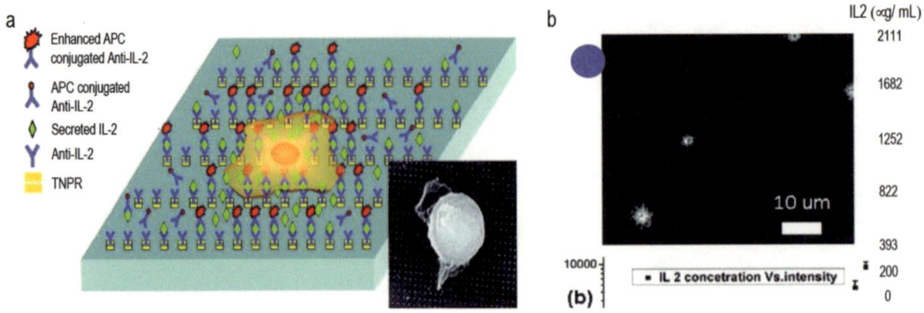

Figure 5.
Demonstration of quantitative high spatial resolution mapping of IL-2 secretion from individual Jurkat T cells. (a) Schematic of high-resolution mapping of cytokine secretion by a TNPR-enhanced in situ immunoassay. ATNPR array fabricated by NIL was incubated with anti-IL-2 antibody, and after Jurkat T cell plating, stimulation, and removal, a portion of the secreted IL-2 was captured by the antibodies on TNPR. Fluorescence-conjugated anti- bodies were applied to detect the secreted IL-2 by forming an antibody- antigen (IL-2)-antibody sandwich on the TNPR surface. Insert: SEM image of a Jurkat T cell adherent to a TNPR array (500 nm pitch). (b) quantitative mapping of Jurkat T cell secretion profiles. Reprinted (adapted) with permission from Ref. [50]. Copyright 2011 American Chemical Society.

it breaks the limit of target-molecular adsorption kinetics, which is controlled by diffusion rates, and exists in majority of immobilized or stationary biosensors [84]. In addition, the regeneration of biosensors can be as simple as removing used beads, and infusing new beads [85]. Son et al. [86] used microcompartments as small as 20 picoliter to confine single cells, suspended antibody-labeled microbeads, and fluorescently-labeled secondary antibody together. The quantitation of secreted cytokines was achieved by tracking the intensity changes of fluorescence on microbeads. They found that the number of microbeads confined within a single microcompartment did not significantly affect the fluorescence enhancement on a single microbead. An et al. [87] utilized a microwell device for cell confinement, and detected the fluorescence changes on functionalized detection beads which are co-incubated with single cells.

Other than the design of microwell, Cui et al. [88] developed an microfluidic immunoassay device that integrated a cell culture chamber, an array of cytokine detection units and an array of active peristaltic mixers for on-chip sample mixing. Cells were isolated, cultured and biochemically stimulated in the same chamber. The detection chambers were loaded with cytometric fluorescent beads. Upon sandwich structure formed after cytokine secretion, the fluorescence intensity changes were analyzed by flow cytometry. The continuous monitoring of cytokine secretion was achieved by the extraction of a small portion of the cytokine-containing culture media to the detection chamber. With this system, the secretion profilings of IL-6, IL-8, and TNF were observed with a detection limit of 20 pg/mL and a sample volume of 160 nl.

3.1.7 Cell-surface affinity sensors

Cell-surface affinity sensors functionalize cell surface to capture secreted molecules from cells. These targets can subsequently be detected by fluorescent labeling. An appealing advantage using this strategy is that, the effect of heterogeneous spatial distribution of secreted molecules is minimized [89, 90]. As secreted molecules release from the cell surface, their diffusion and dilution pose a challenge to the sensitivity of sensors. As the cell surface is turned into sensor surface, these molecules could be captured prior to their diffusion. This immediate interaction enhances the sensitivity of secretion detection. Various cell secretions have been studied previously utilizing cell-surface affinity sensors, including ATP [91, 92], growth factors [93], cytokines [94], and antigens [95]. Liu et al. [96] developed a detection method that utilized fluorescent magnetic nanoparticles labeled secondary antibody, and achieved a detection limit of 0.1 pg/mL. The cell surface was biotinylated, and functionalized by neutravidin and a biotinylated IL-6 capture antibody. Upon the binding of cytokines secreted from cells, fluorescent magnetic nanoparticles labeled secondary antibodies are introduced for indication of the amount of cytokine secretion.

A challenge of cell-surface affinity sensors is the damage and cell viability caused by cell surface modification [97]. Due to the high background signal from free labeled secondary antibody, the cells after secretion have to undergo wash steps to remove free secondary antibodies. This limits its application on the real-time monitoring of cell secretion.

3.1.8 Droplet microfluidics

Droplet microfluidic techniques involve mixture of the aqueous phase and oil phase, and generation of water-in-oil microdroplets in the microfluidic chips [98]. Droplet shape offers encapsulation of a single cell in a picoliter droplet, which confines individual cell and entraps its secretion, restrains the interference from surrounding environment. To achieve real-time monitoring of cell secretion, droplets microfluidic techniques are conventionally integrated with cell-surface affinity sensors or bead-based biosensors. Qiu et al. [94] developed a membrane-anchored aptamer sensor and combined it with droplet microfluidics for IFN-γ detection. This aptamer sensor has a hairpin structure, resulting in quenched fluorescence. Upon binding with IFN-γ, the aptamer switches on the fluorescence signal by aptamer structure change. The limit of detection was approximately 10.0 nM. Due to the proximity of the aptamer sensor to the cell surface, this method achieved monitoring of cytokine secretion at a single-cell level. Chokkalingam et al. [99] took advantage of free capture beads in droplets to detect the secreted cytokines from cells. The cytokine capture step and fluorescent detection step were separated by the gelation of droplets, and de-emulsification. Wei et al. [100] combined LSPR with droplet technique, developing a sensor with a detection limit of 6–7 ng/ml for VEGF and IL-8. The LSPR spectrum shift was obtained by dark-field spectroscope. Due to the advantages of droplet technique, the plasmonic droplets in a continuous flow allow high-throughput detection of 600–1800 droplets/min, 100–150 cells/min.

4. Challenges and future trends

Isolated cell culture in a confined environment for subsequent secretion detection allows good flexibility in the selection of sensing techniques, but such module-based strategy has not been achieved for real-time detection of individual cell secretion. Meanwhile, the integration of cell culture and secretion detection has shown promising results in real-time monitoring single cell secretion by physically presenting the target cells in close proximity to the sensing region. However, there are still significant challenges and difficulties ahead as indicated below.

1. Cell secretion dynamics are found associated with cell states, therefore, it is important for the sensor systems to precisely quantify the cell secretion. An obstacle for current methodology is that, the molecule secretion and molecule detection are both dynamic process occurring at the same time.

The concentrations of target molecules in solution are constantly changing, such that an equilibrium-state based calibration curves are difficult to obtain. Therefore, on one hand, novel or improved detection methods with more rapidly reached equilibrium state are required to minimize the effect of detection process. On the other hand, a comprehensive dynamic model involving secretion and detection dynamics is necessary to understand this complex process and precisely quantify the cell secretion [101, 102].

2. The real-time imaging process requires highly specific and selective responses from sensors. Since the specificity and selectivity of biosensors might be compromised by non-specific binding in complex biological media used in experiments, significant efforts are needed to eliminate the matrix effect. Several blocking strategies that instantaneously passivate the sensor surface and do not affect the recognition chemistry are developed, including protein (like BSA), detergent (Tween, etc.), or different polymer blockers. In imaging experiments, a thoroughly optimized blocking strategy should be applied.

3. It is important to investigate the effects of important experiment conditions for the detection. Previous works mainly focused on the innovation of methodology, improvement of the sensitivity, enhancement of the capability of multiplex detection, etc. However, the influence of multiple important experimental conditions are lack of attention. For instance, in previous works, cells during their secretion were manipulated in various status, including suspended in media, immobilized on the ceiling of microwells, or directly absorbed on sensor surface. These distinct distances between sensing surface and cells are expected to influence the local concentrations of secretions on sensor surface, leading to considerate impact on detection sensitivity.

4. In current stage, multiplex real-time imaging of cell secretion is a great challenge. Though the fluorescence based barcode chip has demonstrated its capability in profiling up to 42 types of proteins secreted from a single cell, the real-time imaging of these proteins is incapable due to the lag between cell secretion and protein detection, and intensive wash steps which require several hours. Nanoplasmonic biosensors and SPR imaging have difficulty to broaden their multiplexity owing to their label-free characteristic. Therefore, to achieve the multiplex real-time imaging, the integration of these techniques might provide promising opportunities.

5. Current studies focus on the secretion of single type cells. The interactions of different cells, and their intercellular communication through proteins such as cytokines demand comprehension and further exploration. Therefore, a platform capable of monitoring of multiple cells' real-time secretion is demanded.

5. Conclusions

In the past two decades, cell secretion monitoring has gained increasing attention. To understand the heterogeneity of protein secretion in single cell level, various optic methods have been developed including labelling and label-free techniques. The label-free techniques such as plasmonic sensors, PCR, EOT, are able to recognize the secreted proteins by sensing the changes of refractive index on the sensor interfaces. The limit of detection differs from 20 pg/mL to 50 ng/mL. The signal transduction during the analyte-ligand interaction does not require the involvement of any additional materials, therefore, the label-free techniques allow simple operation and fast response, suitable for real-time imaging. The labelling techniques such as fluorescence microscopy utilize fluorophore-labeled bioreceptors to recognize the proteins. Different from the label-free techniques, the fluorescence based methods conventionally use two recognition elements to form a sandwich complex, one of them as the capture element, the other as the signal transducer (the fluorophore-labeled bioreceptor). The limit of detection differs from 0.1 pg/mL to 20 ng/mL. Even though the two recognition element approaches involve additional processing and washing steps, which prolong the response time, the extraordinary sensitivity and low background improve the reliability and allow multiplex detection, making it very attractive to some applications.

For instance, TIRFM has demonstrated its possibilities on real-time imaging of protein secretion from single cells by utilizing both high sensitivity from fluorescence microscopy, and wash-free process due to the evanescent field created by total internal reflection. In spite of the achievements mentioned above, intensive work is demanded in future such as understanding of cell secretion dynamics, improving the detection specificity, developing multiplex real-time imaging platform, and investigating the interactions of different cells, and their intercellular communication.

Acknowledgements

This research was supported by the NIH MIRA R35GM133795 and NSF CAREER CBET-1943302 (P. Chen). Additionally, this material is based upon work supported ALS while serving at the National Science Foundation. Any opinion, findings, and conclusions or recommendations expressed in this material are those of the author(s) and do not necessarily reflect the views of the National Science Foundation.

Conflict of interest

The authors declare no conflict of interest.

Author details

Lang Zhou, Pengyu Chen and Aleksandr Simonian*
Materials Research and Education Center, Department of Mechanical Engineering, Auburn University, Auburn, AL 36849, USA

*Address all correspondence to: als@auburn.edu

References

[1] Cavalli G, Cenci S. Autophagy and Protein Secretion. J Mol Biol [Internet]. 2020 Apr 3 [cited 2020 Sep 22];432(8):2525-45. Available from: https://www.sciencedirect.com/science/article/pii/S002228362030067X

[2] Uhlén M, Karlsson MJ, Hober A, Svensson A-S, Scheffel J, Kotol D, et al. The human secretome. Sci Signal [Internet]. 2019 Nov 26 [cited 2020 Sep 22];12(609). Available from: http://www.ncbi.nlm.nih.gov/pubmed/31772123

[3] Brandi J, Pozza ED, Dando I, Biondani G, Robotti E, Jenkins R, et al. Secretome protein signature of human pancreatic cancer stem-like cells. J Proteomics [Internet]. 2016 Mar 16 [cited 2020 Sep 22];136:1-12. Available from: https://www.sciencedirect.com/science/article/pii/S1874391916300203

[4] Baberg F, Geyh S, Waldera-Lupa D, Stefanski A, Zilkens C, Haas R, et al. Secretome analysis of human bone marrow derived mesenchymal stromal cells. Biochim Biophys Acta - Proteins Proteomics [Internet]. 2019 Apr 1 [cited 2020 Sep 22];1867(4):434-41. Available from: https://www.sciencedirect.com/science/article/pii/S1570963919300263

[5] Štrbák V. Pancreatic Thyrotropin Releasing Hormone and Mechanism of Insulin Secretion. Cell Physiol Biochem [Internet]. 2018 [cited 2020 Sep 22];50:378-84. Available from: www.karger.com/cpbwww.karger.com/cpb

[6] Ponpuak M, Mandell MA, Kimura T, Chauhan S, Cleyrat C, Deretic V. Secretory autophagy. Curr Opin Cell Biol [Internet]. 2015 Aug 1 [cited 2020 Sep 22];35:106-16. Available from: https://www.sciencedirect.com/science/article/pii/S0955067415000563

[7] Al-Qudah MA, Al-Dwairi A. Mechanisms and regulation of neurotrophin synthesis and secretion. Neurosciences (Riyadh) [Internet]. 2016 Oct [cited 2020 Sep 22];21(4):306-13. Available from: http://www.ncbi.nlm.nih.gov/pubmed/27744458

[8] Rabouille C. Pathways of Unconventional Protein Secretion. Trends Cell Biol [Internet]. 2017 Mar 1 [cited 2020 Sep 22];27(3):230-40. Available from: https://www.sciencedirect.com/science/article/pii/S0962892416302057

[9] Fujita-Yoshigaki J, Yokoyama M, Katsumata-Kato O. Determinants for selective transport of exogenously expressed cargo proteins into regulated and constitutive secretory pathways. J Oral Biosci [Internet]. 2017 May 1 [cited 2020 Sep 22];59(2):87-91. Available from: https://www.sciencedirect.com/science/article/pii/S1349007917300221?via%3Dihub

[10] Labunskyy VM, Gerashchenko M V., Delaney JR, Kaya A, Kennedy BK, Kaeberlein M, et al. Lifespan Extension Conferred by Endoplasmic Reticulum Secretory Pathway Deficiency Requires Induction of the Unfolded Protein Response. Kim SK, editor. PLoS Genet [Internet]. 2014 Jan 2 [cited 2020 Sep 22];10(1):e1004019. Available from: https://dx.plos.org/10.1371/journal.pgen.1004019

[11] Kienzle C, von Blume J. Secretory cargo sorting at the trans-Golgi network. Trends Cell Biol [Internet]. 2014 Oct 1 [cited 2020 Sep 22];24(10):584-93. Available from: https://www.sciencedirect.com/science/article/pii/S0962892414000725

[12] Ponnambalam S, Baldwin SA. Constitutive protein secretion from the trans -Golgi network to the plasma membrane (Review). Mol Membr Biol [Internet]. 2003 Jan 9 [cited 2020 Aug 22];20(2):129-39. Available from:

http://www.tandfonline.com/doi/full/10.1080/0968768031000084172

[13] Simpson JC, Joggerst B, Laketa V, Verissimo F, Cetin C, Erfle H, et al. Genome-wide RNAi screening identifies human proteins with a regulatory function in the early secretory pathway. Nat Cell Biol [Internet]. 2012 Jul 3 [cited 2020 Aug 22];14(7):764-74. Available from: http://www.nature.com/articles/ncb2510

[14] Li W, Li D. Fluorescent probes for monitoring regulated secretion. Curr Opin Chem Biol [Internet]. 2013 Aug 1 [cited 2020 Aug 22];17(4):672-81. Available from: https://www.sciencedirect.com/science/article/pii/S136759311300077X

[15] Meldolesi J. Exosomes and Ectosomes in Intercellular Communication. Curr Biol [Internet]. 2018 Apr 23 [cited 2020 Sep 22];28(8):R435-44. Available from: https://www.sciencedirect.com/science/article/pii/S0960982218300927

[16] Diegeler S, Hellweg CE. Intercellular Communication of Tumor Cells and Immune Cells after Exposure to Different Ionizing Radiation Qualities. Front Immunol [Internet]. 2017 Jun 7 [cited 2020 Sep 22];8:664. Available from: http://journal.frontiersin.org/article/10.3389/fimmu.2017.00664/full

[17] Kveler K, Starosvetsky E, Ziv-Kenet A, Kalugny Y, Gorelik Y, Shalev-Malul G, et al. Immune-centric network of cytokines and cells in disease context identified by computational mining of PubMed. Nat Biotechnol [Internet]. 2018 Aug 18 [cited 2020 Sep 22];36(7):651-9. Available from: http://www.nature.com/articles/nbt.4152

[18] Altan-Bonnet G, Mukherjee R. Cytokine-mediated communication: a quantitative appraisal of immune complexity. Nat Rev Immunol [Internet]. 2019 Apr 15 [cited 2020 Sep 22];19(4):205-17. Available from: http://www.nature.com/articles/s41577-019-0131-x

[19] Kulkarni A, Chen J, Maday S. Neuronal autophagy and intercellular regulation of homeostasis in the brain. Curr Opin Neurobiol [Internet]. 2018 Aug 1 [cited 2020 Sep 22];51:29-36. Available from: https://www.sciencedirect.com/science/article/pii/S0959438818300011

[20] Kudryashova I V., Stepanichev MY, Gulyaeva N V. Neonatal Proinflammatory Stress and the Maturation of Intercellular Communication in the Hippocampus. Neurosci Behav Physiol [Internet]. 2020 Jul 5 [cited 2020 Sep 22];50(6):730-42. Available from: http://link.springer.com/10.1007/s11055-020-00971-6

[21] Osipova ED, Semyachkina-Glushkovskaya O V., Morgun A V., Pisareva N V., Malinovskaya NA, Boitsova EB, et al. Gliotransmitters and cytokines in the control of blood-brain barrier permeability. Rev Neurosci [Internet]. 2018 Jul 26 [cited 2020 Sep 22];29(5):567-91. Available from: http://www.degruyter.com/view/j/revneuro.2018.29.issue-5/revneuro-2017-0092/revneuro-2017-0092.xml

[22] Patel BG, Lenk EE, Lebovic DI, Shu Y, Yu J, Taylor RN. Pathogenesis of endometriosis: Interaction between Endocrine and inflammatory pathways. Best Pract Res Clin Obstet Gynaecol [Internet]. 2018 Jul 1 [cited 2020 Sep 22];50:50-60. Available from: https://www.sciencedirect.com/science/article/pii/S1521693418300233

[23] Tan C, Hu W, He Y, Zhang Y, Zhang G, Xu Y, et al. Cytokine-mediated therapeutic resistance in breast cancer. Cytokine [Internet]. 2018 Aug 1 [cited 2020 Sep 22];108:151-9. Available from: https://www.sciencedirect.com/science/article/pii/S1043466618301066

[24] Esquivel-Velázquez M, Ostoa-Saloma P, Palacios-Arreola MI, Nava-Castro KE, Castro JI, Morales-Montor J. The Role of Cytokines in Breast Cancer Development and Progression. J Interf Cytokine Res [Internet]. 2015 Jan 13 [cited 2020 Sep 22];35(1):1-16. Available from: http://www.liebertpub.com/doi/10.1089/jir.2014.0026

[25] Balderman SR, Calvi LM. Biology of BM failure syndromes: role of microenvironment and niches. Hematology [Internet]. 2014 Dec 5 [cited 2020 Aug 22];2014(1):71-6. Available from: https://ashpublications.org/hematology/article/2014/1/71/20496/Biology-of-BM-failure-syndromes-role-of

[26] Clapes T, Lefkopoulos S, Trompouki E. Stress and Non-Stress Roles of Inflammatory Signals during HSC Emergence and Maintenance. Front Immunol [Internet]. 2016 Nov 7 [cited 2020 Aug 22];7:487. Available from: http://journal.frontiersin.org/article/10.3389/fimmu.2016.00487/full

[27] Cooper GM. The cell : a molecular approach [Internet]. ASM Press; 2000 [cited 2020 Aug 22]. 689 p. Available from: https://www.ncbi.nlm.nih.gov/books/NBK9839/

[28] Lu Y, Chen JJ, Mu L, Xue Q, Wu Y, Wu P-H, et al. High-Throughput Secretomic Analysis of Single Cells to Assess Functional Cellular Heterogeneity. Anal Chem [Internet]. 2013 Feb 19 [cited 2020 Aug 22];85(4):2548-56. Available from: https://pubs.acs.org/doi/10.1021/ac400082e

[29] Ma C, Fan R, Ahmad H, Shi Q, Comin-Anduix B, Chodon T, et al. A clinical microchip for evaluation of single immune cells reveals high functional heterogeneity in phenotypically similar T cells. Nat Med [Internet]. 2011 Jun 22 [cited 2020 Aug 22];17(6):738-43. Available from: http://www.nature.com/articles/nm.2375

[30] Deng Y, Zhang Y, Sun S, Wang Z, Wang M, Yu B, et al. An Integrated Microfluidic Chip System for Single-Cell Secretion Profiling of Rare Circulating Tumor Cells. Sci Rep [Internet]. 2015 May 16 [cited 2020 Aug 22];4(1):7499. Available from: http://www.nature.com/articles/srep07499

[31] Whiteside TL. The tumor microenvironment and its role in promoting tumor growth. Oncogene. 2008

[32] da Cunha BR, Domingos C, Buzzo Stefanini AC, Henrique T, Polachini GM, Castelo-Branco P, et al. Cellular interactions in the tumor microenvironment: The role of secretome. Journal of Cancer. 2019

[33] Liu W, Kin T, Ho S, Dorrell C, Campbell SR, Luo P, et al. Abnormal regulation of glucagon secretion by human islet alpha cells in the absence of beta cells. EBioMedicine [Internet]. 2019 Dec 1 [cited 2020 Aug 22];50:306-16. Available from: https://www.sciencedirect.com/science/article/pii/S2352396419307674

[34] Del Prato S, Bianchi C, Daniele G. Abnormalities of Insulin Secretion and β-Cell Defects in Type 2 Diabetes. In: Textbook of Diabetes [Internet]. Chichester, UK: John Wiley & Sons, Ltd; 2016 [cited 2020 Aug 22]. p. 161-73. Available from: http://doi.wiley.com/10.1002/9781118924853.ch12

[35] Showalter A, Limaye A, Oyer JL, Igarashi R, Kittipatarin C, Copik AJ, et al. Cytokines in immunogenic cell death: Applications for cancer immunotherapy. Cytokine [Internet]. 2017 Sep 1 [cited 2020 Aug 22];97:123-32. Available from: https://www.sciencedirect.com/science/article/pii/S1043466617301539

[36] Tong L, Wei H, Zhang S, Xu H. Recent Advances in Plasmonic Sensors. Sensors [Internet]. 2014 May

5 [cited 2020 Sep 22];14(5):7959-73. Available from: http://www.mdpi.com/1424-8220/14/5/7959

[37] Kazanskiy NL, Khonina SN, Butt MA. Plasmonic sensors based on Metal-insulator-metal waveguides for refractive index sensing applications: A brief review. Phys E Low-dimensional Syst Nanostructures [Internet]. 2020 Mar 1 [cited 2020 Sep 22];117:113798. Available from: https://www.sciencedirect.com/science/article/pii/S1386947719311336

[38] Barizuddin S, Bok S, Gangopadhyay S. Plasmonic Sensors for Disease Detection - A Review. J Nanomed Nanotechnol [Internet]. 2016 [cited 2020 Sep 22];7:373. Available from: http://dx.doi.org/10.4172/2157-7439.1000373

[39] Sharma AK, Pandey AK, Kaur B. A Review of advancements (2007-2017) in plasmonics-based optical fiber sensors. Opt Fiber Technol [Internet]. 2018 Jul 1 [cited 2020 Sep 22];43:20-34. Available from: https://www.sciencedirect.com/science/article/pii/S1068520018300324

[40] Jeon TY, Kim DJ, Park S-G, Kim S-H, Kim D-H. Nanostructured plasmonic substrates for use as SERS sensors. Nano Converg [Internet]. 2016 Dec 1 [cited 2020 Sep 22];3(1):18. Available from: http://nanoconvergencejournal.springeropen.com/articles/10.1186/s40580-016-0078-6

[41] Wang J, Lin W, Cao E, Xu X, Liang W, Zhang X. Surface Plasmon Resonance Sensors on Raman and Fluorescence Spectroscopy. Sensors [Internet]. 2017 Nov 24 [cited 2020 Sep 22];17(12):2719. Available from: http://www.mdpi.com/1424-8220/17/12/2719

[42] Wang D-S, Fan S-K. Microfluidic Surface Plasmon Resonance Sensors: From Principles to Point-of-Care Applications. Sensors [Internet]. 2016 Jul 27 [cited 2020 Sep 22];16(8):1175. Available from: http://www.mdpi.com/1424-8220/16/8/1175

[43] Jackman JA, Yorulmaz Avsar S, Ferhan AR, Li D, Park JH, Zhdanov VP, et al. Quantitative Profiling of Nanoscale Liposome Deformation by a Localized Surface Plasmon Resonance Sensor. Anal Chem [Internet]. 2017 Jan 17 [cited 2020 Sep 22];89(2):1102-9. Available from: https://pubs.acs.org/doi/10.1021/acs.analchem.6b02532

[44] Kim H-M, Park J-H, Jeong DH, Lee H-Y, Lee S-K. Real-time detection of prostate-specific antigens using a highly reliable fiber-optic localized surface plasmon resonance sensor combined with micro fluidic channel. Sensors Actuators B Chem [Internet]. 2018 Nov 10 [cited 2020 Sep 22];273:891-8. Available from: https://www.sciencedirect.com/science/article/pii/S0925400518312449

[45] Blanchard-Dionne A-P, Meunier M. Sensing with periodic nanohole arrays. Adv Opt Photonics [Internet]. 2017 Dec 31 [cited 2020 Sep 22];9(4):891. Available from: https://www.osapublishing.org/abstract.cfm?URI=aop-9-4-891

[46] Jackman JA, Linardy E, Yoo D, Seo J, Ng WB, Klemme DJ, et al. Plasmonic Nanohole Sensor for Capturing Single Virus-Like Particles toward Virucidal Drug Evaluation. Small [Internet]. 2016 Mar 1 [cited 2020 Sep 22];12(9):1159-66. Available from: http://doi.wiley.com/10.1002/smll.201501914

[47] Schasfoort R, Abali F, Stojanovic I, Vidarsson G, Terstappen L. Trends in SPR Cytometry: Advances in Label-Free Detection of Cell Parameters. Biosensors [Internet]. 2018 Oct 30 [cited 2020 Aug 22];8(4):102. Available from: http://www.mdpi.com/2079-6374/8/4/102

[48] Liu C, Lei T, Ino K, Matsue T, Tao N, Li C-Z. Real-time monitoring biomarker expression of carcinoma

cells by surface plasmon resonance biosensors. Chem Commun [Internet]. 2012 Sep 26 [cited 2020 Aug 20];48(84):10389. Available from: http://xlink.rsc.org/?DOI=c2cc34853e

[49] Milgram S, Cortes S, Villiers MB, Marche P, Buhot A, Livache T, et al. On chip real time monitoring of B-cells hybridoma secretion of immunoglobulin. Biosens Bioelectron. 2011 Jan 15;**26**(5):2728-2732

[50] Wu C, He J, Li B, Xu Y, Gu D, Liu H, et al. Real-time monitoring of T-cell-secreted interferon-γ for the diagnosis of tuberculosis. Biotechnol Biotechnol Equip [Internet]. 2018 Jul 4 [cited 2020 Mar 2];32(4):993-8. Available from: https://www.tandfonline.com/doi/full/10.1080/13102818.2018.1432416

[51] Stojanović I, van der Velden TJG, Mulder HW, Schasfoort RBM, Terstappen LWMM. Quantification of antibody production of individual hybridoma cells by surface plasmon resonance imaging. Anal Biochem [Internet]. 2015 Sep 15 [cited 2020 Aug 20];485:112-8. Available from: https://www.sciencedirect.com/science/article/pii/S0003269715003115

[52] Stojanović I, Baumgartner W, van der Velden TJG, Terstappen LWMM, Schasfoort RBM. Modeling single cell antibody excretion on a biosensor. Anal Biochem [Internet]. 2016 Jul 1 [cited 2020 Aug 20];504:1-3. Available from: https://www.sciencedirect.com/science/article/pii/S0003269716300094

[53] Puiu M, Bala C. SPR and SPR Imaging: Recent Trends in Developing Nanodevices for Detection and Real-Time Monitoring of Biomolecular Events. Sensors [Internet]. 2016 Jun 14 [cited 2020 Aug 22];16(6):870. Available from: http://www.mdpi.com/1424-8220/16/6/870

[54] Homola J. Surface Plasmon Resonance Sensors for Detection of Chemical and Biological Species. 2008 [cited 2020 Aug 22]; Available from: https://pubs.acs.org/doi/full/10.1021/cr068107d

[55] Spoto G, Minunni M. Surface Plasmon Resonance Imaging: What Next? J Phys Chem Lett [Internet]. 2012 Sep 20 [cited 2020 Aug 22];3(18):2682-91. Available from: https://pubs.acs.org/doi/10.1021/jz301053n

[56] Wang D, Loo J, Chen J, Yam Y, Chen S-C, He H, et al. Recent Advances in Surface Plasmon Resonance Imaging Sensors. Sensors [Internet]. 2019 Mar 13 [cited 2020 Aug 22];19(6):1266. Available from: https://www.mdpi.com/1424-8220/19/6/1266

[57] Bryce P. Nelson, Anthony G. Frutos, Jennifer M. Brockman and, Corn* RM. Near-Infrared Surface Plasmon Resonance Measurements of Ultrathin Films. 1. Angle Shift and SPR Imaging Experiments. 1999 [cited 2020 Aug 22]; Available from: https://pubs.acs.org/doi/abs/10.1021/ac990517x

[58] Mukherji S, Shukla G. Nanoplasmonic biosensors: current perspectives. Nanobiosensors Dis Diagnosis [Internet]. 2015 Sep 10 [cited 2020 Aug 22];4:75. Available from: https://www.dovepress.com/nanoplasmonic-biosensors-current-perspectives-peer-reviewed-article-NDD

[59] Mazzotta F, Johnson TW, Dahlin AB, Shaver J, Oh S-H, Höök F. Influence of the Evanescent Field Decay Length on the Sensitivity of Plasmonic Nanodisks and Nanoholes. ACS Photonics [Internet]. 2015 Feb 18 [cited 2020 Aug 22];2(2):256-62. Available from: https://pubs.acs.org/doi/10.1021/ph500360d

[60] Peixoto de Almeida M, Pereira E, Baptista P, Gomes I, Figueiredo S, Soares L, et al. Gold Nanoparticles as (Bio)Chemical Sensors. Compr Anal

Chem [Internet]. 2014 Jan 1 [cited 2020 Aug 22];66:529-67. Available from: https://www.sciencedirect.com/science/article/pii/B9780444632852000134

[61] Jackman JA, Rahim Ferhan A, Cho N-J. Nanoplasmonic sensors for biointerfacial science. Chem Soc Rev [Internet]. 2017 Jun 19 [cited 2020 Aug 22];46(12):3615-60. Available from: http://xlink.rsc.org/?DOI=C6CS00494F

[62] Zhu C, Luo X, Espulgar WV, Koyama S, Kumanogoh A, Saito M, et al. Real-Time Monitoring and Detection of Single-Cell Level Cytokine Secretion Using LSPR Technology. Micromachines [Internet]. 2020 Jan 19 [cited 2020 Feb 19];11(1):107. Available from: https://www.mdpi.com/2072-666X/11/1/107

[63] Oh B-R, Chen P, Nidetz R, McHugh W, Fu J, Shanley TP, et al. Multiplexed Nanoplasmonic Temporal Profiling of T-Cell Response under Immunomodulatory Agent Exposure. ACS Sensors [Internet]. 2016 Jul 22 [cited 2020 Aug 20];1(7):941-8. Available from: https://pubs.acs.org/doi/10.1021/acssensors.6b00240

[64] Faridi A, Yang W, Kelly HG, Wang C, Faridi P, Purcell AW, et al. Differential Roles of Plasma Protein Corona on Immune Cell Association and Cytokine Secretion of Oligomeric and Fibrillar Beta-Amyloid. Biomacromolecules [Internet]. 2019 Nov 11 [cited 2020 Aug 20];20(11):4208-17. Available from: https://pubs.acs.org/doi/10.1021/acs.biomac.9b01116

[65] Ahmad Mohamed Ali R, Mita D, Espulgar W, Saito M, Nishide M, Takamatsu H, et al. Single Cell Analysis of Neutrophils NETs by Microscopic LSPR Imaging System. Micromachines [Internet]. 2019 Dec 31 [cited 2020 Aug 20];11(1):52. Available from: https://www.mdpi.com/2072-666X/11/1/52

[66] Raphael MP, Christodoulides JA, Delehanty JB, Long JP, Byers JM. Quantitative Imaging of Protein Secretions from Single Cells in Real Time. Biophys J [Internet]. 2013 Aug 6 [cited 2020 Aug 20];105(3):602-8. Available from: https://www.sciencedirect.com/science/article/pii/S0006349513007017

[67] Escobedo C, Brolo AG, Gordon R, Sinton D. Flow-Through vs Flow-Over: Analysis of Transport and Binding in Nanohole Array Plasmonic Biosensors. Anal Chem [Internet]. 2010 Dec 15 [cited 2020 Aug 22];82(24):10015-20. Available from: https://pubs.acs.org/doi/10.1021/ac101654f

[68] Li X, Soler M, Özdemir CI, Belushkin A, Yesilköy F, Altug H. Plasmonic nanohole array biosensor for label-free and real-time analysis of live cell secretion. Lab Chip. 2017 Jun 27;**17**(13):2208-2217

[69] Li X, Soler M, Szydzik C, Khoshmanesh K, Schmidt J, Coukos G, et al. Label-Free Optofluidic Nanobiosensor Enables Real-Time Analysis of Single-Cell Cytokine Secretion. Small [Internet]. 2018 Jun 27 [cited 2020 Feb 20];14(26):1800698. Available from: http://doi.wiley.com/10.1002/smll.201800698

[70] Pitruzzello G, Krauss TF. Photonic crystal resonances for sensing and imaging. J Opt [Internet]. 2018 Jul 1 [cited 2020 Aug 22];20(7):073004. Available from: https://iopscience.iop.org/article/10.1088/2040-8986/aac75b

[71] Triggs GJ, Fischer M, Stellinga D, Scullion MG, Evans GJO, Krauss TF. Spatial Resolution and Refractive Index Contrast of Resonant Photonic Crystal Surfaces for Biosensing. IEEE Photonics J [Internet]. 2015 Jun [cited 2020 Aug 22];7(3):1-10. Available from: http://ieeexplore.ieee.org/document/7110507/

[72] Juan-Colás J, Hitchcock IS, Coles M, Johnson S, Krauss TF. Quantifying

single-cell secretion in real time using resonant hyperspectral imaging. Proc Natl Acad Sci U S A. 2018 Dec 26;**115**(52):13204-13209

[73] Young G, Kukura P. Interferometric Scattering Microscopy. Annu Rev Phys Chem [Internet]. 2019 Jun 14 [cited 2020 Aug 22];70(1):301-22. Available from: https://www.annualreviews.org/doi/10.1146/annurev-physchem-050317-021247

[74] Park J-S, Lee I-B, Moon H-M, Joo J-H, Kim K-H, Hong S-C, et al. Label-free and live cell imaging by interferometric scattering microscopy. Chem Sci [Internet]. 2018 Mar 7 [cited 2020 Aug 22];9(10):2690-7. Available from: http://xlink.rsc.org/?DOI=C7SC04733A

[75] McDonald MP, Gemeinhardt A, König K, Piliarik M, Schaffer S, Völkl S, et al. Visualizing Single-Cell Secretion Dynamics with Single-Protein Sensitivity. Nano Lett. 2018 Jan 10;**18**(1):513-519

[76] Crotty S, Aubert RD, Glidewell J, Ahmed R. Tracking human antigen-specific memory B cells: a sensitive and generalized ELISPOT system. J Immunol Methods [Internet]. 2004 Mar 1 [cited 2020 Aug 21];286(1-2):111-22. Available from: https://www.sciencedirect.com/science/article/pii/S0022175904000031

[77] Janetzki S, Rueger M, Dillenbeck T. Stepping up ELISpot: Multi-Level Analysis in FluoroSpot Assays. Cells [Internet]. 2014 Nov 27 [cited 2020 Aug 22];3(4):1102-15. Available from: http://www.mdpi.com/2073-4409/3/4/1102

[78] Han Q, Bradshaw EM, Nilsson B, Hafler DA, Love JC. Multidimensional analysis of the frequencies and rates of cytokine secretion from single cells by quantitative microengraving. Lab Chip [Internet]. 2010 May 18 [cited 2020 Aug 22];10(11):1391. Available from: http://xlink.rsc.org/?DOI=b926849a

[79] Bradshaw EM, Kent SC, Tripuraneni V, Orban T, Ploegh HL, Hafler DA, et al. Concurrent detection of secreted products from human lymphocytes by microengraving: Cytokines and antigen-reactive antibodies. Clin Immunol [Internet]. 2008 Oct 1 [cited 2020 Aug 21];129(1):10-8. Available from: https://www.sciencedirect.com/science/article/pii/S1521661608006888

[80] Fan R, Vermesh O, Srivastava A, Yen BKH, Qin L, Ahmad H, et al. Integrated barcode chips for rapid, multiplexed analysis of proteins in microliter quantities of blood. Nat Biotechnol [Internet]. 2008 Dec 16 [cited 2020 Aug 22];26(12):1373-8. Available from: http://www.nature.com/articles/nbt.1507

[81] Lu Y, Xue Q, Eisele MR, Sulistijo ES, Brower K, Han L, et al. Highly multiplexed profiling of single-cell effector functions reveals deep functional heterogeneity in response to pathogenic ligands. Proc Natl Acad Sci U S A [Internet]. 2015 Feb 17 [cited 2020 Aug 21];112(7):E607-15. Available from: http://www.ncbi.nlm.nih.gov/pubmed/25646488

[82] Shirasaki Y, Yamagishi M, Suzuki N, Izawa K, Nakahara A, Mizuno J, et al. Real-time single-cell imaging of protein secretion. Sci Rep [Internet]. 2015 May 22 [cited 2020 Aug 22];4(1):4736. Available from: http://www.nature.com/articles/srep04736

[83] Wang S, Ota S, Guo B, Ryu J, Rhodes C, Xiong Y, et al. Subcellular resolution mapping of endogenous cytokine secretion by nano-plasmonic-resonator sensor array. Nano Lett. 2011 Aug 10;**11**(8):3431-3434

[84] Cohen N, Sabhachandani P, Golberg A, Konry T. Approaching near real-time biosensing: Microfluidic microsphere based biosensor for real-time analyte detection. Biosens

Bioelectron [Internet]. 2015 Apr 15 [cited 2020 Aug 22];66:454-60. Available from: https://www.sciencedirect.com/science/article/pii/S0956566314009075

[85] Son KJ, Gheibi P, Stybayeva G, Rahimian A, Revzin A. Detecting cell-secreted growth factors in microfluidic devices using bead-based biosensors. Microsystems Nanoeng [Internet]. 2017 Dec 3 [cited 2020 Aug 22];3(1):17025. Available from: http://www.nature.com/articles/micronano201725

[86] Son KJ, Rahimian A, Shin D-S, Siltanen C, Patel T, Revzin A. Microfluidic compartments with sensing microbeads for dynamic monitoring of cytokine and exosome release from single cells. Analyst [Internet]. 2016 Jan 4 [cited 2020 Aug 22];141(2):679-88. Available from: http://xlink.rsc.org/?DOI=C5AN01648G

[87] An X, Sendra VG, Liadi I, Ramesh B, Romain G, Haymaker C, et al. Single-cell profiling of dynamic cytokine secretion and the phenotype of immune cells. Ahlenstiel G, editor. PLoS One [Internet]. 2017 Aug 24 [cited 2020 Aug 22];12(8):e0181904. Available from: https://dx.plos.org/10.1371/journal.pone.0181904

[88] Cui X, Liu Y, Hu D, Qian W, Tin C, Sun D, et al. A fluorescent microbead-based microfluidic immunoassay chip for immune cell cytokine secretion quantification. Lab Chip. 2018 Jan 30;**18**(3):522-531

[89] Wimmers F, Subedi N, van Buuringen N, Heister D, Vivié J, Beeren-Reinieren I, et al. Single-cell analysis reveals that stochasticity and paracrine signaling control interferon-alpha production by plasmacytoid dendritic cells. Nat Commun [Internet]. 2018 Dec 20 [cited 2020 Aug 22];9(1):3317. Available from: http://www.nature.com/articles/s41467-018-05784-3

[90] Qiu L, Zhang T, Jiang J, Wu C, Zhu G, You M, et al. Cell Membrane-Anchored Biosensors for Real-Time Monitoring of the Cellular Microenvironment. J Am Chem Soc [Internet]. 2014 Sep 24 [cited 2020 Aug 22];136(38):13090-3. Available from: https://pubs.acs.org/doi/10.1021/ja5047389

[91] Lobas MA, Tao R, Nagai J, Kronschläger MT, Borden PM, Marvin JS, et al. A genetically encoded single-wavelength sensor for imaging cytosolic and cell surface ATP. Nat Commun [Internet]. 2019 Dec 12 [cited 2020 Aug 22];10(1):711. Available from: http://www.nature.com/articles/s41467-019-08441-5

[92] Beigi R, Kobatake E, Aizawa M, Dubyak GR. Detection of local ATP release from activated platelets using cell surface-attached firefly luciferase. https://doi.org/101152/ajpcell19992761C267 [Internet]. 1999 [cited 2020 Aug 22]; Available from: https://journals.physiology.org/doi/full/10.1152/ajpcell.1999.276.1.C267

[93] Zhao W, Schafer S, Choi J, Yamanaka YJ, Lombardi ML, Bose S, et al. Cell-surface sensors for real-time probing of cellular environments. Nat Nanotechnol [Internet]. 2011 Aug 17 [cited 2020 Aug 22];6(8):524-31. Available from: http://www.nature.com/articles/nnano.2011.101

[94] Qiu L, Wimmers F, Weiden J, Heus HA, Tel J, Figdor CG. A membrane-anchored aptamer sensor for probing IFNγ secretion by single cells. Chem Commun [Internet]. 2017 Jul 13 [cited 2020 Aug 22];53(57):8066-9. Available from: http://xlink.rsc.org/?DOI=C7CC03576D

[95] Zhang J, Jin R, Jiang D, Chen H-Y. Electrochemiluminescence-Based Capacitance Microscopy for Label-Free Imaging of Antigens on the Cellular Plasma Membrane. J Am Chem Soc

[Internet]. 2019 Jul 3 [cited 2020 Aug 22];141(26):10294-9. Available from: https://pubs.acs.org/doi/10.1021/jacs.9b03007

[96] Liu G, Bursill C, Cartland SP, Anwer AG, Parker LM, Zhang K, et al. A Nanoparticle-Based Affinity Sensor that Identifies and Selects Highly Cytokine-Secreting Cells. iScience [Internet]. 2019 Oct 25 [cited 2020 Aug 22];20:137-47. Available from: https://www.sciencedirect.com/science/article/pii/S2589004219303578?via%3Dihub

[97] Hernandez-Fuentes MP, Warrens AN, Lechler RI. Immunologic monitoring. Immunol Rev [Internet]. 2003 Dec 1 [cited 2020 Aug 22];196(1):247-64. Available from: http://doi.wiley.com/10.1046/j.1600-065X.2003.00092.x

[98] Rotem A, Ram O, Shoresh N, Sperling RA, Goren A, Weitz DA, et al. Single-cell ChIP-seq reveals cell subpopulations defined by chromatin state. Nat Biotechnol [Internet]. 2015 Nov 12 [cited 2020 Aug 22];33(11):1165-72. Available from: http://www.nature.com/articles/nbt.3383

[99] Chokkalingam V, Tel J, Wimmers F, Liu X, Semenov S, Thiele J, et al. Probing cellular heterogeneity in cytokine-secreting immune cells using droplet-based microfluidics. Lab Chip [Internet]. 2013 Nov 12 [cited 2020 Aug 22];13(24):4740. Available from: http://xlink.rsc.org/?DOI=c3lc50945a

[100] Wei S-C, Hsu MN, Chen C-H. Plasmonic droplet screen for single-cell secretion analysis. Biosens Bioelectron [Internet]. 2019 Nov 1 [cited 2020 Aug 22];144:111639. Available from: https://www.sciencedirect.com/science/article/pii/S0956566319307183

[101] Stephens DC, Osunsanmi N, Sochacki KA, Powell TW, Taraska JW, Harris DA. Spatiotemporal organization and protein dynamics involved in regulated exocytosis of MMP-9 in breast cancer cells. J Gen Physiol [Internet]. 2019 Dec 2 [cited 2020 Aug 22];151(12):1386-403. Available from: https://rupress.org/jgp/article/151/12/1386/132562/Spatiotemporal-organization-and-protein-dynamics

[102] Chen Z, Lu Y, Zhang K, Xiao Y, Lu J, Fan R. Multiplexed, Sequential Secretion Analysis of the Same Single Cells Reveals Distinct Effector Response Dynamics Dependent on the Initial Basal State. Adv Sci [Internet]. 2019 May 13 [cited 2020 Aug 22];6(9):1801361. Available from: https://onlinelibrary.wiley.com/doi/abs/10.1002/advs.201801361

Chapter 10

Novel Biosensing Strategies for the *in Vivo* Detection of microRNA

Junling Zhang, Shanshan Zhao and Jikui Wu

Abstract

As a regulatory molecule of post-transcriptional gene expression, microRNA (miRNA) is a class of endogenous, non-coding small molecule RNAs. MiRNA detection is essential for biochemical research and clinical diagnostics but challenging due to its low abundance, small size, and sequence similarities. In this chapter, traditional methods of detecting miRNA like polymerase chain reaction (PCR), DNA microarray, and northern blotting are introduced briefly. These approaches are usually used to detect miRNA *in vitro*. Some novel strategies for sensing miRNAs *in vivo*, including hybridization probe assays, strand-displacement reaction (SDR), entropy-driven DNA catalysis (EDC), catalytic hairpin assembly (CHA), hybridization chain reaction (HCR), DNAzyme-mediated assays, and CRISPR-mediated assays are elaborated in detail. This chapter describes the principles and designs of these detection technologies and discusses their advantages as well as their shortcomings, providing guidelines for the further development of more sensitive and selective miRNA sensing strategies *in vivo*.

Keywords: microRNA, hybridization probe assays, strand-displacement reaction (SDR), entropy-driven DNA catalysis (EDC), catalytic hairpin assembly (CHA), hybridization chain reaction (HCR), CRISPR

1. Introduction

MicroRNA (miRNA) is a kind of endogenous non-coding RNA with a length of 18–25 nucleic acid sequences. It is usually integrated into the RNA-induced silencing complex (RISC) to execute its biological function of degrading mRNA or inhibiting transcription. MicroRNA is highly conservative and has strict temporal and spatial specificity. It plays a key regulatory role in the development of animals and plants, cell proliferation, differentiation and apoptosis, immunity and metabolism, angiogenesis, tumor invasion, and metastasis. Mature miRNA has the disadvantages of small fragment, no poly (A), high similarity among family members, and low expression level. As a result, it is difficult to sensitively and accurately detect miRNA. Therefore, it is very important to establish fast and simple methods with high sensitivity and specificity for miRNA detection [1].

Many miRNA analysis methods, including polymerase chain reaction (PCR), DNA Microarray, and Northern blotting have been developed. Although these traditional strategies are the gold standard methods for miRNA identification, detection, and analysis *in vitro*, it is very difficult for them to achieve accurate and sensitive spatio-temporal information of miRNA in living organisms. Therefore, in this chapter, we summarize the novel strategies for biosensing miRNAs *in vivo* including hybridization probe assays, strand-displacement reaction (SDR), entropy-driven DNA catalysis (EDC), catalytic hairpin assembly (CHA), hybridization chain reaction (HCR), DNAzyme-mediated assays and CRISPR-mediated assays. These contents involve their principles and methods, including their advantages and shortcomings, in order to provide important help for the further study of related detection technology.

2. Overview of traditional miRNA detection methods

2.1 Northern blotting

Northern blotting, invented by Alwine in 1979, is the first established method to identify and detect miRNA. It is widely used to detect the expression of miRNAs of various sizes from long primitive miRNAs to mature miRNAs. In the process, the miRNA was separated by polyacrylamide gel electrophoresis in total RNA, then transferred to the imprinted membrane, hybridized with the radionuclide labeled probe. The RNA molecule of interest is detected by the signal of labeled probe. This method can detect both the quantity and the length of miRNA, but it has some defects such as cumbersome operation, low sensitivity, time-consuming, and large sample consumption, which limits its application in clinical diagnosis.

To improve the detection sensitivity, Válóczi *et al.* [2] employed locked nucleic acid (LNA) probe instead of traditional oligonucleotide probe to enhance the affinity and stability of the nucleotide double strand. Pall *et al.* [3] utilized 1-(3-Dimethylaminopropyl)-3-ethylcarbodiimide hydrochloride crosslinking method instead of the traditional UV crosslinking method to improve the binding efficiency of miRNA and nylon membrane. The method of biotin labeling instead of isotope labeling was used to conduct chemiluminescence detection and reduce radioactive pollution [4].

2.2 Microarray

The microarray, developed in the early 1990s, enables the high-throughput miRNA detection in a parallel fashion. In this method, the target miRNA is incubated and hybridized with multiple probes (complementary to the target miRNA sequence) on a chip. After removing the non-hybridized part, the signal can be detected and analyzed by fluorescence scanning or northern blotting [5]. DNA probe-based microarray usually consumes a large amount of samples, and has disadvantages such as low sensitivity and specificity and false positives caused by cross-reactions. However, LNA probe can reduce the consumption of starting materials and improve the sensitivity and accuracy of microarray [6]. Furthermore, liquid suspension microsphere hybridization can effectively avoid cross-reaction in the solid chip to decrease the occurrence of false positives.

2.3 qRT-PCR

Quantitative real-time polymerase chain reaction (qRT-PCR) is one of the main methods to detect low abundance miRNA with high sensitivity and accuracy [7]. The principle of this method is to reversely transcribe miRNA into the corresponding cDNA that is used as a template to initiate real-time PCR, and then indirectly analyze miRNA by detecting the signal of amplified products [8].

Because the miRNA sequence is short (18 ~ 25 nt) and similar to the length of PCR primers, researchers overcome this shortcoming by introducing stem-ring primers for reverse transcription [9] or adding poly (A) into RNA to initiate reverse transcription and dyeing with SYBR Green. Besides, pri-miRNA and pre-miRNA can be introduced into qRT-PCR, causing inaccurate quantification [10]. qRT-PCR usually requires complex primer design and precise reaction temperature control, thereby greatly increasing the cost and complexity of the experiment.

Although the traditional miRNA detection methods are widely used in miRNA detection, there are still some shortcomings such as complex operation, low sensitivity, poor specificity, and large sample consumption. These shortcomings greatly limited the application of these methods in clinical diagnosis and treatment. Importantly, these approaches are only applied to the *in vitro* measurement of miRNA.

3. Emerging sensing techniques in microRNA detection *in Vivo*

3.1 Hybridization probe assay

Hybridization probe assay is a simple and direct detection method without amplification of target miRNA. The principle of this method is as follows: firstly, miRNA is fixed in the tissue or cell. Secondly, signal-labeled nucleic acid probes are added and hybridized with the miRNA based on the principle of complementary pairing. Finally, the position of target miRNA to be detected in the tissue or cell is displayed by certain detection means.

With the principle of hybridization, Wang *et al.* [11] combined the excellent fluorescence-quenching ability of Ti_3C_2 nanosheets with a double-labeled DNA fluorescent probes to design a chimeric DNA-functionalized Ti_3C_2 nanoprobe. When this probe crosses the cell membrane, TAMRA-labeled plasma membrane glycoprotein MUC1 aptamer interacted with MUC1 and peeled off from Ti_3C_2, lighting up red fluorescence. In the cytoplasm, FAM-tagged hairpin DNA hybridized with miR-21, leading to green fluorescence recovery. This strategy can perform *in vitro* measurement of miR-21 and MUC1 with nanomolar sensitivity and *in situ* simultaneous imaging of dual biomarkers in living cells. Although Ti_3C_2 greatly reduces the fluorescence background, the sensitivity of the probe is still limited because one target miRNA only restore the fluorescence of one fluorescent molecule.

To further improve the detection and imaging sensitivity, fluorescence double-labeling and double-quenching strategy is undoubtedly a good design. Molecular beacon (MB) is hairpin-structure DNA probe. Its two ends are labeled with two identical fluorescent molecules. When MB is in a close state, self-quenching effect between two fluorescent molecules occurs. Graphene oxide (GO) is a good fluorescence quencher. The electrostatic interaction between DNA probe and GO also quenches effectively the fluorescence of DNA probe. Based on the aforementioned properties of MB and GO, Yang *et al.* [12] designed a MB-GO fluorescent sensor for sensitive imaging of intracellular miRNA (**Figure 1**). Two Cy5 fluorophores were tagged at the both ends of MB. MB was electrostatically adsorbed on the surface of GO through the π-π stacking effect. Two Cy5 fluorophores was quenched through their self-quenching effect and cy5-GO resonance energy transfer, which greatly reduced the fluorescence background of sensing system. Once target miRNA hybridize with MB probes, hairpin-structure MBs were unfolded to separate two Cy5 molecules and the MB-miRNA complex with rigid structure was released from the surface of GO, recovering fluorescence signal and significantly enhancing the detection sensitivity (Limit of detection, LOD = 30 pM). This method also visualized miRNA-21 in cancer cells and three xenograft tumor models.

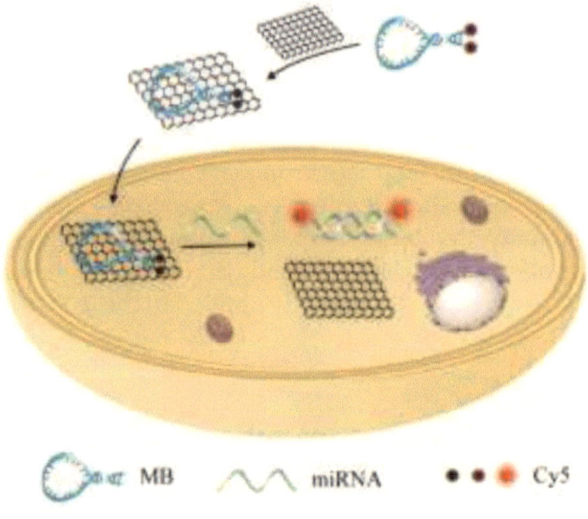

Figure 1.
Illustration of 2Cy5-MB-GO complex sensing miRNA in living cells. Reprinted with permission from ref 12. Copyright 2018 American Chemical Society.

Another approach to enhance the sensitivity of hybridization probe assay is to use the plasmon coupling effect of assembled nanostructures, especially, dissymmetric nanostructures. Xu *et al.* [13] developed a plasmonic nanorod probe by miR-21-directed *in situ* self-assembly of DNA-modified Gold nanorods (AuNR) in living cells. The formation of NR@PS-PAA dimers gives rise to intense chiroplasmonic signal and surface-enhanced Raman scattering (SERS). The LOD were 0.081 fmol/10μg·RNA (CD signal) and 1.12 fmol/10μg·RNA (SERS signal), respectively. Highly sensitive quantitative analysis and *in situ* imaging of microRNA in cells are achieved.

Although the introduction of nanomaterials (gold nanoparticles, graphene oxide, upconversion nanoparticles, MnO_2 nanosheets, quantum dots, silver nanoparticles, noble metal nanoclusters, and silica nanoparticles) remarkably enhanced the sensitivity of hybridization probe assay, the lack of signal amplification limits its practical application in the sensitive detection of intracellular miRNA.

3.2 Strand displacement reaction (SDR)

Strand displacement reaction (SDR) is a dynamic process of hybridization-driven DNA strand exchange accompanied by branch migration [14]. In this process, a single-stranded reactant (input, target miRNA) reacts with multi-stranded DNA complex and releases another single-stranded product (output signal) and a new DNA complex. This process operates autonomously through a series of reversible DNA hybridization and dissociation steps to produce numerous output strands, thereby generating cascaded signal amplification [15, 16].

Using SDR, Wang *et al.* [17] constructed a double-stranded fuel catalyzed DNA molecular machine. The machine was divided into two parts: the first part was composed of the Cy5-labeled signal strand and BHQ-2 labeled complementary quenching strand. The second part was double-strand fuel (DSF), consisting of fuel strand and protected fuel. The target miRNA bound to the quenched strand and triggered the first SDR to obtain the miRNA-quenching double-strand, releasing the signal strand to recover the fluorescence. At this time, DSF initiated the second SDR, the dominated fuel hybridized with quencher strand, replacing miRNA to produce double-stranded waste and intermediated miRNA protected fuel. The new signal strand can combine with the protected fuel to release miRNA again and repeated the above-mentioned cycle reaction. Thus, the target miRNA was continuously released from intermediate 2 and circularly participated in the subsequent reaction to achieve signal amplification. This method has high sensitivity, strong signal amplification ability, and relatively low background signal.

Ma *et al.* [18] similarly developed an artificial intelligence signal amplification system (AISA). The system also consists of a fluorescence-quenching double-strand and fuel-protection double strand. It underwent three-steps reaction: miRNA replaced signal strand and combined with quenching strand, fuel strand replaced miRNA and combined with quenching strand, and new signal strand replaced miRNA to achieve the reuse of it (the last two steps of reaction could be recycled to produce amplified signal). Based on this principle, they built two AISA systems to detect Hsa-miR-100 and Hsa-miR-484, respectively. Their versatility and feasibility were proved to be actively used in disease diagnosis and treatment, evaluation, stem cell tracking, and other fields, but the design of the probe was cumbersome.

In recent years, the combination of SDR and nanomaterials for miRNA detection has become a hot spot. Li *et al.* [19] constructed dsDNA-AuNPs nanoprobes by means of using toehold strand displacement reaction (TSDR) to attain the amplification detection of trace let-7a in living cells (**Figure 2**). The molecular catalytic machine contained dsDNA-AuNPs nanoprobes and DNA fuel strands, while the dsDNA contained an unfolded hairpin sequence labeled with FAM and TAMRA at both ends. Binding to the linker strand of the dsDNA, the target miRNA replaced the hairpin to restore its folded structure. Forster resonance energy transfer (FRET) signal occurred between the fluorescent groups. At the same time, the target miRNA was recycled by cascaded strand displacement reactions realizing the amplification and detection signal of the target miRNA. Zhang *et al.* [20] developed a kind of dendritic mesoporous silica nanoparticles encapsulated by tumor cell

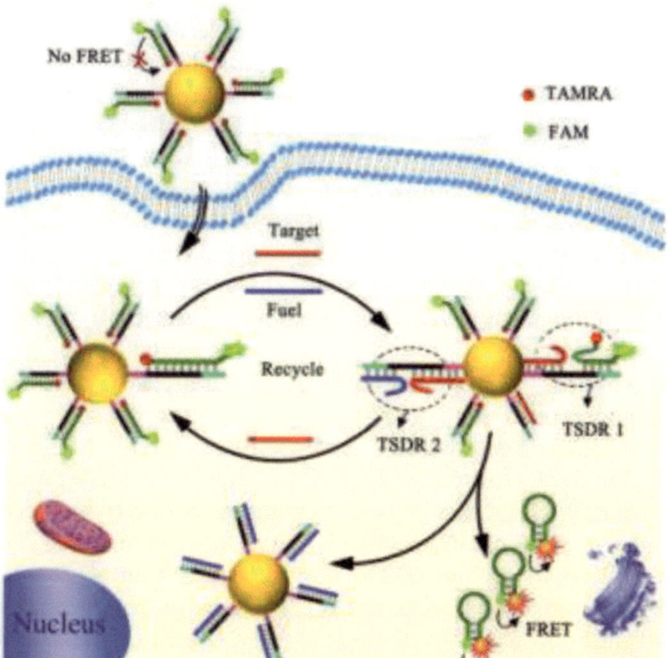

Figure 2.
Mechanism of in vivo imaging microRNA of the DNA-fueled and catalytic molecular machine. Reprinted with permission from ref 19. Copyright 2017 American Chemical Society.

(MCF-7) membrane (DMSN-DP@CM) and simultaneously modified with DNA photoacoustic probe and fuel strand. The target miRNA triggered the release of the near-infrared fluorescence strand from the quenched strand and the fuel strand further replaced the target miRNA. The alternate replacement of target miRNA and DNA fuel strand generated an amplified photoacoustic signal ratio to realize the miRNA detection.

Surface-enhanced Raman spectroscopy (SERS) refers to that when molecules approach the metal surface of nanostructures, the Raman signal of molecules is enhanced. Gold nanoparticles with the core-satellite structure are important SERS substrate structures, which are composed of a single Au (or Ag) inside and multiple Au (or Ag) linked outside. The core-satellite structure is combined with SDR to detect miRNA and produce the SERS signal.

Li *et al.* [21] designed the core-satellite plasma rulers (PRs) for the quantitative determination of miRNA-21 in living cells. Several small gold nanoparticles were assembled on large gold nanoparticles with dsDNA to form a core-satellite. MiRNA-21 initiated a single hybridization event, leading to the destruction of core-satellite structural components. The plasma displacement between the core and the satellite initiated the wavelength changing of scattering intensity. The expression and the amount of miRNA-21 could be detected via statistical analysis of the wavelength signal. This method enabled highly sensitive detection of the intracellular miRNA without side effect.

Gold nanorods have strong and controllable plasma resonance properties, which can be widely used in photothermal therapy and amplification detection of miRNA. Qu *et al.* [22] used the assembly of Ag_2S on the surface of platinum (Pt)-modified gold nanorods (AuNR-Pt) to form a nuclear-satellite structure (AuNR-Pt@Ag2S). The probe can complete the near-infrared imaging of miRNA *in vivo*. Target miRNA bound to the complementary DNA sequence and released the strand modified with Ag_2S, thereby destroying the core-satellite structure and recovering the fluorescence. The LOD was 0.0082 amol ng_{RNA}^{-1}, providing a multifunctional nanoplatform for tumor diagnosis and treatment *in vivo*.

Inspired by Qu's work, Yan *et al.* [23] utilized the electrostatic interaction between polyethylenimine (PEI)-modified gold nanorod and nucleic acid probe to construct a Fuel Improved miRNA Explorer (FIRE) sensing platform. The detection system included a double-strand DNA labeled with BHQ-2, Cy5 fluorescence-quenching group and a fuel strand that realizing the cycling of miRNA for signal amplification. The target miRNA triggered the release of dsDNA to recover fluorescence. In this design, the preparation of FIRE is simple via electrostatic interactions. Moreover, AuNRs enhanced the photoacoustic imaging and real-time monitoring capabilities of FIRE, resulting in sensitive detection of miRNA and effective tumor treatment effect.

In addition to the strand displacement reaction catalyzed by fuel strand, toehold-mediated strand displacement is another commonly used amplification strategy. A novel catalytic self-assembly nanosensor based on quantum dots was constructed [24] to detect miRNA *in vivo*. As an efficient catalyst, miRNA triggered the toehold-mediated strand displacement cascade reaction to produce multiple Cy5/biotin double-labeled dsDNA, which were assembled on a 605QD surface, resulting in significant FRET signal. The nanosensor was simple to operate and has high specificity and sensitivity. Also, the synergistic effect between telomerase and the catalytic strand was helpful to distinguish cancer cells from normal cells, which provided a valuable method for clinical diagnosis.

Enzyme-mediated strand displacement reaction enables the exponential accumulation of DNA products through the continuous polymerization-nicking-displacement cycle process catalyzed by polymerases. Based on the amplification methods, Yang *et al.* [25] proposed a novel strategy by utilizing branched DNA ligation enhanced isothermal strand displacement polymerization (B-ICSDP) for *in vitro* quantitation and intracellular miRNA imaging. This internal Y-shaped DNA structure consisted of a circular DNA scaffold and three repeatable molecular beacons (MB). MiRNA triggered the conformation conversion of MB and recovered the fluorescence. Additionally, polymerase-based cyclic SDR produced a large number of extended Y-type DNA structures (one DNA scaffold could hybridize with three MBs), thus generating amplified signals. This method had the advantages of high sensitivity, high specificity, and simple design. Besides, it could be used to detect single or multiple target miRNAs in living cells.

Peng's team [26] developed a telomerase-catalyzed FRET ratio probe for accurate miRNA detection. AuNPs were modified with capture probe containing recognition sequence and telomerase primer located at the 5′ of capture probe strand. The detection probe (a molecular beacon labeled with donor FAM and acceptor TARMA) hybridized with the capture probe, separating the fluorescent donor and acceptor and causing low FRET signal. Once miRNA specifically recognized and hybridized the capture probe. The detection probe was then replaced by miRNA to form a stem-ring structure. Thus, the FAM and TAMRA were brought in close proximity to produce high FRET signal. In addition, the capture probe was extended with telomerase primers and hybridized with the catalytic strand to displace target miRNA. The released miRNA also triggered the above-mentioned detection system. This method had low background signal and can detect low abundance miRNA molecules in living cells.

3.3 Catalytic hairpin assembly (CHA)

Catalytic hairpin assembly (CHA) is an enzyme-free, hairpin fuel-driven, and automomous nucleic acid amplification technology. A CHA system needs to design two hairpin structures according to the sequence of target miRNA [27]. One segment of the first hairpin is complementary to the target miRNA sequence [28]. Its hairpin structure can be unfolded by miRNA, and then form a complementary structure with another hairpin probe. The target miRNA will be replaced and dissociated, which can further catalyze CHA between other hairpin probes, forming a cycle to generate amplification signal. The catalytic hairpin assembly has been widely used in nucleic acid detection due to its enzyme-free and target-recyclable advantages.

Like SDR, CHA usually employs nanomaterials as a scaffold and carrier to deliver DNA probes into living cells. As shown in **Figure 3**, Liu *et al.* [29] developed a core-satellite nanoprobe (AuNPs-AuNDs CS). Hairpin1 (H1) was immobilized on the Au nanoparticle surface (AuNPs-H1, satellites) and hairpin2 (H2) was assembled on the surface of the plasmonic gold nanodumbbells (AuNDs-H2, core) via Au − S bonds. MiRNA triggered CHA by targeting AuNPs-H1 (AuNPs-H1-miRNA). AuNDs-H2 then hybridized with AuNPs-H1-miRNA to form a core-satellite nanostructure, whereas target miRNA was displaced from AuNPs-H1-miRNA. The released miRNA originated the next assembly of AuNPs-AuNDs CS, generating an amplified signal. This design engineered metallic nanoparticle aggregates to increase electromagnetic hot spots, thereby realizing the highly-sensitive SERS detection of low abundant miRNA.

Wang *et al.* [30] modified the fluorescence-labeled hairpin H1 to the surface of AuNPs. The fluorescence of H1 was quenched by AuNPs. When the probes delivered into cells, the hybridization between H1 and miRNA unfolded H1. The exposed single-strand domain of H1 induced H2 (hairpin fuel) hybridization and displaced miR-21. The released miR-21 participated in the subsequent reaction cycle. The

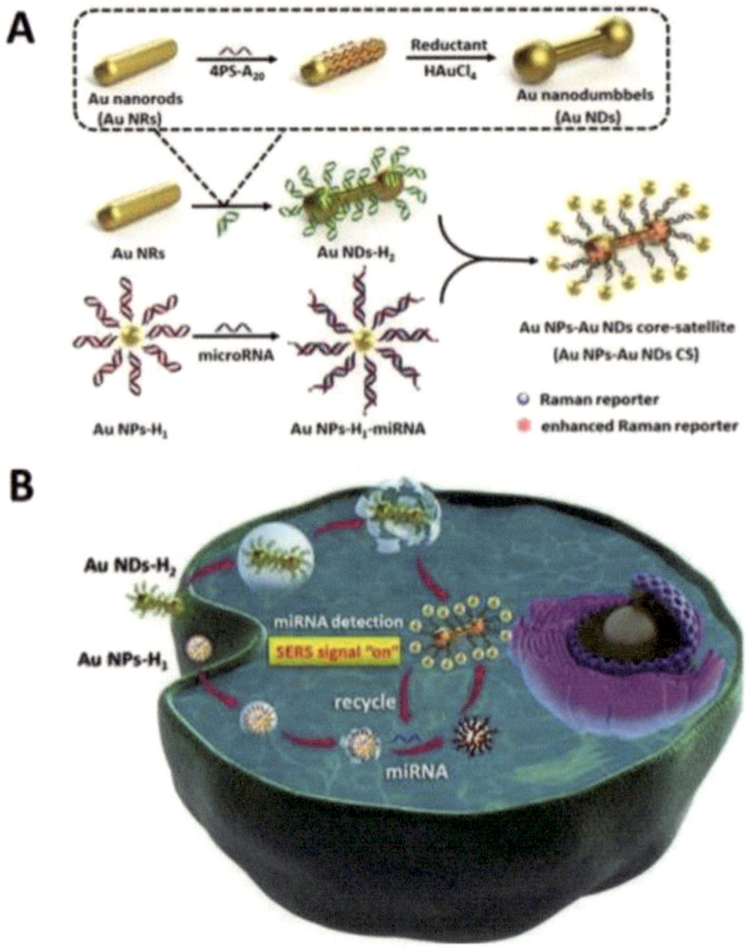

Figure 3.
Schematic representation of (A) the Assembly process of AuNPs-AuNDs-CS and (B) AuNPs-AuNDs-CS sensing miRNA and imaging in living cells. Reprinted with permission from ref 29. Copyright 2018 American Chemical Society.

sensitivity of hairpin-fuelled catalytic nanobeacons is two orders of magnitude lower than that of noncatalytic nanobeacons.

Aruni *et al.* [31] exploited a genetically encoded means to design a RNA-based CHA circuits for imaging miRNA in living cells. In this design, Broccoli, a specific RNA aptamer for DFHBI-1 T, was used as fluorescence reporter. It was split into two non-fluorescent parts (Broc and Coli). Broc was attached to the 5′ end of H1, while Coli was conjugated to the 3′ end of H2. The target miRNA initiated CHA and hybridized with H1. The unfolded H1 then hybridized with H2 to displace target miRNA and form dsDNA. The recombinant Broccoli activated the dye DFHBI-1 T to emit fluorescence, and the target miRNA can be recycled to catalyze the fluorescence of ten to hundreds of broccolis, achieving signal amplification. This strategy provided a new opportunity for the application of gene-encoded RNA circuits in cells.

To improve the kinetics and efficiency of CHA in the complex intracellular environment, inspired by spatial-confinement effects of cells, Liu *et al.* [32] constructed a three-dimensional DNA nanocube to implement the localized hairpin-DNA cascade signal amplification. The hairpin H1 and H2 labeled with Cy3 and Cy5 were modified in the cube, respectively. MiRNA could specifically unfold H1 and then unfold H2. The rapid and efficient imaging of miRNA could be monitored by FRET. This cascade amplifier significantly improved the speed (7 times faster) and efficiency (2.6 times higher) of signal amplification. Furthermore, this probe possesses good cell permeability, good nuclease resistance, and the ability to avoid false-positive signals.

3.4 Hybrid chain reaction (HCR)

The hybridized chain reaction proposed by Dirks and Pierce in 2004 is an isothermal signal amplification technology based on DNA strand displacement reaction [33]. Single strand promoter DNA (target miRNA) binds to the stem-loop nucleic acid probe and causes conformation changing of hairpin DNA. The unfolded hairpin structure can unfold a new DNA hairpin. Two kinds of stem-loop probes were alternately hybridized to form double-stranded DNA containing a large number of repeat units [34]. This method has the advantages of constant temperature, efficient signal amplification, and without the requirement of enzyme. It has been applied to the detection of DNA or RNA.

Wang *et al.* [35] combined CHA with HCR to design a sensing system with six DNA hairpins (**Figure 4**). Target miRNA first catalyzed CHA and formed numerous double-stranded products (H1•H2) containing initiator sequences to initiate downstream HCR circuit. The resultant dsDNA products then triggered subsequently autonomous cross-hybridization reactions to form HCR copolymer (H3•H4•H5•H6). The resultant HCR copolymer carries many donor-acceptor pairs that can generate FRET signal. The synergistic amplification effect of CHA-HCR system significantly increased the selectivity and sensitivity of miRNA detection.

Exploiting the signal amplification function of protein with multiple binding sites, Huang *et al.* [36] used streptavidin (SA) as a protein scaffold and four biotinylated hairpin DNA probes to construct a DNA tetrads probe. When miRNA was

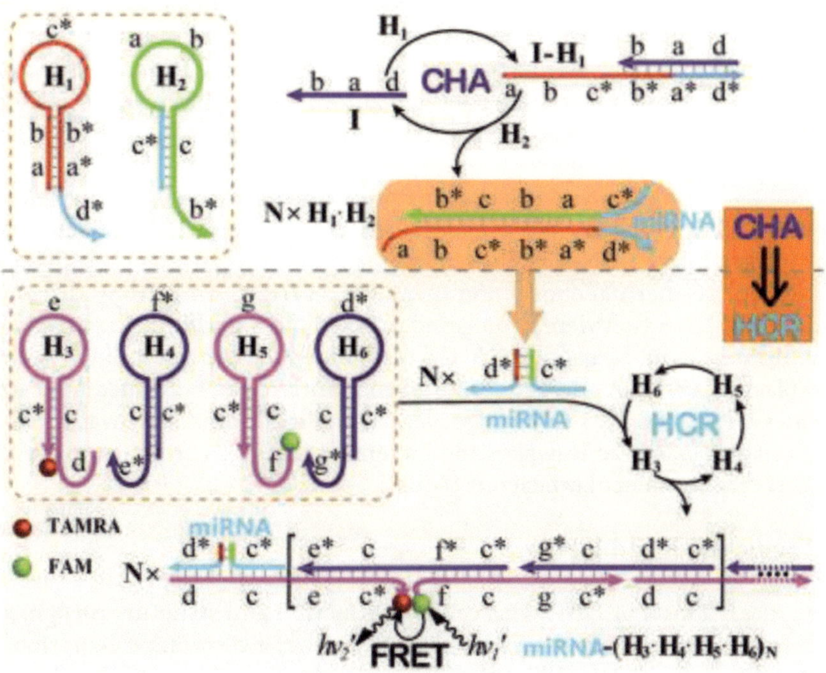

Figure 4.
Schematic of the isothermal CHA–HCR cascaded circuit for miRNAs assay. Adapted with permission from ref 35. Copyright 2018 Royal Society of Chemistry.

present, miRNA unfolded the Cy3-labeled hairpin H1, triggered HCR, and hybridized with Cy5-labeled H2 to form a cross-linked hydrogel network, generating the signal. It is proved that the DNA tetrad was a highly robust delivery agent and could realize the sensitive imaging of miRNA.

To improved the stability of miRNA sensing system, Wu and coworkers [37] designed a DNA probe composed of tripartite Y-shaped DNA structures, folate probe FAP and hairpin probe H1, H2. MiRNA triggered H1 and H2 hairpin probes to assemble HCR, separating Cy5 and BHQ-2 labeled on H1 to recover fluorescence signal. This method was proved to have high sensitivity with a sub-picomolar limit *in vitro*, and the probe had high stability *in vivo*.

3.5 Entropy-driven DNA catalysis (EDC)

Entropy-driven DNA catalysis (EDC) exponentially amplifies DNA signal by target-induced entropy change of pre-design sensing system [38]. EDC is a simple, rapid, and enzyme-free isothermal signal amplification technology based on toehold exchange mechanism and adaptable to different low-abundance targets due to its modular design and tunability.

A EDC system usually is composed of a three-strand substrate complex (output strand and signal strand are complementary with link strand) and a fuel strand [39]. In the absence of targets, the sensing system does not work because the toehold domain in substrate that binds to the fuel strand has been protected. As a catalyst, miRNA can combine with the substrate link strand to replace the signal strand, and then the fuel strand replaced miRNA to be recycled. The production of liberated molecules leads to the increase of entropy, repeating the abovementioned strand displacement reaction to generate amplified signals.

Liang *et al.* [40] constructed an entropy-driven DNA nanomachine. A three-stranded substrate complex (A/B/C) and an affinity ligand (L) were modified on the AuNP surface, respectively. Target miRNA hybridized with L to replace B from C. A fuel strand (F) bound to C and the C-F complex departed from the AuNP surface, restoring the fluorescence of the FAM-labeled C strand. Thus, such entropy-driven catalytic DNA nanomachine operated automatically and progressively to realize signal amplification. The assay had superior sensitivity (LOD = 8 pM) due to the accelerated intramolecular reaction.

To avoiding the addition of external enzyme or fuel transfection, Lu *et al.* [41] developed a NIR-controlled DNA sensing system based on entropy-driven catalysis to detect intracellular miRNA. Hollow copper sulfide nanoparticle (HCuSNPs) served as the photothermal conversion agent and a carrier. An entropy-driven DNA probe and DNA fuel were conjugated to HCuSNPs. Under the irradiation of the near-infrared laser, target miRNA-155 recognized toe1 and combined with the probe, replaced Cy3-DNA and exposed toe2 that initiates toehold-mediated strand displacement reactions. Cy3-DNA was released and its fluorescence was recovered. This method possessed facile design and its sensitivity is two orders of magnitude higher than that of molecular beacons (MBs).

3.6 DNAzyme-mediated assays

DNAzyme is a kind of DNA with catalytic function and structure recognition ability. It was screened by Breaker and Joyce through the systematic evolution of ligands by exponential enrichment (SELEX) technology in 1994. The single strand, simulating the function of enzymes *in vivo*, can catalyze different chemical reactions, including nucleic acid cleavage, nucleic acid ligation, phosphorylation, porphyrin metallization enzyme activity, and peroxidase activity. It has high catalytic efficiency, simple modification of fluorescent dyes, and strong chemical stability. Also, compared with the traditional protease, DNAzyme can be denaturated repeatedly and renatured without loss of enzyme activity. DNAzyme catalytic amplification technology is a constant temperature amplification technology, which is especially suitable for high sensitivity detection of intracellular targets.

Wu *et al.* [42] constructed a signal-enhanced split DNAzyme probe loaded on gold nanoparticles for miRNA detection in living cells. They split Mg^{2+}-dependent DNAzyme into two nucleic acid strands, which were hybridized with the substrate to form a complex. The fluorescence of the complex was quenched without target miRNA. In the presence of miRNA, two split strands hybridized with target miRNA to form a secondary structure with catalytic activity, cleaving the substrate to separate fluorescence reporter and quenching groups and restoring fluorescence. The released miRNA targeted the next DNAzyme probe and switched on recognition-cleavage-release cycles to produce signal amplification. In this experiment, split DNAzyme serves as both recognition element and signal reporter. As a carrier, gold nanoparticles increase the biological affinity of nanoprobe and avoid the degradation of the nucleic acid probe in the process of transport into cells. This method improved the detection sensitivity and specificity. Additionally, it had low cytotoxicity, high enzymatic degradation resistance which is effective for detection in living cells.

Yang *et al.* [43] integrated DNAzyme, its substrate, and recognition strand into a FAM-labeled hairpin-locked-DNAzyme probe. The probe was immobilized on surface of gold nanoparticles. The catalytic activity of DNAzyme was inhibited and the fluorescence of FAM was quenched by gold nanoparticles. When target miRNA hybridized with the hairpin probe, the change of the probe structure activated the DNAzyme to cleave the substrate strand and made the FAM-labeled substrate strand emit fluorescence. After the miRNA was released, it entered the next cycle and generated amplification signals. This design significantly reduced fluorescent background signal. The detection limit of the target miRNA was 25 pM. It can be applied to the *in vivo* detection of different types of miRNA.

Although AuNP-DNA probes are highly sensitive and selective, they suffer from the aggregation of AuNPs in the complex intracellular environment. To overcome this limitation, there is highly desirable for homogeneous DNA (composed entirely of DNAs) sensing system. Xue *et al.* [44] utilized a Y-shaped backbone-rigidified triangular DNA scaffold (YTDS) to develop a self-powered DNAzyme walker (**Figure 5**). This sensing platform consists of YTDS (carrier), nuclide aptamer (transportation), and a locked M-DNAzyme-substrate complex (recognition and signal reporter). The binding of miRNA trigger DNAzyme walker to perform self-powered stepwise walking and amplify the signal at the same time. The detection platform has the advantages of efficient delivery without any transfection agent and amplification of output signal without any protein enzyme.

To effectively protect the probe from degradation by nuclease and greatly improve its cell permeability, Li *et al.* [45] constructed a DNAzyme probe based on the tetrahedral nanostructure. FAM and Dabcyl were labeled the linker strand and partial complementary strand, respectively. Catalytic activity of DNAzyme was effectively silenced by the locking strand in the absence of target miRNA. The target miRNA hybridized with the locking strand to release DNAzyme. With the assist of Na^{+} cofactor, the substrate strand was cleaved and the fluorescence was recovered. Activated DNAzyme could compete with inactive DNAzyme for the next locking strand, starting the next hybridization, and generating amplified signals circularly. The LOD of the DNAzyme probe is 16 pM. It possessed high specificity and distinguished target miRNA from its family members.

The catalytic activity of DNAzyme depends on the concentration of its cofactor Mg^{2+}. However, the content of Mg^{2+} in the cell is too low to support the long-time

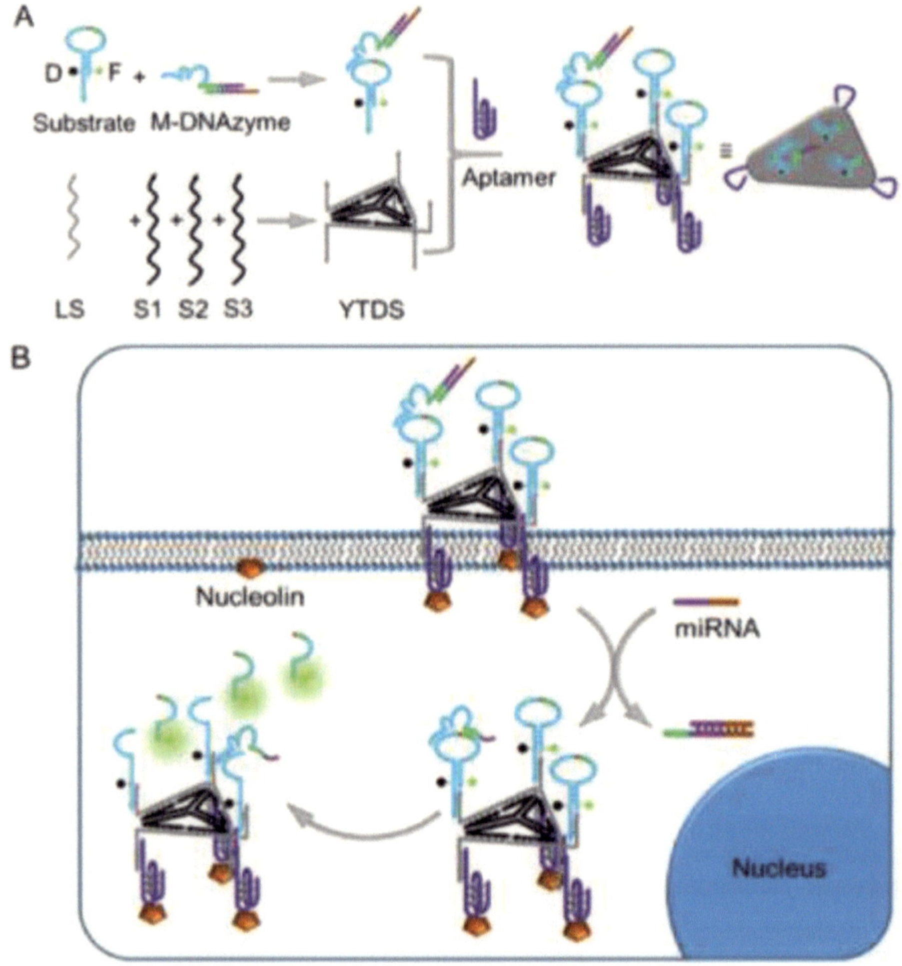

Figure 5.
(A) The preparation routes of Ap-YTDS-DzW. (B) Ap-YTDS-DzW imaging of miRNAs in vivo. Reprinted with permission from ref 44. Copyright 2019 American Chemical Society.

catalytic reactions used for the signal amplification. To circumvent this limitation, Wei *et al.* [46] constructed a smart autocatalytic DNAzyme imaging machinery to execute magnetic resonance imaging (MRI) of miRNA *in vivo*. The imaging system composed of honeycomb-like MnO_2 nanosponge (hMNS), HCR, and autocatalytic DNAzyme. In this system, hMNS act as three roles, that is, nanocarrier, DNAzyme cofactors, and MRI agents. The multifunctional hMNS effectively delivered the system into the cells and was degraded into Mn^{2+} by intracellular glutathione (GSH) as a DNAzyme cofactor. MiR-21 activates HCR amplification to produce DNAzyme nanowires, mediating the automatic catalytic accumulation of the new trigger and the retroaction to the original HCR sensor. This robust assay can accurately locate miRNAs *in vivo* and enhance the amplification signal.

3.7 CRISPR-mediated assays

CRISPR/Cas9 system is a new gene-editing technology based on the bacterial adaptive immune defense system. It can insert or delete genes accurately to knock out target genes [47]. CRISPR/Cas9 system consists of CRISPR RNA, transactivating crRNA, and endonuclease Cas9. Cas9 is specific to the protospacer adjacent motif with the guidance of crRNA and tracrRNA to form RNA–DNA complex. Cas9 can cut double-stranded DNA to complete gene editing.

For the convenience of operation, scientists fused the mature tracrRNA-crRNA dual structure into a sgRNA, its 5′ strand sequence is complementary to the target miRNA, and the 3′ stranded structure could bind to Cas9. Therefore, only one sgRNA needs to be designed to edit the related genes. This method has some advantages such as simple operation, high efficiency, low cost, and no introduction of foreign genes. So far, it has become the most popular gene-editing technology. Similarly, this method has been applied to the detection of miRNA.

Wang *et al.* [48] constructed a CRISPR–Cas9 sensing platform based on a miRNA-mediated sgRNA releasing strategy. The sensing approach successfully realized miRNA imaging and cell-specific regulation of the CRISPR gene editing system. The sensing system was divided into two parts. One part was composed of Cas9 or Cas9 mutant fusion protein to edit or inhibit gene expression, the other was sgRNA with miRNA binding site without activity, mediating the binding of Cas9 protein in a specific position of the genome. As a result, only specific miRNA could finish cleavage reaction, producing mature sgRNA, and starting CRISPR system. The system could sense two kinds of miRNAs in the same cell and turn on red or green fluorescence respectively. It was proved that the detection platform could accomplish precise regulation of different gene sites by multiple miRNAs, and provided new ideas for other gene therapy technologies.

4. Conclusions

An ideal method for detecting intracellular miRNA should possess high throughput, high specificity, high detection sensitivity, wide detection range, and low detection cost. To achieve this goal, a variety of miRNA detection methods have been developed, but there are many shortcomings, and the technology needs to be improved. The additionally introduced nanomaterials is self-aggregated and enriched in different tissues in a complex living environment. Hybridization probe assay lacks signal amplification capabilities. SDA, HCR, and CHA need to avoid high background signal caused by probe leakage. DNAzyme-mediated assays usually require exogenous cofactors to initiate signal amplification. Therefore, EDC and CRISPR-mediated assays are the most promising detection methods of miRNA *in vivo* in the future. The establishment of an ideal miRNA detection technology still needs the efforts of scientists and the continuous progress of related science and technology.

Acknowledgements

The authors gratefully acknowledge the National Natural Science Foundation of China (No. 31972772) and the Laboratory for Marine Fisheries Science and Food Production Processes, Qingdao National Laboratory for Marine Science and Technology, China (ZZ-A11).

Conflict of interest

There are no conflicts to declare.

Author details

Junling Zhang[1,2], Shanshan Zhao[1,2] and Jikui Wu[3,4*]

1 Key Laboratory of Exploration and Utilization of Aquatic Genetic Resources, Ministry of Education, Shanghai Ocean University, Shanghai, China

2 Shanghai Collaborative Innovation for Aquatic Animal Genetics and Breeding, Shanghai Ocean University, Shanghai, China

3 Laboratory of Quality and Safety Risk Assessment for Aquatic Products on Storage and Preservation (Shanghai), Ministry of Agriculture, Shanghai Ocean University, Shanghai, China

4 National R&D Branch Center for Freshwater Aquatic Products Processing Technology (Shanghai), Shanghai Ocean University, Shanghai, China

*Address all correspondence to: jkwu@shou.edu.cn

References

[1] Cissell K A, Shrestha S, Deo S K. MicroRNA detection: challenges for the analytical chemist. Analytical Chemistry.2007;79:4754-4761. DOI: 10.1021/ac0719305

[2] Válóczi A, Hornyik C, Varga N, Burgyán J, Kauppinen S, Havelda Z. Sensitive and specific detection of microRNAs by northern blot analysis using LNA-modified oligonucleotide probes. Nucleic Acids Research. 2004;32:e175. DOI: 10.1093/nar/gnh171

[3] Pall G S, Codony-Servat C, Byrne J, Ritchie L, Hamliton A. Carbodiimide-mediated cross-linking of RNA to nylon membranes improves the detection of siRNA, miRNA and piRNA by northern blot. Nucleic Acids Research. 2007;35:e60. DOI: 10.1093/nar/gkm112

[4] Sugatani T, Hruska K A. Impaired microRNA pathways diminish osteoclast differentiation and function. Journal of Biological Chemistry. 2009;284:4667-4678. DOI: 10.1074/jbc.m805777200

[5] Thomson J M, Parker J, Perou C M, Hammond S M. A custom microarray platform for analysis of microRNA gene expression. Nature Methods. 2004;1:47-53. DOI: 10.1038/nmeth704

[6] Castoldi M, Schmidt S, Benes V, Noerholm M, Kulozik A E, Hentze M W, Muckenthaler M U. A sensitive array for microRNA expression profiling (miChip) based on locked nucleic acids (LNA). RNA. 2006;12:913-920. DOI: 10.1261/rna.2332406

[7] Schmittgen T D, Lee E J, Jiang J, Sarkar A, Yang L Q, Elton T S, Chen C F. Real-time PCR quantification of precursor and mature microRNA. Methods. 2008;44:31-38. DOI: 10.1016/j.ymeth.2007.09.006

[8] Kroh E M, Parkin R K, Mitchell P S, Tewari M. Analysis of circulating microRNA biomarkers in plasma and serum using quantitative reverse transcription-PCR (qRT-PCR). Methods. 2010;50:298-301. DOI: 10.1016/j.ymeth.2010.01.032

[9] Raymond C K, Roberts B S, Garrett-Engele P, Lim L P, Johnson J M. Simple, quantitative primer-extension PCR assay for direct monitoring of microRNAs and short-interfering RNAs. RNA. 2005; 11:1737-1744.DOI: 10.1261/rna.2148705

[10] Pieter M, Pieter V V, An D W, Daniel M, Frank W, Frank P, Jo V. A novel and universal method for microRNA RT-qPCR data normalization. Genome Biology. 2009;10:R64.1-10. DOI: 10.1186/gb-2009-10-6-r64

[11] Wang S, Wei S H, Wang SG, Zhu X H, Lei C Y, Huang Y, Nie Z, Yao S Z. A chimeric DNA-functionalized titanium carbide MXenes for simultaneous mapping of dual cancer biomarkers in living cells. Analytical Chemistry. 2019;91:1651-1658. DOI: 10.1021/acs.analchem.8b05343

[12] Yang L M, Liu B, Wang M M, Li J, Pan W, Gao X N, Li N, Tang B. A highly sensitive strategy for fluorescence imaging of microRNA in living cells and in vivo based on graphene oxide-enhanced signal molecules quenching of molecular beacon. ACS Applied Materials & Interfaces. 2018;10:6982-6990. DOI: 10.1021/acsami.7b19284

[13] Xu L, Gao Y, Hua K. Xu LG, Gao Y F, Kuang H, Luis M L, Xu C L.MiRNA-directed intracellular self-assembly of chiral nanorod dimers. Angewandte Chemie International Edition. 2018;57:10544-10548. DOI: 10.1002/anie.201805640

[14] Qian L L, Winfree E, Bruck J. Neural network computation with DNA

strand displacement cascades. Nature. 2011;475:368-372. DOI: 10.1038/nature10262

[15] Simmel F C, Yurke B, Singh H R. Principles and applications of nucleic acid strand displacement reactions. Chemical Reviews. 2019;119:6326-6369. DOI: 10.1021/acs.chemrev.8b00580

[16] Zhang D Y, Seelig G. Dynamic DNA nanotechnology using strand-displacement reactions. Nature Chemistry. 2011;3:103-113. DOI: 10.1038/nchem.957

[17] Wang X J, Yan N, Song T J, Wang B, Wei B, Lin L, Chen X S, Tian H Y, Liang H J. Robust fuel catalyzed DNA molecular machine for *in vivo* microRNA detection. Advanced Biosystems. 2017;1:1700060. DOI: 10.1002/adbi.201700060

[18] Ma X B, Chen L, Yang Y C, Zhang W Q, Wang P X, Zhang K, Zheng B, Zhu L, Sun Z, Zhang S, Guo Y K, Liang M M, Wang H Y, Tian J. An artificial intelligent signal amplification system for *in vivo* detection of miRNA. Frontiers in Bioengineering and Biotechnology. 2019;7:330. DOI: 10.3389/fbioe.2019.00330

[19] Li D X, Zhou W J, Yuan R, Xiang Y. A DNA-fueled and catalytic molecule machine lights up trace under-expressed microRNAs in living cells. Analytical Chemistry. 2017;89:9934-9940. DOI: 10.1021/acs.analchem.7b02247

[20] Zhang K, Meng X D, Yang Z, Cheng Y R, Wang D D, Lu H T, Shi Z J, Dong H F, Zhang X J. Cancer cell membrane camouflaged nanoprobe for catalytic ratio metric photoacoustic imaging of microRNA in living mice. Advanced Materials. 2019;31:1807888. DOI: 10.1002/adma.201807888

[21] Li M X, Zhao W, Wang H, Li X L, Xu C H, Chen H Y, Xu J J. Dynamic single molecular rulers: toward quantitative detection of microRNA-21 in living cells. Analytical chemistry. 2018;90:14255-14259. DOI: 10.1021/acs.analchem.8b03322

[22] Qu A H, Xu L G, Sun M Z, Liu L Q, Kuang H, Xu C L. Photoactive hybrid AuNR-Pt@Ag2S core-satellite nanostructures for near-infrared quantitive cell imaging. Advanced Functional Materials. 2017;27:1703408. DOI: 10.1002/adfm.201703408

[23] Yan N, Wang X J, Lin L, Song T J, Sun P J, Tian H Y, Liang H J, Chen X S. Gold nanorods electrostatically binding nucleic acid probe for *in vivo* microRNA amplified detection and photoacoustic imaging-guided photothermal therapy. Advanced Functional Materials. 2018;28:1800490. DOI: 10.1002/adfm.201800490

[24] Ma F, Zhang Q, Zhang C Y. Catalytic self-assembly of quantum-dot-based microRNA nanosensor directed by toehold-mediated strand displacement cascade. Nano Letters. 2019;19:6370-6376. DOI: 10.1021/acs.nanolett.9b02544

[25] Yang Z, Zhang S B, Zhao H, Niu H M, Wu Z S, Zhang H T. Branched DNA junction-enhanced isothermal circular strand displacement polymerization for intracellular imaging of microRNAs. Analytical chemistry. 2018;90:13891-13899. DOI: 10.1021/acs.analchem.8b03063

[26] Xian L M, Ge H Y, Xu F, Xu N, Fan J L, Shao K, Peng X J. Intracellular microRNA imaging using telomerase-catalyzed FRET ratioflares with signal amplification. Chemical Science. 2019;10:7111-7118. DOI: 10.1039/c9sc02301a

[27] Zhuang J Y, Lai W Q, Chen G N, Tang D P. A rolling circle amplification-based DNA machine for miRNA screening coupling catalytic hairpin assembly with DNAzyme

formation. Chemical Communications. 2014;50:2935-2938. DOI: 10.1039/c3cc49873e

[28] Wei Q M, Huang J, Li J, Wang J L, Yang X H, Liu J B, Wang K M. A DNA nanowire based localized catalytic hairpin assembly reaction for microRNA imaging in live cells. Chemical Science. 2018;9:7802-7808. DOI: 10.1039/c8sc02943a

[29] Liu C H, Chen C, Li S Z, Dong H F, Dai W H, Xu T L, Liu Y, Yang F, Zhang X J. Target-triggered catalytic hairpin assembly-induced core-satellite nanostructures for high-sensitive "Off-to-On" SERS detection of intracellular microRNA. Analytical chemistry. 2018;90:10591-10599. DOI: 10.1021/acs.analchem.8b02819

[30] Wang J L, Huang J, Quan K, Li J, Wu Y, Wei Q M, Yang X H, Wang K M. Hairpin-fuelled catalytic nanobeacons for amplified microRNA imaging in live cells. Chemical Communications. 2018;54:10336-10339. DOI: 10.1039/c8cc06298f

[31] Aruni K M, Yu Q K, Mark A L, Zhao B, Wu R, You M X. Genetically encoded catalytic hairpin assembly for sensitive RNA imaging in live cells. Journal of the American Chemical Society. 2018;140:8739-8745. DOI: 10.1021/jacs.8b03956

[32] Liu L, Rong Q M, Ke G L, Zhang M, Li J, Li Y Q, Liu Y C, Chen M, Zhang X B. Efficient and reliable microRNA imaging in living cells via a FRET-based localized hairpin-DNA cascade amplifier. Analytical chemistry. 2019;91:3675-3680. DOI: 10.1021/acs.analchem.8b05778

[33] Dirks R M, Pierce N A. Triggered amplification by hybridization chain reaction. Proceedings of the National Academy of Sciences of USA. 2004;101:15275-15278. DOI: 10.1073/pnas.0407024101

[34] Kim H, Kang S, Park K S, Park H G. Enzyme-free and label-free miRNA detection based on target-triggered catalytic hairpin assembly and fluorescence enhancement of DNA-silver nanoclusters. Sensors & Actuators B Chemical. 2018; 260:140-145. DOI: 10.1016/j.snb.2017.12.137

[35] Wang H M, Li C X, Liu X Q, Zhou X, Wang F. Construction of an enzyme-free concatenated DNA circuit for signal amplification and intracellular imaging. Chemical Science. 2018;9:5842-5849. DOI: 10.1039/c8sc01981a

[36] Huang D J, Huang Z M, Xiao H Y, Wu Z K, Tang L J, Jiang J H. Protein scaffolded DNA tetrads enable efficient delivery and ultrasensitive imaging of miRNA through crosslinking hybridization chain reaction. Chemical Science. 2018;9:4892-4897. DOI: 10.1039/c8sc01001c

[37] Wu H, Chen T T, Wang X N, Ke Y G, Jiang J H. RNA imaging in living mice enabled by an *in vivo* hybridization chain reaction circuit with a tripartite DNA probe. Chemical Science. 2020;11:62-69. DOI:10.1039/c9sc03469b

[38] Zhang D Y, Turberfield A J, Yurke B, Winfree E. Engineering entropy-driven reactions and networks catalyzed by DNA. Science. 2007;318:1121-1125. DOI: 10.1126/science.1148532

[39] Eckhoff G, Codrea V, Ellington A D, Chen X. Beyond allostery: Catalytic regulation of a deoxyribozyme through an entropy-driven DNA amplifier. Journal of Systems Chemistry. 2010;1: 1-6. DOI: 10.1186/1759-2208-1-13

[40] Liang C P, Ma P Q, Liu H, Guo X G, Yin B C, Ye B C. Rational engineering of dynamic, entropy-driven DNA nanomachine for intracellular microRNA imaging. Angewandte Chemie International Edition.

2017;56:9077-9081. DOI: 10.1002/anie.201704147

[41] Lu H T, Yang F, Liu B H, Zhang K, Cao Y, Dai W B, Li W J, Dong H F. Intracellular low-abundance microRNA imaging by a NIR-assisted entropy-driven DNA system. Nanoscale Horizons. 2019;4:472-479. DOI:10.1039/c8nh00330k

[42] Wu Y, Huang J, Yang X H, Yang Y J, Quan K, Xie N L, Li J, Ma C B, Wang K M. Gold nanoparticle loaded split-DNAzyme probe for amplified miRNA detection in living cells. Analytical Chemistry. 2017;89:8377-8383. DOI:10.1021/acs.analchem.7b01632

[43] Yang Y J, Huang J, Yang X H, He X, Quan K, Xie N L, Ou M, Wang K M. Gold nanoparticle based hairpin-locked-DNAzyme probe for amplified miRNA imaging in living cells. Analytical Chemistry. 2017;89:5850-5856. DOI: 10.1021/acs.analchem.7b00174

[44] Xue C, Zhang S B, Li C, Yu X, Ouyang C H, Lu Y, Wu Z S. Y-shaped backbone-rigidified triangular DNA scaffold-directed stepwise movement of a DNAzyme walker for sensitive microRNA imaging within living cells. Analytical Chemistry. 2019;91:15678-15685. DOI: 10.1021/acs.analchem.9b03784

[45] Li C, Xue C, Wang J, Luo M X, Shen Z F, Wu Z S. Oriented tetrahedron-mediated protection of catalytic DNA molecular-scale detector against *in vivo* degradation for intracellular miRNA detection. Analytical Chemistry. 2019;91:11529-11536. DOI: 10.1021/acs.analchem.9b00860

[46] Wei J, Wang H M, Wu Q, Gong X, Ma K, Liu X Q, Wang F. A smart, autocatalytic, DNAzyme biocircuit for *in vivo*, amplified, microRNA imaging. Angewandte Chemie International Edition. 2020;59:5965-5971. DOI: 10.1002/ange.201911712

[47] Bassett A R, Tibbit C, Ponting C P, Liu J L. Highly efficient targeted mutagenesis of *drosophila* with the CRISPR/Cas9 system. Cell Reports. 2013;4:220-228. DOI:10.1016/j.celrep.2013.06.020

[48] Wang X W, Hu L F, Hao J, Liao L Q, Chiu Y T, Shi M, Wang Y M. A microRNA-inducible CRISPR–Cas9 platform serves as a microRNA sensor and cell-type-specific genome regulation tool. Nature Cell Biology. 2019;21:522-530. DOI: 10.1038/s41556-019-0292-7

Chapter 11

Electrochemical Response of Cells Using Bioactive Plant Isolates

Elvis K. Tiburu, Richard Asiamah, Bernard O. Asimeng, Samuel Kojo Kwofie, Emmanuel Nyankson and William N. Gblerkpor

Abstract

Traditional herbal medical practices continue to be part of the healthcare needs of the world especially residents of sub-Sahara Africa (sSA). However, the mechanism of action of the plant metabolites to elicit their potency continue to be a mystery due to the lack of standardized methods. The mechanism of plant bioactive compounds to cause cell death is gradually being linked to membrane polarization and depolarization behaviour. The current work seeks to probe the electrochemical response of model cells using bioactive compounds captured in bio-zeolites or membrane mimetics. The voltage and current fluctuations emanating from such studies will establish a correlation between cell death and membrane depolarization. It will be a useful biological interface sensing material with the potential to identify plant metabolites that can selectively detect and destroy diseased cells. Several model membranes have already been developed for biomedical applications and this new paradigm will elevate the usefulness of these model systems. The concept was investigated using extracts from *Dioclea reflexa (DR)* hook which belongs to the leguminous family. There are certain class of compounds in *Dioclea reflexa (DR)* that have clinical usefulness in both temperate and tropical regions, however the identity of the bioactive compounds responsible for inducing cell death continue to be a major challenge.

Keywords: model membrane, electrochemical, bioactive, polarization, depolarization, bio-zeolites

1. Introduction

Living organisms use small molecules including membrane targeted drugs to enhance membrane fluidity and permeability to elicit their potency in signal transduction as well as in the treatment of various diseases including cancer, fungal and microbial pathogens. Electrochemical signaling from reactive oxygen species (ROS) is a major mechanism used to regulate different cancer-related processes including cell proliferation, migration, invasion, metastasis and vascularization. The key players in the redox microenvironment of the cancer and neighboring cells are superoxide (O^2), hydrogen peroxide (H_2O_2), nitric oxide (NO) and ions which are produced or regulated by membrane bound nicotinamide adenine dinucleotide phosphate (NADPH), oxidases known as NOX and by the dual oxidases (DUOX), or nitric oxide synthases. For example studies using scanning electrochemical microscopy (SECM) and fluorescence microscopy confirmed the release of ROS from prostate cancer (PC3) cells [1, 2].

Among the ion channels that are membrane bound include voltage-gated Na_+ channels that selectively allow the passage of Na^+ ions into cells resulting in membrane depolarization leading to generation of action potential in excitable cells including neurons, heart and skeletal tissues. It is known that strongly metastatic prostate cancer cell lines such as PC3 cells demonstrate significantly higher expression of voltage-gated Na^+ channels (Nav1.9 alpha subunit). Studies have shown that inhibiting specific voltage-gated Na^+ channels activity have helped to reduce cell proliferation and therefore such channels including K^+, Ca^{2+}, and Cl^- may emerge as novel biomarkers and therapeutic targets for certain cancer treatments. The concept is to develop small molecular probes or nanoparticles that are either delivery vehicles or the nanoparticle itself having the potential to specifically block a particular ion channel to prevent the movement of ions across the membrane which is key critical step for tumor cell survival.

Saccharomyces cerevisiae (SC) cells are single-celled eukaryotes and model organisms for studying cellular mechanisms including DNA damage and repair as well as systematic fungal infections. Additionally, *S. cerevisiae* shares the complex internal cell structure of animals without the high percentage of non-coding DNA that can confound research in higher eukaryotes. Three of the most extensively used antibiotic drugs for studying SC is amphotericin B (Amp B), rifampicin and fluconazole [3, 4]. The antibiotics target different cellular organs to elicit their antimicrobial and antifungal effects. For example, Amp B is membrane mediated thereby increasing the permeability of ions and small molecules by binding more strongly to ergosterol, the principal fungi sterol found in SC [5]. Rifampicin and fluconazole on the other hand have broad antibacterial and antifungal influence with rifampicin targeting different forms of mycobacteria by inhibiting DNA-dependent RNA polymerase activities, whereas fluconazole is used for a number of fungal infections including candidiasis as well as other fungal diseases. Since Amp B and rifampicin are redox mediators that can interact with eukaryotic cell membrane thereby increasing redox activity by creating pores or inhibiting the synthesis of ergosterol respectively, it will be interesting to compare their redox activity with fluconazole. These antifungal drugs were used as model drugs because they have been extensively used for various *in vitro* and *in vivo* studies of model cells.

Based on the background outlined, it is obvious that there are essentially two pathways (lipid-mediated and diffusion porins) through which both hydrophobic and hydrophilic plant metabolites or drugs elicit their potency at the cellular level. It is obvious that the degree of permeation of the cell membrane has a major impact on the redox activity. In addition, the presence of a hydrophobic drug within the complex architecture of the membrane, enhances easy access of small ions through pores which can be detected electrochemically. Non-membrane-mediated drugs diffuse freely through the membrane and may not necessarily destabilize the membrane architecture; thereby limiting ionic flow that can be captured by electrochemical detection techniques. In the current work, an entrapment strategy was developed using aluminosilicate minerals to selectively pool plant metabolites using different pH conditions and evaluating the polarization and depolarization of model cells using electrochemical sensing techniques. For membrane targeted bioactive compounds, the fluctuation in the redox signals will reveal important lead bioactive compounds for further investigation.

Several biopolymers and aluminosilicate minerals derived composite drug delivery carriers have been reported from several laboratories. For example halloysites natural tubules (HNTs) are aluminosilicate minerals composed of different proportions of aluminum, silicon, hydrogen and oxygen often with the chemical formula $Al_2Si_2O_5(OH)_4.nH_2O$ [6, 7]. They are empty cylinders with widths of about 100 nanometers and consist of two structures; the anhydrous structure with an interlayer dispersing of approximately 7 Å and the hydrated structure with an augmented interlayer dividing of 10 Å, due to the presence of water in the lamellar spaces [8–10]. In each layer of the halloysite nanotube, the SiOH groups are found on the outer surface whiles the AlOH groups are situated on the inner surfaces making the outer and inner surfaces to have different charges [11–13]. The positive charge of the internal lumen is a consequence of protonation of the AlOH group at low pH whereas the SiOH groups have overall negative charge due to the coordination of the atoms. When the halloysites nanotubes are modified with biopolymer such as chitosan new functional materials with improved physicochemical properties are generated. The composite materials can serve as effective drug carriers.

The charge disparity of halloysites has also drawn interest from the research community whereby overall negatively charged proteins taken above their isoelectric points are mostly loaded into the positively charged nanotube lumen [14]. Therefore, in a pool of organic compounds, halloysites nanotubes can facilitate the formation of a transient bond between selected bioactive compounds and the AlOH or SiOH as a function of pH conditions and can be very effective as a nano drug carrier for different applications [15–19].

Traditional herbal medical practices continue to be part of the healthcare needs of the world especially residents of sub-Sahara Africa (sSA) [20–23]. However, the mechanism of action of the plant metabolites to illicit their potency continues to be a mystery due to the lack of standardized methods. Electrochemical detection of drugs interacting with most biological systems is an important strategy to understand cellular stresses that causes cell death [24–26]. Evidence emanating from previous findings, indicate that there are several membrane redox centers in most eukaryotic cells that can be targeted to monitor redox activities in the presence of certain drugs including plant metabolites [27–29].

The concept is investigated using extracts from *Dioclea reflexa (DR)* hook which belongs to the leguminous family. There are certain class of compounds in *Dioclea reflexa (DR)* that have clinical usefulness in both temperate and tropical regions [30–33]. Extract of *DR* seed has been shown to boost hematological parameters and antioxidant activities which protect the kidney and blood from oxidative and related injuries under acute and chronic toxicological challenges [30, 31, 33–37]. Also, the aqueous extract of the seeds produces 100% mortality in third stage mosquito larvae of *Aedes aegypti*. The seed is a potential food source which contains around 14% protein, 8% fats and 58% carbohydrates [32]. Though these metabolites continue to show promise in disease treatment, there is very limited data in the literature of the properties of single isolates and their medicinal relevance, albeit due to the difficulties in pursuing systematic separation of the complex mixtures in a single separation method. Thus, the current work describes the use of a simplified method to systematically pool bioactive compound mixtures from *DR* and test their inhibitory effects on breast (MCF-7) cancer cells and *Saccharomyces cerevisiae* (SC) cells. The rationale is that the larger surface area coupled with the differential polarity of the lumen and the surface of the halloysites nanotubes will be sufficient to bind selectively with the plant metabolites in the crude extracts of *DR*. The evidence of the entrapped species on the halloysites nanotubes was monitored using X-ray diffractometry (XRD) and Fourier transform infrared spectroscopy (FTIR) to determine the degree of aluminol (AlOH) and the siloxane (SiOH) groups modification since these two functional groups will be key sites for bioactive compounds interaction. pH-dependent eluted samples were then tested on breast (MCF-7) cancer cell lines to investigate their inhibitory effects and the mechanism of inhibition were determined using cyclic voltammetry and flow cytometry analyses [38–41]. The results are reported here and show evidence of differential inhibitory effects of the bioactive compounds from the various pH conditions.

2. Methods

2.1 Extraction of bioactive compounds

Dioclea reflexa seeds were obtained from the District of Jaman North in the Brong Ahafo region of Ghana (7°57′1.8" North and 2°41′52.08" West). The content of the seeds was dried in the sun, and the cotyledon ground into powder using a laboratory mortar and pestle. The drugs used for the study were obtained from a Company (Sigma-Aldrich, Saint Louis, MO, USA). 5 gram of *Dioclea reflexa* Seed powder was dissolved in 30 mL of 70% ethanol. 5 mL of the supernatant was used for immobilization using 10, 50, 75, 100, 150 and 200 mg of HNTs. 200 mg gave the best entrapment. The loaded HNTs were released with a buffer with pH ranging from 4 to 9 and the contents vacuum dried followed by dissolution in 1% dimethyl sulfoxide (DMSO) to give a final concentration of 3.2 mg/mL.

2.2 Cell viability and electrochemical detection

The methods used for preparing stock solution of the drug are previously described [23]. Cells were treated with the drugs or the extracts to study the effects at prescribe time interval followed by estimating cell death. A correlation of cell death to electrochemical behavior was conducted using cyclic voltammetry under steady-state conditions as previously described [17].

3. Results

The stepwise procedure in this work probes the mechanism of action of standard drugs for treating microbial infections and the results compared to plant bioactive metabolites and chitosan nanocomposites. Two classes of standard drugs were used for comparison; anti-microbial drugs that include amphotericin B, rifampicin and fluconazole as well as cancer drugs which included curcumin and gossypol. Whereas the plant metabolites were derived from *Dioclea reflexa (DR)*. The therapeutic effect of nanocomposites were also tested. Chitosan nanocomposites were synthesized using chitosan as the base material and Tetraethyl orthosilicate (TEOS) as well as acetic acid as modifiers. Our hypothesis stipulated that drug candidate target membrane environment of cells leading to polarization or depolarization. The outcome in this case would enhance ionic mobility across membranes which could be captured through electrochemical detection as shown in **Figure 1**.

The various standardized drugs, plant metabolites as well as the synthesized nanocomposites used to investigate the electrochemical behaviour of the cells are displayed in **Table 1**. The cell lines and their sources are also indicated in **Table 2**. First, the electrochemical behaviour of *S. cerevisiae* cells was investigated using the standard antimicrobial drugs, amphotericin B, fluconazole and rifampicin. As shown in **Figure 2**, fluconazole and rifampicin exhibited very limited changes in the anodic peak potential (**Figure 2A** and **B**) compared to the amphotericin B doped *S. cerevisiae* cell lines (**Figure 2C**). The results obtained confirmed membrane polarization/depolarization behaviour of the *S. cerevisiae* due to the

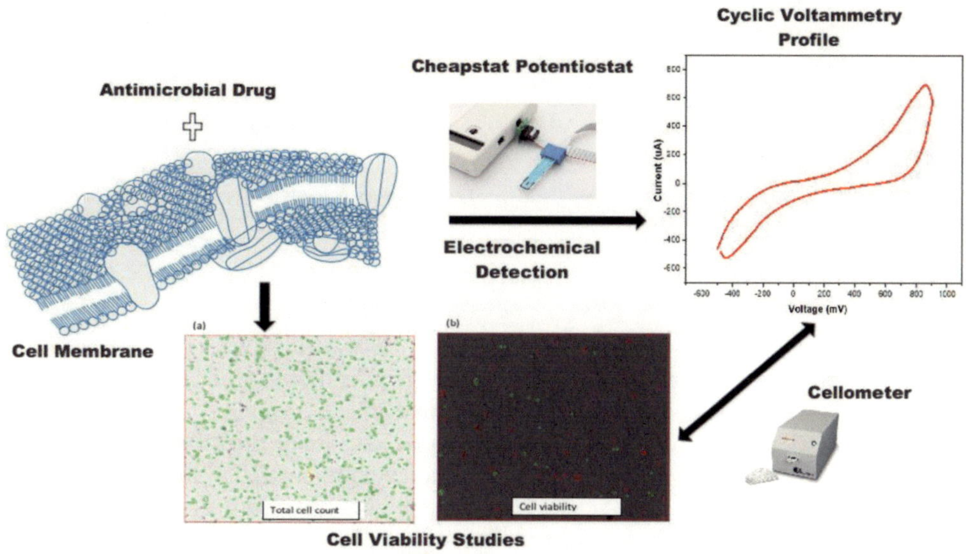

Figure 1.
Schematic illustration of the mechanism of drug interaction with biological membranes and how its electrochemical response (using a miniature electrode) correlates to cell viability as captured by the a cell counting device (Cellometer) [33].

Compound	Source	Structure
Fluconazole	Human milk	Triazole
Rifampicin	Streptomyces	Polyketide
Amphotericin	Streptomyces nodosus	Polyene with seven adjoining trans double bonds
Gossypol	Cotton plant	Natural phenol
Curcumin	*Curcuma longa* plants	Beta-diketone
Chitosan nanocomposite[*,1]	Syntheisized from chitosan and Tetraethyl orthosilicate (TEOS)	Chitosan modified with TEOS in different sequence (no known structures)
Dioclea reflexa Extract[*,2]	Seed	pH dependent elution of plant metabolites from halloysites nanotubes (no known structures)

[*]*Extracted or synthesized and unpurified.*
[1]*The following composites were tested: CT; chitosan modified by TEOS followed by acetic acid, CC; chitosan modified with TEOS/acetic acid mixture, CA; chitosan modified with acetic acid, and CT, chitosan modified with TEOS.*
[2]*Plant metabolites obtained from pH ~4.1–9.6.*

Table 1.
List of compounds used for the study.

presence of amphotericin B leading to increase ionic mobility. Fluconazole and rifampicin which are not directly linked to membrane destabilization as the former are mainly responsible for RNA synthesis inhibition and rifampicin being responsible for inhibition of ergosterol synthesis.

A correlation between cell death and electrochemical response was established using *S. cerevisiae* cell lines and MTT assay detection. Although the result indicated cell death in the presence of the antimicrobial drugs, Amphotericin B exhibited

Cell lines	Source	Redox behavior	Cell viability
Prostate cancer (PC3)	ATCC (Manassas, VA)	Cyclic Voltammetry	Trypan blue and MTT assays
Breast (MCF-7) cancer	ATCC (Manassas, VA)	Cyclic Voltammetry	Trypan blue and MTT assays
S. cerevisiae	(ATCC/LGC Standards, Teddington, UK)	Cyclic Voltammetry	MTT assay

Table 2.
Cell lines and Detection methods used for Investigating membrane mediated effects.

enhanced cell death probably due to the high degree of membrane permeability of ions as indicated in the voltammograms in **Figure 2C**.

To test the electrochemical behaviour and redox activity of the *Dioclea reflexa* extracts, cyclic voltammetry analysis was conducted using interdigitated gold electrodes (IDEs), (Metrohm, DropSens). The current from the quasi-reversible oxidation curve was plotted against concentration of the plant metabolites.
Figure 3A (*control, black*) indicated insignificant redox mechanism, however, the extracts showed quasi-reversible oxidation values ranging from 0.25 to 0.70 mA at a scan rate of 10 mV/s. The water extract (SWE) had higher redox potential compared to those of the ethanol extract (SEE). The water extract (SWE) *(red)* demonstrated the most cell death followed by methanol extract (SME) (*purple*) and ethanol extract (SEE) (*blue*) respectively with the control cells *(black)* exhibiting the least cell death at higher concentrations and extended incubation time periods. *SWE* (*red*) revealed cell death of about 57%, whereas *SME (purple), SEE (blue*) recorded about 31 and 22% respectively at the same concentration. It was concluded that the extracts caused membrane porosity to initiate reactive oxygen species release leading to cell death.

Another important strategy in plant phytochemical studies is to develop local immobilization materials that can capture bioactive plant metabolites and release the cargo steadily onto diseased cells. Optimization parameters were developed to capture plant metabolites from *Dioclea Reflexa (DR)* seed extracts on halloysites nanotubes (HNTs). An encapsulating capacity of 13% was obtained when approximately 5 g of *DR* extracts was immobilized onto about 1 g of HNTs. Evidence of plant metabolites entrapment was monitored with FTIR and X-ray diffraction methods. As shown in **Figure 4A**, changes in the FTIR signatures peak intensities of the halloysite nanotubes (HNTs) revealed all the functional groups present in the empty halloysites nanotubes (black). The inner Al-OH and outer Si-OH groups have characteristic stretching peaks at 3624 and 3691 cm^{-1}, respectively. Bending vibrations of Al-OH and Si-O revealed absorption peaks at 907 cm^{-1}. In addition, the uneven stretching vibrations of the Si-O bond gives a strong absorption peak at 1005 cm^{-1}. There was a significant reduction of the transmission peak after immobilization of the *DR* extracts on the halloysites nanotubes (blue) and this indicated a modification of the nanotubes with the plant metabolites. Following the release of the bioactive compounds from the nanotubes, the transmission peaks reverted to the original peaks of the empty nanotubes (red). Similarly, **Figure 4B**, showed the characteristics 2θ ° peak positions of the nanotubes which occurs at 11.7, 20.5, 24.8, 37.5, 43.3 and 64.4° (red). After immobilization of the *DR* extract on the nanotubes, there was dramatic reduction of peak intensities at the same 2θ ° positions and that indicated chemical modifications of the nanotubes by the bioactive constituents in *DR* extract (black). The bioactive constituents were eluted with 70% ethanol and resulted in the reversal of the nanotubes peaks as shown in **Figure 4B** (blue). The characteristic peak intensities reverted to those observed in the control.

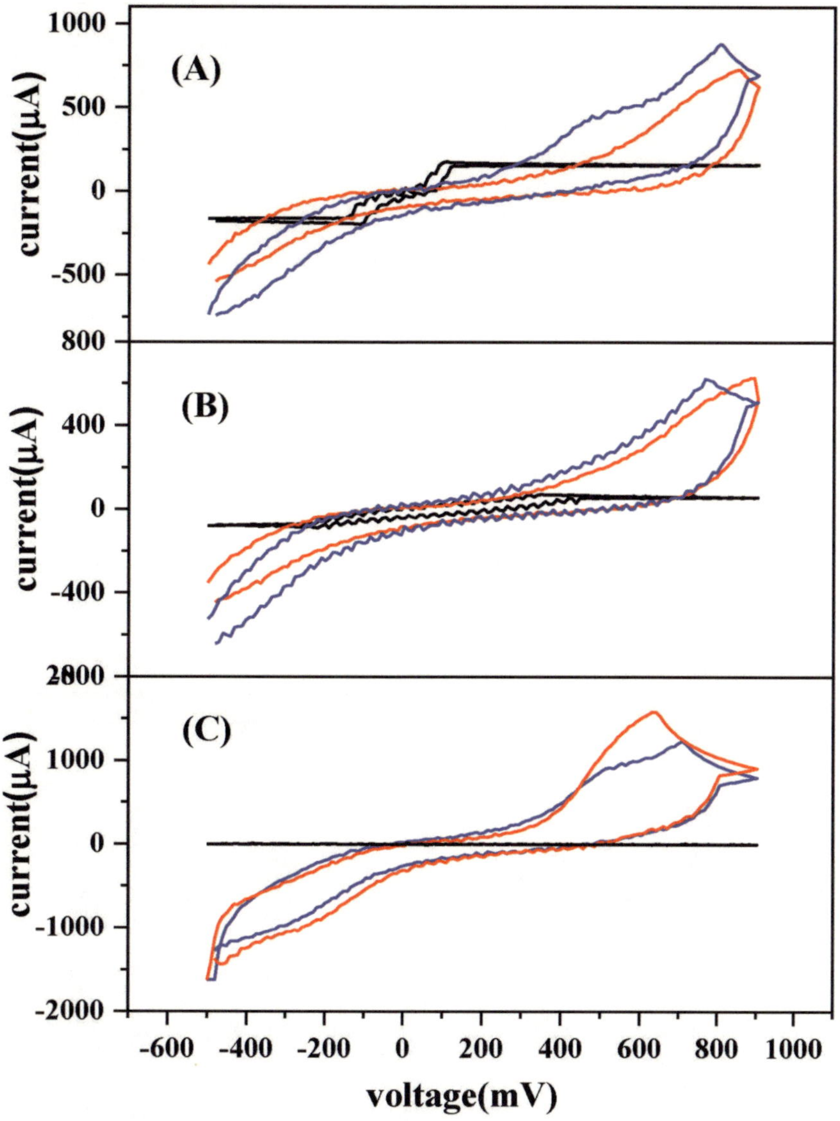

Figure 2.
Cyclic voltammetry response of S. Cerevisiae *in the presence of (A) rifampicin, (B) fluconazole, and (C) amphotericin B on IDE electrode (Colour code: black, antibiotic; red, cells and blue, cell + antibiotic).*

The antiproliferative activity of the crude extracts did not reveal significant inhibitory effects on breast (MCF-7) cancer cells, however, the pH-dependent eluted metabolites revealed that the acidic pH samples exhibited profound antiproliferative effects on the cancer cells compared to the basic pH metabolites using both trypan blue dye exclusion assay and MTT viability test as shown in **Table 3**. pH ~ 5.2 demonstrated IC_{50} of 0.8 mg and a cyclic voltammetry oxidation peak potential and current of 234 mV and 0.45 μA respectively indicating membrane polarization/depolarization of the cancer cells as shown in **Figure 5**. It was confirmed through fluorescence-activated cell sorting (FACS) studies that the plant metabolites influenced breast cancer apoptotic signaling pathways of cell death as shown in **Figure 6**. The studies proved that plant metabolites could be captured using simplified screening procedures for rapid drug discovery purposes. Such procedures, however, would require the integration of affordable analytical tools to isolate individual metabolites

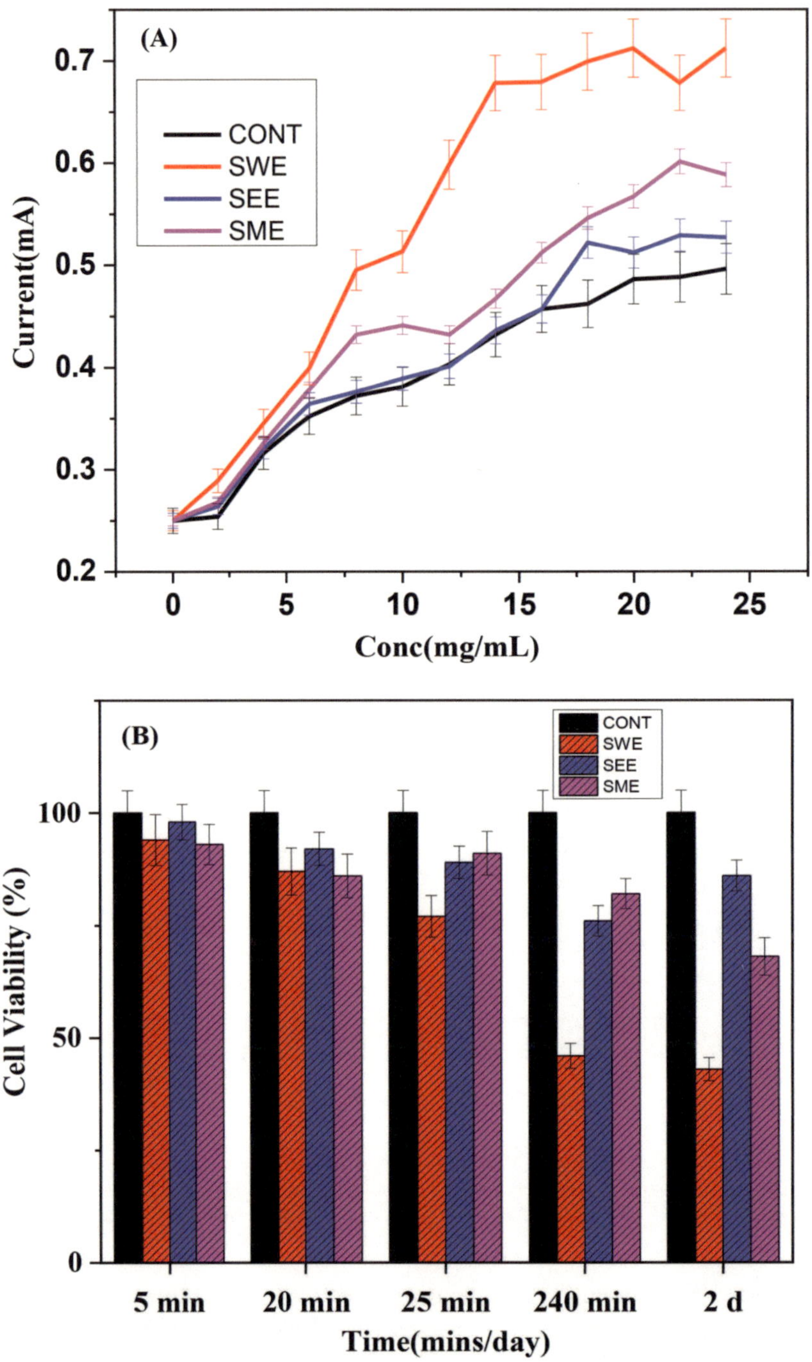

Figure 3.
(A) A graph of current versus concentration of plant extracts revealed the water extract generated highest current, followed by the methanol extract, ethanol extract and the control cells in that order. (B) Investigating cell death as a function time. The water extract revealed significant cell death (red) *after 2 days of incubation, followed by the methanol extract, ethanol extract and control in that order.*

for testing. Our approach could be an important strategy to create plant metabolite database based on pH values.

Biopolymers such as chitosan, gelatin and cellulose have been used with different additives in order to modify their surfaces for biomedical application. In the

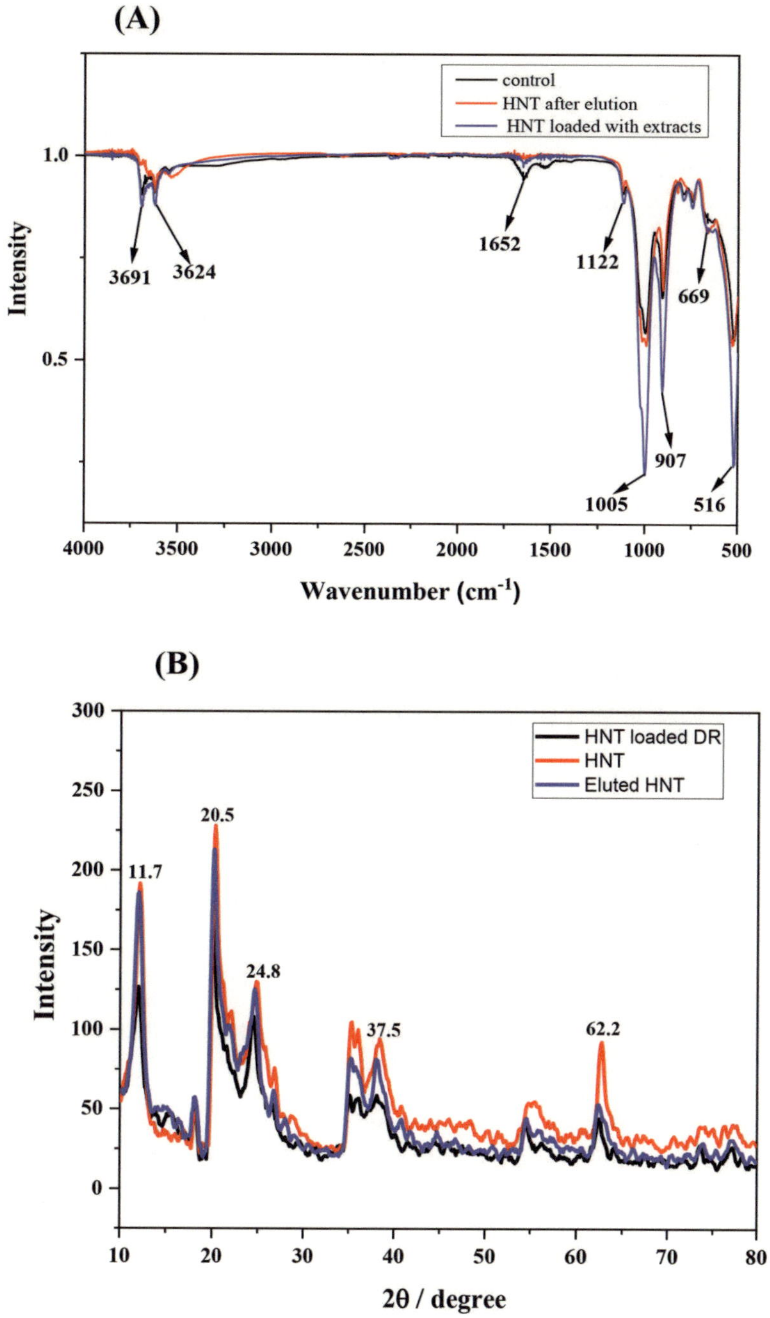

Figure 4.
(A) Characterization of HNTs and loaded HNTs with plant metabolites using FTIR techniques. Reduction in IR transmittance indicates OH on the HNTs are functionalized by at least one bioactive. (B) XRD spectra of the entrapped metabolites showing the signature peaks at two theta position of HNTs and loaded HNTs with plant metabolites. Intensity has inverse relationship to surface area. Larger area due to immobilization will cause a decrease peak intensity.

next paragraph, a description of the synthesis of chitosan nanocomposites using tetraorthosilicate (TEOS) and acetic acid (AA) to study their influence on prostate cancer (PC3) cell lines would be described. The particles synthesized for the study include *SC*; chitosan modified by TEOS followed by acetic acid, *CC*; chitosan modified with TEOS/acetic acid mixture, CA; chitosan modified with acetic acid, and

		Normalized
Sample/Dry extract	IC_{50} (mg)	R squared value
Water	33.3	0.959
Ethanol	1.6	0.991
pH 4.1	1.4	0.967
pH 5.2	0.8	0.998
pH 6.4	1.6	0.975
pH 7.4	1.9	0.983
pH 8.1	2.3	0.948
pH 9.6	3.1	0.994

Table 3.
Experimental IC_{50} values of the extracts eluted at different pH conditions all measured in milligram quantities of the seed extract.

CT, chitosan modified with TEOS. As shown in **Figure 7A** and **B**, The electrochemical response of normal cells and prostate cancer cells (PC3) when treated with the particles revealed the latter showed modest response whereas the PC3 cells anodic peak currents changed dramatically with the treatment with the nanocomposites especially the *SC* nanoparticles. The cell viability studies revealed a corresponding decrease in cell viability as measured by a cell counting device. The normal cells again showed no significant difference in cell viability after 24–48 hours of cell growth as shown in **Figure 7C** and **D**. The results were compared with a standard drug used to treat cancers, gossypol (GP).

4. Discussion

In the current work, a systematic approach was undertaken to carefully investigate standard drugs, plant metabolites and chitosan nanoparticles on the electrochemical behaviour of selected cell lines and also to correlate their electrochemistry to cell viability.

It is becoming evident that taking advantage of the numerous redox mediators, scientists could develop biosensors from many biological systems. For example, *S. Cerevisiae* has several Redox centers which could be exploited using hydrophilic/hydrophobic molecules as extensively discussed previously by *Rawson et al.* [1, 2]. The fact that Electrochemical behavior could be monitored using membrane targeted drugs [42–45], opens avenue for future development of a biosensor for identifying potential drug candidate from plant sources. For example, the famous antifungal drug, Amp B has been used to treat fungal infection effectively and its mechanism of action has been well characterized [46, 47]. It is established that the antifungal drug binds to ergosterol in the cell membrane to enhance leakage of ions leading to depolarization of the membrane [48]. Increase in ions leakage across membrane could ultimately increase the oxidation potential across membranes. Such source of ions can be detected through electrochemical techniques as already observed in our studies as well as studies from other groups [2].

The fact that Amp B and the plant extracts behave similarly on *S. cerevisiae* cell viability supported a general claim that Amp B and the plant extracts exhibited a common mechanism leading to cell death. Hence, due to the quasi-reversible oxidation process observed in the anodic response, it was concluded that membrane

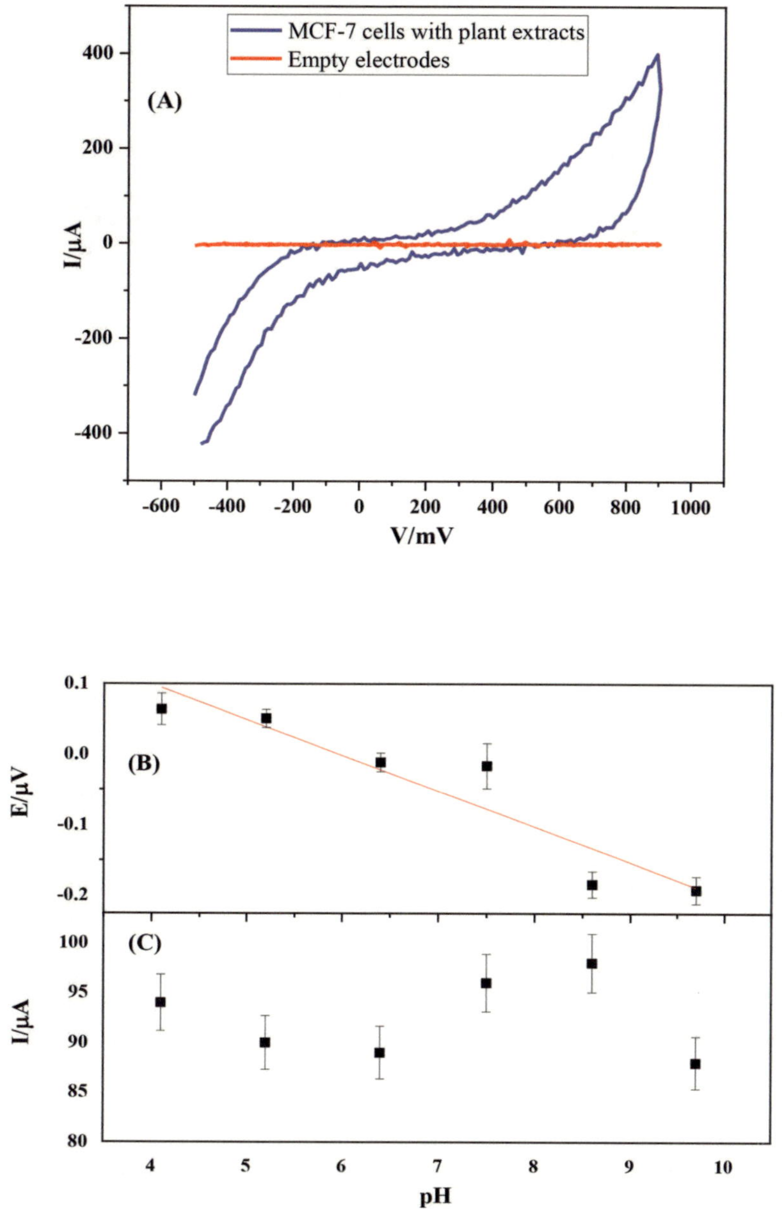

Figure 5.
(A) Effects of the bioactive compounds from the pH ~5.2 on the depolarization potential of the MCF-7 cells. (B) The influence of the voltage on current of the MCF-7 cells as a function of pH. The cyclic voltammogram measurements conditions were: Scanning from 690 mV to 970 mV at a scan rate of 10 mV s^{-1}. MCF-7 cancer cell viability studies of the bioactive compounds extracted at pH ~ 5.2 at cell concentration of 1 x10^6 cells/well [submitted results for publication, Scientific Reports].

polarization/depolarization leading to ionic leakage might have been the mechanism through which one or more of the organic bioactive molecules illicit their action. This correlation had highlighted an important opportunity that could be further exploited for identifying bioactive plant metabolites in the natural product field.

We used pH dependent elution of the *DR* bioactive compounds from the halloysites nanotubes to further validate the activity of the captured metabolites on electrochemical behaviour and cell death. Halloysite nanotubes have SiOH and AlOH

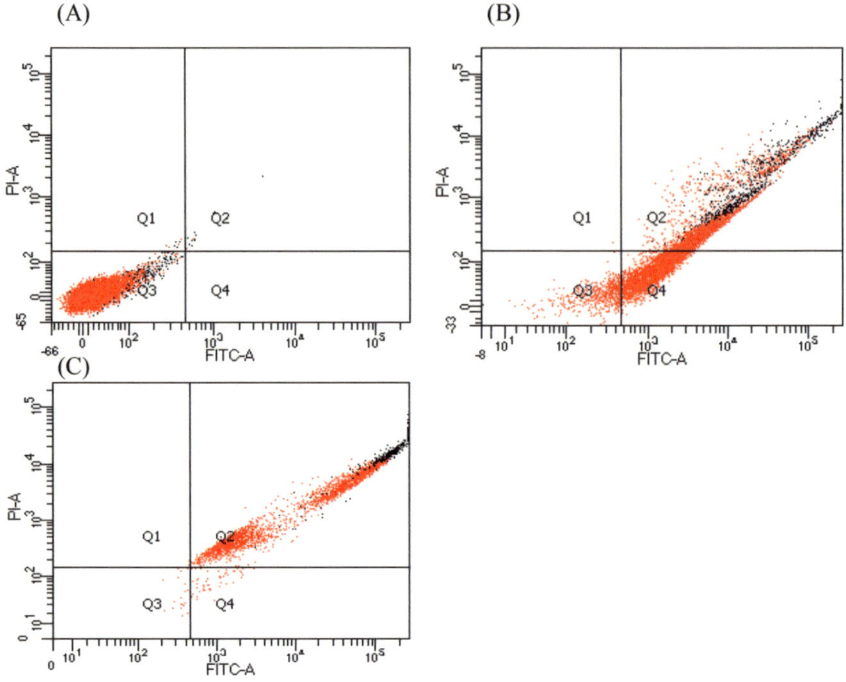

Figure 6.
Fluorescence activated cell sorting (FACS) analysis of the inhibitory effects of breast (MCF-7) cancer cells using bioactive extracts at pH ~ 5.2 (best IC_{50} concentration). The results were compared to the inhibitory effects of a Commercially available cancer drug, cucurmin. (A) untreated cells, (B) cells treated with extract and (C) cells treated with curcumin all at cell concentration of 1 x10^6 cells/well.

groups which are found on the outer surface and the inner surface making the outer and inner surfaces to have different charges respectively [10, 49, 50]. Thus, depending on the pH conditions, aluminol (AlOH) and the siloxane (SiOH) groups could either be protonated or deprotonated leading to different affinities towards certain macromolecules and organic compounds. Our hypothesis was that partially positive metabolites will be weakly attracted to SiOH groups whereas negatively charged metabolites would prefer the latter. The pH dependent release of the metabolites from the HNT were not statistically different after determining the amount in milligram quantities and expressing the entrapment efficiency as a percentage value. However, when tested against the breast (MCF-7) cancer cell lines, the acidic pH elution demonstrated significant anti-proliferative activity against the cancer cell lines compared to the basic pH metabolites. The most profound activity was found in the pH ~ 5.2 which was supported by IC_{50} calculated values.

Depolarization is an indicator of mitochondrial dysfunction in most cancer cells and therefore investigating polarization and depolarization could inform the mechanism of cell death [51]. In this work, Cyclic voltammetry measurements were used to probe the extent of polarization and depolarization by relating the voltage to current surge using electrochemical methods. The results revealed that the metabolites exhibited quasi-reversible redox behavior and concentration dependent reduction in the applied voltage [52]. The currents also showed a triangular modulation with a rise in oxidation current at lower pH, followed by another rise beyond acidic pH and further reduction to the strongly basic pH. Metabolites from the pH ~ 5.2 extract required a higher voltage application to generate the minimum amount of current in the cells indicating cell membrane polarization in the presence of the metabolite was achieved. The extracts from pH ~ 7.4 and pH ~ 8.1, even though gave higher IC_{50} values, the voltage required to initiate cell depolarization

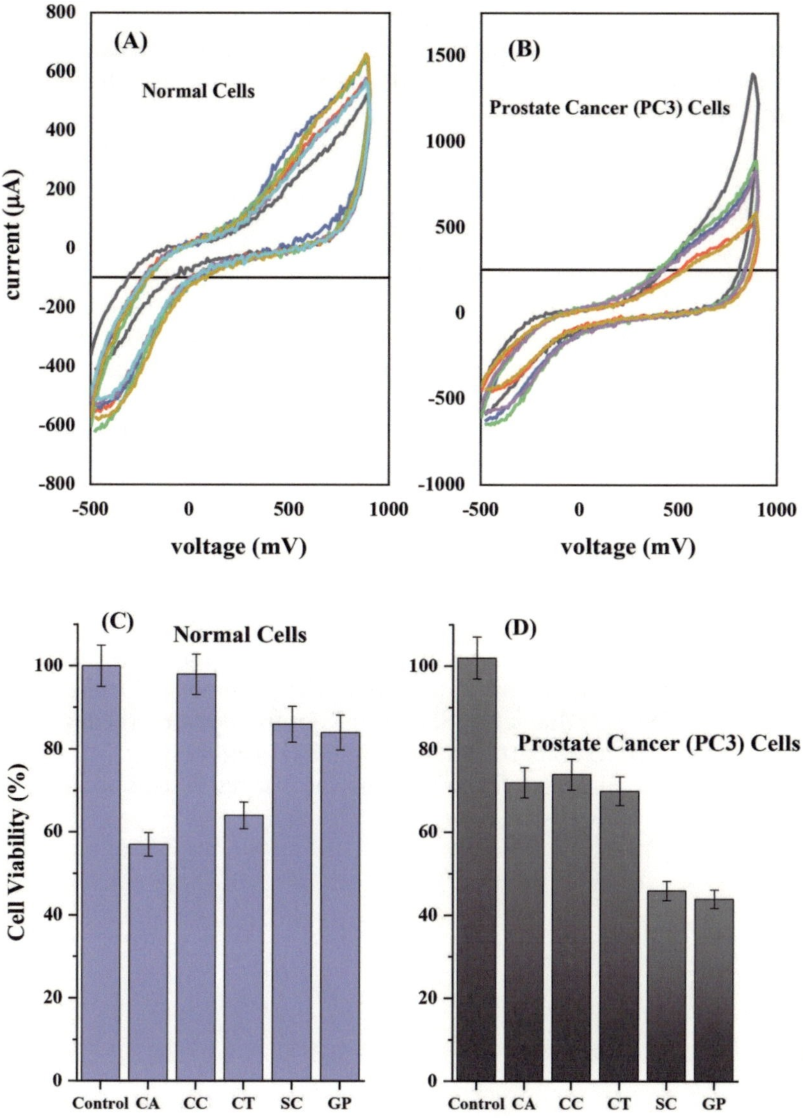

Figure 7.
Correlation electrochemical response of the (A) normal cells and (B) prostate cancer cells (PC3) as a function of chitosan composite treatment. SC*; chitosan modified by TEOS followed by acetic acid,* CC*; chitosan modified with TEOS/acetic acid mixture,* CA*; chitosan modified with acetic acid, and* CT*, chitosan modified with TEOS The corresponding cell viability as measured by the cell counting device. (C) normal cells and (D) cancer cells.*

in the cells was at a minimum as indicated in the maximum current generation. The results highlighted that the metabolites could cause cell death through a polarization/depolarization mechanism as documented by other researchers in the literature [53]. Flow cytometer-based analysis showed that the metabolites showed dose-dependent apoptosis of MCF-7 cells. It was noted that exposure of 2 mgmL^{-1} concentrations of the metabolites led to greater than two-fold increase in apoptosis in comparison to the untreated cells. Curcumin is a well-known polyphenol and widely used for its anti-oxidative and anti-cancerous application. Curcumin effects on the breast cancer cells were also investigated and compared with the result from the metabolites. It was observed that curcumin improved cell death significantly without going through the apoptotic phase indicating synergistic effect could be developed when both metabolites and curcumin are used to treat cancer. Finally, the chitosan nanoparticles also demonstrated that membrane polarization and depolarization could also be used to monitor particle permeation into cell membrane to induce varied cell behaviour.

5. Conclusion

In conclusion, electrochemical behaviour of cells in the presence of plant metabolites if carefully pursued could help establish a database with fundamental information on herbal medicine isolation and characterization to serve the scientific community in future studies of herbal medicine. It is also simple, robust and required a specific protocol that could be adopted for understanding the medicinal plants behaviour for easy characterization. It has to be emphasized that further work needs to be pursued to understand the mechanism of these membrane targeted behaviours.

Acknowledgements

We will like to thank the West African Center for Cell Biology of Infectious Pathogens (WACCBIP) for support in providing the facilities and technical assistants for the work. We also thank Mr. Solomon Katu for assisting the team conducting the experiments in the Department of Biomedical engineering. Mr. Ayirebaje Azuponga and Mr. Kwasi Obeng for processing the images for this book.

Author details

Elvis K. Tiburu[1*], Richard Asiamah[1], Bernard O. Asimeng[1], Samuel Kojo Kwofie[1], Emmanuel Nyankson[2] and William N. Gblerkpor[3]

1 Department of Biomedical Engineering, University of Ghana, Legon, Ghana

2 Department of Material Science and Engineering, University of Ghana, Legon, Ghana

3 Department of Archaeology and Heritage Studies, University of Ghana, Legon, Ghana

*Address all correspondence to: etiburu@ug.edu.gh

References

[1] Rawson FJ, Cole MT, Hicks JM, Aylott JW, Milne WI, Collins CM, Jackson SK, Silman NJ, Mendes PM: Electrochemical communication with the inside of cells using micro-patterned vertical carbon nanofibre electrodes. Sci Rep 2016, 6: 37672. doi: 10.1038/srep05216.

[2] Rawson FJ, Downard AJ, Baronian KH: Electrochemical detection of intracellular and cell membrane redox systems in Saccharomyces cerevisiae. Sci Rep 2014, 4:5216. doi: 10.1038/srep05216.

[3] Robbins N, Spitzer M, Yu T, Cerone RP, Averette AK, Bahn YS, Heitman J, Sheppard DC, Tyers M, Wright GD: An Antifungal Combination Matrix Identifies a Rich Pool of Adjuvant Molecules that Enhance Drug Activity against Diverse Fungal Pathogens. Cell Rep 2015, 13(7):1481-1492. doi: 10.1016/j.celrep.2015.10.018. Epub 2015 Nov 5.

[4] Hartland CL, Pu J, Krysan D, Didone L, Moquist PN, Dandapani S, Munoz B, Palmer M, Schreiber S: Discovery and Evaluation of Fungicidal Anti-Cryptococcal Molecules. In: *Probe Reports from the NIH Molecular Libraries Program.* Bethesda (MD); 2010.

[5] Ibragimova V, Alieva I, Kasumov K, Khutorsky V: Transient permeability induced by alkyl derivatives of amphotericin B in lipid membranes. Biochim Biophys Acta 2006, 1758(1):29-37. doi:10.1016/j.bbamem.2005.12.011 doi: 10.1016/j.bbamem.2005.12.011

[6] Gianni E, Avgoustakis K, Papoulis D: Kaolinite group minerals: applications in cancer diagnosis and treatment. Eur J Pharm Biopharm 2020. doi:10.1016/j.ejpb.2020.07.030

[7] Saif MJ, Asif HM, Naveed AM: Properties and modification methods of Halloysite nanotubes: a state-of-the- art review. J Chil Chem Soc 2018, 63. doi: 10.4067/s0717-97072018000304109

[8] Park K, Lee J, Chang JH, Hwang KH, Lee Y: Characterization of Surface-Modified Halloysite Nanotubes by Thermal Treatment Under Reducing Atmosphere. J Nanosci Nanotechnol 2020, 20(7):4221-4226.doi: 10.1016/j.biopha.2018.10.186

[9] Tas CE, Sevinis Ozbulut EB, Ceven OF, Tas BA, Unal S, Unal H: Purification and Sorting of Halloysite Nanotubes into Homogeneous, Agglomeration-Free Fractions by Polydopamine Functionalization. ACS Omega 2020, 5(29):17962-17972.doi: 10.1021/acsomega.0c01057

[10] Jang SH, Jang SR, Lee GM, Ryu JH, Park SI, Park NH: Halloysite Nanocapsules Containing Thyme Essential Oil: Preparation, Characterization, and Application in Packaging Materials. J Food Sci 2017, 82(9):2113-2120.doi: 10.1111/1750-3841.13835

[11] Lisuzzo L, Cavallaro G, Milioto S, Lazzara G: Halloysite Nanotubes Coated by Chitosan for the Controlled Release of Khellin. Polymers (Basel) 2020, 12(8). doi:10.3390/polym12081766

[12] Fizir M, Dramou P, Dahiru NS, Ruya W, Huang T, He H: Halloysite nanotubes in analytical sciences and in drug delivery: A review. Mikrochim Acta 2018, 185(8):389. doi:10.1007/s00604-018-2908-1

[13] Jana S, Kondakova AV, Shevchenko SN, Sheval EV, Gonchar KA, Timoshenko VY, Vasiliev AN: Halloysite nanotubes with immobilized silver nanoparticles for anti-bacterial application. Colloids Surf B Biointerfaces 2017, 151:249-254. doi. 10.1016/j.colsurfb.2016.12.017

[14] Tully J, Yendluri R, Lvov Y: Halloysite Clay Nanotubes for Enzyme Immobilization. Biomacromolecules 2016, 17(2):615-621. doi:10.1021/acs.biomac.5b01542

[15] Barman M, Mahmood S, Augustine R, Hasan A, Thomas S, Ghosal K: Natural halloysite nanotubes/chitosan based bio-nanocomposite for delivering norfloxacin, an anti-microbial agent in sustained release manner. Int J Biol Macromol 2020. doi:10.1016/j.ijbiomac.2020.08.060

[16] Bonifacio MA, Gentile P, Ferreira AM, Cometa S, De Giglio E: Insight into halloysite nanotubes-loaded gellan gum hydrogels for soft tissue engineering applications. Carbohydr Polym 2017, 163:280-291. doi:10.1016/j.carbpol.2017.01.064

[17] Bottino MC, Yassen GH, Platt JA, Labban N, Windsor LJ, Spolnik KJ, Bressiani AH: A novel three-dimensional scaffold for regenerative endodontics: materials and biological characterizations. J Tissue Eng Regen Med 2015, 9(11):E116-123. doi: 10.1002/term.1712

[18] De Oliveira T, Guegan R, Thiebault T, Milbeau CL, Muller F, Teixeira V, Giovanela M, Boussafir M: Adsorption of diclofenac onto organoclays: Effects of surfactant and environmental (pH and temperature) conditions. *J Hazard Mater* 2017, 323(Pt A):558-566. doi:10.1016/j.jhazmat.2016.05.001.

[19] Li W, Liu D, Zhang H, Correia A, Makila E, Salonen J, Hirvonen J, Santos HA: Microfluidic assembly of a nano-in-micro dual drug delivery platform composed of halloysite nanotubes and a pH-responsive polymer for colon cancer therapy. Acta Biomater 2017, 48:238-246. doi: 10.1016/j.actbio.2016.10.042

[20] Nguyen-Vo TH, Nguyen L, Do N, Nguyen TN, Trinh K, Cao H, Le L: Plant Metabolite Databases: From Herbal Medicines to Modern Drug Discovery. J Chem Inf Model 2020, 60(3):1101-1110. doi:10.1021/acs.jcim.9b00826

[21] Tajadini H, Divsalar K, Mehrabani M, Haghdoost AA, Esmaili Z, Shadkam M, Moradi M: The frequency of using herbal medicines among patients with hypertension in Kerman, Iran, 2012-2013. J Evid Based Complementary Altern Med 2015, 20(3):199-202. doi: 10.1177/2156587215573141

[22] Zhang X, Schmitter S, Van de Moortele PF, Liu J, He B: From complex B(1) mapping to local SAR estimation for human brain MR imaging using multi-channel transceiver coil at 7T. IEEE Trans Med Imaging 2013, 32(6):1058-1067. doi: 10.1109/TMI.2013.2251653

[23] Wang X, Han L, Li G, Peng W, Gao X, Klaassen CD, Fan G, Zhang Y: From the Cover: Identification of Natural Products as Inhibitors of Human Organic Anion Transporters (OAT1 and OAT3) and Their Protective Effect on Mercury-Induced Toxicity. Toxicol Sci 2018, 161(2):321-334. doi:10.1093/toxsci/kfx216

[24] Nikitin M, Deych K, Grevtseva I, Girsova N, Kuznetsova M, Pridannikov M, Dzhavakhiya V, Statsyuk N, Golikov A: Preserved Microarrays for Simultaneous Detection and Identification of Six Fungal Potato Pathogens with the Use of Real-Time PCR in Matrix Format. *Biosensors (Basel)* 2018, 8(4). doi: 10.3390/bios8040129

[25] Antunes RS, Ferraz D, Garcia LF, Thomaz DV, Luque R, Lobon GS, Gil ES, Lopes FM: Development of a Polyphenol Oxidase Biosensor from Jenipapo Fruit Extract (Genipa americana L.) and Determination of Phenolic Compounds in Textile Industrial Effluents. Biosensors (Basel) 2018, 8(2). doi:10.3390/bios8020047

[26] Anderson DE, Balapangu S, Fleischer HNA, Viade RA, Krampa FD, Kanyong P, Awandare GA, Tiburu EK: Investigating the Influence of Temperature on the Kaolinite-Base Synthesis of Zeolite and Urease Immobilization for the Potential Fabrication of Electrochemical Urea Biosensors. *Sensors (Basel)* 2017, 17(8). doi.org/10.3390/s17081831

[27] Holzmann C, Kilch T, Kappel S, Dorr K, Jung V, Stockle M, Bogeski I, Peinelt C: Differential Redox Regulation of Ca(2)(+) Signaling and Viability in Normal and Malignant Prostate Cells. Biophys J 2015, 109(7):1410-1419. doi: 10.1016/j.bpj.2015.08.006

[28] Martino T, Kudrolli TA, Kumar B, Salviano I, Mencalha A, Coelho MGP, Justo G, Costa PRR, Sabino KCC, Lupold SE: The orally active pterocarpanquinone LQB-118 exhibits cytotoxicity in prostate cancer cell and tumor models through cellular redox stress. Prostate 2018, 78(2):140-151. doi: 10.1002/pros.23455

[29] Sajjadi M, Karimi E, Oskoueian E, Iranshahi M, Neamati A: Galbanic acid: Induced antiproliferation in estrogen receptor-negative breast cancer cells and enhanced cellular redox state in the human dermal fibroblasts. J Biochem Mol Toxicol 2019, 33(11):e22402. doi:10.1002/jbt.22402

[30] Pinto-Junior VR, Osterne VJ, Santiago MQ, Correia JL, Pereira-Junior FN, Leal RB, Pereira MG, Chicas LS, Nagano CS, Rocha BA *et al*: Structural studies of a vasorelaxant lectin from Dioclea reflexa Hook seeds: Crystal structure, molecular docking and dynamics. Int J Biol Macromol 2017, 98:12-23. doi: 10.1016/j.ijbiomac.2017.01.092

[31] Pinto-Junior VR, Correia JL, Pereira RI, Pereira-Junior FN, Santiago MQ, Osterne VJ, Madeira JC, Cajazeiras JB, Nagano CS, Delatorre P *et al*: Purification and molecular characterization of a novel mannose-specific lectin from Dioclea reflexa hook seeds with inflammatory activity. J Mol Recognit 2016, 29(4):134-141. doi: 10.3390/molecules180910857

[32] Ajatta MA, Akinola SA, Otolowo DT, Awolu OO, Omoba OS, Osundahunsi OF: Effect of Roasting on the Phytochemical Properties of Three Varieties of Marble Vine (Dioclea reflexa) Using Response Surface Methodology. Prev Nutr Food Sci 2019, 24(4):468-477. doi: 10.3746/pnf.2019.24.4.468

[33] Arthur PK, Yeboah AB, Issah I, Balapangu S, Kwofie SK, Asimeng BO, Foster EJ, Tiburu EK: Electrochemical Response of Saccharomyces cerevisiae Corresponds to Cell Viability upon Exposure to Dioclea reflexa Seed Extracts and Antifungal Drugs. Biosensors (Basel) 2019, 9(1). doi: 10.3390/bios9010045

[34] Kazenel MR, Debban CL, Ranelli L, Hendricks WQ, Chung YA, Pendergast THt, Charlton ND, Young CA, Rudgers JA: A mutualistic endophyte alters the niche dimensions of its host plant. AoB Plants 2015, 7. doi: 10.1093/**aobpla**/plv005

[35] Saqib Z, Mahmood A, Naseem Malik R, Mahmood A, Hussian Syed J, Ahmad T: Indigenous knowledge of medicinal plants in Kotli Sattian, Rawalpindi district, Pakistan. *J Ethnopharmacol* 2014, 151(2):820-828. doi: 10.1016/j.jep.2013.05.035

[36] Pal DK, Mandal M, Senthilkumar GP, Padhiari A: Antibacterial activity of Cuscuta reflexa stem and Corchorus olitorius seed. Fitoterapia 2006, 77(7-8):589-591. doi: 10.1016/j.fitote.2006.06.015

[37] Mazumder UK, Gupta M, Pal D, Bhattacharya S: Chemical and toxicological evaluation of methanol

extract of Cuscuta reflexa Roxb. stem and Corchorus olitorius Linn. seed on hematological parameters and hepatorenal functions in mice. Acta Pol Pharm 2003, 60(4):317-323. doi: 10.3742/OPEM.2009.9.1.049

[38] Munge BS, Stracensky T, Gamez K, DiBiase D, Rusling JF: Multiplex Immunosensor Arrays for Electrochemical Detection of Cancer Biomarker Proteins. Electroanalysis 2016, 28(11):2644-2658. doi: 10.1002/elan.201600183

[39] Nejadnik MR, Deepak FL, Garcia CD: Adsorption of Glucose Oxidase to 3-D Scaffolds of Carbon Nanotubes: Analytical Applications. Electroanalysis 2011, 23(6):1462-1469. doi:10.1002/elan.201000758

[40] Szigeti Z, Vigassy T, Bakker E, Pretsch E: Approaches to Improving the Lower Detection Limit of Polymeric Membrane Ion-Selective Electrodes. Electroanalysis 2006, 18(13-14):1254-1265. doi:10.1002/elan.200603539

[41] de Oliveira LA, Soares RO, Buzzi M, Mourao C, Kawase T, Kuckelhaus SAS: Cell and platelet composition assays by flow cytometry: basis for new platelet-rich fibrin methodologies. J Biol Regul Homeost Agents 2020, 34(4). doi: 10.23812/20-278-A

[42] Hashkavayi AB, Raoof JB, Ojani R, Kavoosian S: Ultrasensitive electrochemical aptasensor based on sandwich architecture for selective label-free detection of colorectal cancer (CT26) cells. Biosens Bioelectron 2017, 92:630-637. doi: 10.1016/j.bios.2016.10.042

[43] Haupt A, Campetelli A, Bonazzi D, Piel M, Chang F, Minc N: Electrochemical regulation of budding yeast polarity. PLoS Biol 2014, 12(12):e1002029. doi:10.1371/journal.pbio.1002029

[44] Hudcova K, Trnkova L, Kejnovska I, Vorlickova M, Gumulec J, Kizek R, Masarik M: Novel biophysical determination of miRNAs related to prostate and head and neck cancers. Eur Biophys J 2015, 44(3):131-138. doi: 10.1007/s00249-015-1008-y

[45] Nguyen HV, Richtera L, Moulick A, Xhaxhiu K, Kudr J, Cernei N, Polanska H, Heger Z, Masarik M, Kopel P *et al*: Electrochemical sensing of etoposide using carbon quantum dot modified glassy carbon electrode. Analyst 2016, 141(9):2665-2675. doi:10.1039/c5an02476e

[46] Huang W, Zhang Z, Han X, Tang J, Wang J, Dong S, Wang E: Ion channel behavior of amphotericin B in sterol-free and cholesterol- or ergosterol-containing supported phosphatidylcholine bilayer model membranes investigated by electrochemistry and spectroscopy. *Biophys J* 2002, 83(6):3245-3255Uno B. doi: 10.1016/S0006-3495(02)75326-5

[47] Gray KC, Palacios DS, Dailey I, Endo MM, E, Wilcock BC, Burke MD: Amphotericin primarily kills yeast by simply binding ergosterol. Proc Natl Acad Sci U S A 2012, 109(7):2234-2239. doi: 10.1073/pnas.1117280109

[48] Fang J, Palanisami A, Rajapakshe K, Widger WR, Miller JH: Nonlinear dielectric spectroscopy as an indirect probe of metabolic activity in thylakoid membrane. Biosensors (Basel) 2011, 1(1):13-22. doi: 10.3390/bios1010013

[49] Santos AC, Ferreira C, Veiga F, Ribeiro AJ, Panchal A, Lvov Y, Agarwal A: Halloysite clay nanotubes for life sciences applications: From drug encapsulation to bioscaffold. Adv Colloid Interface Sci 2018, 257:58-70. doi: 10.1016/j.cis.2018.05.007

[50] Vergaro V, Lvov YM, Leporatti S: Halloysite clay nanotubes for resveratrol

delivery to cancer cells. Macromol Biosci 2012, 12(9):1265-1271. doi:10.1002/mabi.201200121

[51] Wang B, Zhang X, Wang C, Chen L, Xiao Y, Pang Y: Bipolar and fixable probe targeting mitochondria to trace local depolarization via two-photon fluorescence lifetime imaging. Analyst 2015, 140(16):5488-5494. doi:10.1039/c5an01063b

[52] Kuralay F, Dukar N, Bayramli Y: Poly-L-lysine Coated Surfaces for Ultrasensitive Nucleic Acid Detection. Electroanalysis 2018, 30(7):1556-1565. doi:10.3390/jfb11040071

[53] Verhoeven HA, van Griensven LJ: Flow cytometric evaluation of the effects of 3-bromopyruvate (3BP) and dichloracetate (DCA) on THP-1 cells: a multiparameter analysis. J Bioenerg Biomembr 2012, 44(1):91-99. doi: 10.1007/s10863-012-9414-7